The Gifts of Civilization

The Gifts of Civilization

Germs and Genocide in Hawai'i

O. A. BUSHNELL

UNIVERSITY OF HAWAII PRESS
HONOLULU

Library of Congress Cataloging-in-Publication Data
Bushnell, O. A. (Oswald A.), 1913–
The gifts of civilization : germs and genocide in Hawai'i / O.A.
Bushnell.
p.   cm.
Includes bibliographical references and index.
ISBN 0–8248–1457–6
1. Hawaiians—Health and hygiene—History—18th century.
2. Hawaiians—Health and hygiene—History—19th century.
3. Hawaiians—First contact with Europeans. 4. Hawaiians—Diseases.
RA448.5.H38B87 1993
362.1'089994—dc20   92-40415
CIP

Cover illustration: "An Inland View of Atooi," by John Webber, 1778,
courtesy of Bishop Museum.

Book design by Janet Heavenridge

University of Hawaii Press books are printed on
acid-free paper and meet the guidelines for permanence
and durability of the Council on Library Resources

For *ka poʻe kahiko,*

the people of old,

and for their descendants

who live in Hawaiʻi today

About the Author

O. A. Bushnell, born and raised in Honolulu, received an undergraduate science degree from the University of Hawaii and a doctorate from the University of Wisconsin. He is emeritus professor of medical microbiology and medical history of the John A. Burns School of Medicine at the University of Hawaii. Dr. Bushnell, one of Hawaiʻi's foremost historical novelists, is the author of *The Return of Lono: A Novel of Captain Cook's Last Voyage; Kaʻaʻawa: A Novel about Hawaii in the 1850s; Molokai; The Stone of Kannon;* and *The Water of Kane;* as well as coauthor, with Sister Mary Laurence Hanley, O.S.F., of the biography *Pilgrimage and Exile: Mother Marianne of Molokai.* He has also written numerous articles on subjects in microbiology and medical history and is coauthor of three histories about Hawaiʻi.

CONTENTS

PREFACE

This is not a formal history. Nor is it a textbook. It is, rather, a series of essays, all concerned with the theme stated in the subtitle. The essay form was chosen because it allows a writer great freedom in the manner of presenting information, opinions, and conclusions he wants to share with interested readers.

These essays are part of the harvest from seventy years of thinking about the fate of the native Hawaiian people; from more than fifty years of reading innumerable books, manuscripts, newspapers, scientists' reports, and government documents; and from almost as many years of writing about subjects related to the linking theme.

Some readers may argue that many of the opinions expressed in these essays are "haolecentric." Of course they are. They must be so, because no other point of view is possible or realistic. (One look at Honolulu today, and at despoiled O'ahu around it, will tell you what realism means.)

In presenting such an account as this, a wise writer would be well advised to borrow entire the "Preface by the Author" composed by David Malo for his *Moolelo Hawaii*, or *History of Hawaii*. Written in Hawaiian during the 1830s and 1840s, translated into English in the 1890s (but, during the process, considerably altered, even censored, in some sections), it was published in 1903 as *Hawaiian Antiquities*. His preface is quoted here, not for the pious sentiments that Malo thought he should express, but for the commendable humility that he, being wise, assumed for the occasion:

> I do not suppose the following history to be free from mistakes, in that material for it has come from oral traditions; consequently it is marred by errors of human judgment and does not approach the accuracy of the word of God.

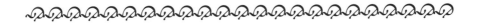

ONE

Life and the Land

The Hawaiian Islands are the most isolated of the world's habitable places, and the most difficult to reach by sea. The Pacific hemisphere's continents and the nearest of its high islands are more than 2,000 miles away. Between them and Hawai'i lies the ocean-moat, broad, deep, and cruel. Of all the places that venturesome men have claimed as home, the islands of Hawai'i probably were the last to be found.

We today do not know who the first Hawaiians were, or when they arrived in these islands. In fact, we can be certain about almost nothing that happened in Hawai'i or to its people before 1778. That is the pivotal time in Hawai'i's history—the beginning not of Hawaiians' history (for of course they had been making their own since the moment they reached these islands), but the beginning of a history that has been preserved and recorded in terms that today's scholars will accept. A few clues from the remote past are helping scientists to guess what might have happened so long ago.

According to the evidence gained from long-buried fishhooks and from C-14 datings of organic compounds taken from shelters and middens found at many different sites, some archaeologists now believe that Polynesian discoverers of Hawai'i came from the Marquesas Islands about 1,500 to 2,000 years ago—that is, sometime during the period between 100 B.C.E. and 500 C.E. Anthropologist P. F. Kirch favored a somewhat later settlement—"by the fourth to the seventh century."[1] However, scientists agree, these datings must be regarded as only tentative, because other sites may yet be found that will suggest even earlier times.

The islands of Hawai'i may have been habitable, useful, even

1

beloved to the people who settled here, but they have not always been as beautiful or as comfortable to live in as they are now. Beauty and comfort, as we define them, are attractions the islands have acquired only during the last hundred years or so. Before that time—except in a few places, such as the green hills and valleys around Waimea on Kaua'i of which Captain Cook approved in 1778, or the tantalizing coast near Hana on Maui toward which Captain de La Pérouse yearned in 1786—the islands were very different from the pleasure gardens they are today. People, not their gods, have transformed all of Hawai'i, Hawai'i *nei:* with much hard work and lavish applications of carelessness, human beings have done to these islands what djinn, angels, and deities are credited with having done for the paradises of humankind's imaginings.

The first people to reach Hawai'i would have found it a grim and brutal land, very different from the southern islands they called home. Barren and inhospitable for the most part, Hawai'i's islands were almost entirely lacking in edible plants and animals, generous only with rocks and stones. The stark beauty of sea-girt cliffs was here, and of the fluted sides and pointed peaks of high mountain ridges—the impassive patient beauty of sculptured lava, ageless, unchanging, and sterile, almost like a landscape on the moon. But the rampant vegetation we see today on foothills and plains, the cool green loveliness of Hawai'i as we think of it now—these were not here when those first Hawaiians came.

On windward coasts, to be sure, where high mountains won rains from clouds and many streams flowed or numerous springs welled up, earth responded with a covering of grasses, shrubs, and trees. Everywhere else, especially along leeward shores and on the mountains' lower slopes, the land was sere and bare, a desert of lava, or of cinders, or of naked dirt. Hawai'i was a place awaiting the touch of people. It was not so much a land grudging of its gifts as a land so poor as to have few gifts to offer. Yet what little it held it was willing to share, and this was kindness enough to those first voyagers who found their way to its shores.

Why they came, those first Hawaiians, we shall never know. Yet they came, borne in narrow outrigger canoes, or perhaps in safer double canoes joined by a stabilizing deck, helped by winds "when good fortune sat in the belly of their sails," or by strong paddlers when the winds fell away. They would have found these islands by accident—and only their gods will know how many Marquesans were lost to the sea before the first Hawaiians reached the new home to which kinder gods directed them.

Perhaps they were explorers searching for such a new home, seafarers as daring as their forefathers had been, who many centuries before had set out from the ancestral homelands in Indonesia and, trusting to their canoes, their guardian deities, and their knowledge of the stars high overhead, discovered one after the other all those far-flung islands in the South Pacific, from New Caledonia and Kapingamarangi in the west to the Marquesas and the Tuamotus in the east—and beyond. Perhaps they were desperate folk who, without having the chance to choose a destination, were forced to leave home by hunger, or tribal conflicts, or the tyranny of chiefs and priests. They may have been a curious group, driven by a very human compulsion to see what lay beyond the horizons near home. Possibly they were only fishermen, or gadabout travelers content with the familiar, who were blown off course by one of those violent storms that sweep so frequently across the southern sea. Such events have happened during recorded history, and they could have happened centuries ago, to begin the story of the people of Hawai'i.

Whatever the reason, they crossed the vast ocean. We cannot know what names they bore, or what Marquesan valley they came from. Because the immense mountains on the island of Hawai'i probably would have given them their first sight of this new discovery, more than likely they beached their canoes on the southernmost shores of that island, in the district now called Ka'ū. Among the oldest habitations that archaeologists have found so far are sand dunes and shallow caves near the tip of the southern cape on Hawai'i. From there the land swells up, like a young mother's full breast. Seeing this, the people would name the place Ka'Ū, "the breast that nursed them."

The island gave the voyagers rest from the sea, fresh water to drink, fern fronds, limpets, crabs, lobsters, edible seaweeds, reef fish, eels, and some birds to eat, but little else. For the seafarers, accustomed to little, grateful for anything, these would have been provender enough. The lonely austere island sustained them, even as it offered the promise of being able to yield much more.

No one can say with certainty what the discoverers did next. Some anthropologists believe that they were content with what they had found and, needing nothing more in order to exist, settled in their new home without making an attempt to return to the old. Other anthropologists, supported by ethnobotanists—and by traditions, which offer less reliable testimony than do fishhooks and plants— believe that they did return home with tidings of the great high islands they had found in the northern sea.

More than likely they did go back, to the southern land from which they had started. The sea would not have daunted them. But memories of the cool green valleys at home, and the knowledge that only through their efforts could the big new islands be made to provide them with the foods for which they hungered, must have urged them to return.

Steering this time by stars newly recognized, they went back. There they gathered willing companions and assembled the stocks of animals and plants which the northern islands lacked. And then, in one of the most wonderful achievements in the history of humankind, they found the way again, across the wide rolling sea, to the islands which were known only to them, to reach the haven that thereafter would be theirs. To those pioneers it was not a paradise— and not only because they had no thought of such a place. To them, children of the sea and of islands risen from the sea, it was to be home. When they returned, the last large habitable lands in the world were empty no longer.

We cannot know how many people embarked upon that first perilous voyage. Perhaps no more than fifty men, women, and children, possibly as many as a hundred, set out in canoes from the island of their birth. One of their largest double canoes—with its high curving prows and the connecting platform bearing masts for sails and a small thatched hut for meager shelter—could have carried twenty or thirty passengers, their few personal possessions, the animals and plants they brought along with supplies of foods to supplement the fish they might draw from the sea, bottle gourds holding stream water from home, and wide-mouthed bowls to catch whatever fresh water the *lauhala*-mat sails might collect from heaven-sent rains. During the 1970s and 1980s, Hawai'i's own *Hōkūle'a,* built according to models of double canoes of earlier centuries, demonstrated these facts of seafaring life in her several voyages to and from central Polynesia. On one of those trips, she sailed from Tahiti to Honolulu in twenty-one days.

The settlers' descendants, in stories they would tell in time, called Hawai'i-loa the leader of that first brave company. Thinking to honor him, they gave his name to the largest island in this northern archipelago. But in the name they were remembering also legendary homelands in Southeast Asia from which their ancestors had sailed centuries before.

They were a forethoughtful folk. On that first planned voyage, and probably on a number of later visits to islands south of the equator, they brought everything they could transport that would help them to live in the land of Hawai'i-loa. They began the process that continues to this day, by which these islands were transformed from little more than comfortless protrusions of rock above the surface of the sea into gardens where food is plentiful—and where, to later visitors from other places in the world, the prospects do resemble their notions of Paradise.

ৼৼৼৼ

So goes, more or less, the generally accepted—certainly romanticized and probably erroneous—reconstruction of Hawaiians' history during the centuries before 1778. The theorizers who first arranged this sequence of events knew very little about those times except the suggestions offered by a few artifacts, the vagaries of traditions, and carefully regulated infusions of imagination. Younger scholars, however, are contending that the idea that these islands were discovered accidentally by only a small number of wandering Polynesians is both naive and mistaken. These modern theorizers, provided with much more information about the past than their precursors could call upon (and also with much larger inputs of imagination), are drastically revising the old scenario. And who can say they are wrong?

Thus, anthropologists Tom Dye of Hawaii Pacific University and Eric Komori of Bernice Pauahi Bishop Museum, in considering the ancient problems, used a wide range of C-14 datings, the latest in statistical techniques, and computer analyses to reach their conclusions. They studied the distribution in time and space of C-14 datings from 606 charcoal samples collected from sites on "every major island except Lāna'i and Ni'ihau." Those charcoal samples, they assumed, represented "permanent habitations" occupied during long periods of datable time, rather than "temporary camps." C-14 data from these specimens showed that the number of cooking fires (and therefore of the people who started them) rose sharply "from about 900 to 1300 A.D." A slower rate of growth occurred in the fifteenth and sixteenth centuries, followed by "a levelling off after . . . 1600."

Employing "a new statistical approach described by Stanford University archaeologist John Rick in 1987," Dye and Komori concluded that the native population before 1778 grew at an average annual rate of 0.27 percent. (For comparison, David Stannard calculated a rate of 0.52 percent and R. C. Schmitt settled on 0.63 percent.) With a growth rate of 0.27 percent, said Dye and Komori, "a population of 100,000 in 1778 would have required an initial Polynesian colonization of about 938 in the year 400 A.D.—or 771 in 300 A.D." These figures mean that generally accepted estimates of 200,000 to 300,000 for the total Hawaiian population in 1778 are far too high. Moreover, Dye added, Stannard's claim that 800,000 to 1 million people "could have been" living here in 1778 is even more extreme: for that number of residents "the founding population had to be around 30,000 people, which we think is unrealistically high."

Finally, according to Dye and Komori, migrations of as many as 938 people in 400 C.E. (or 771 people in 300 C.E.) "indicate that Hawai'i was not settled by 'outcasts' from South Pacific islands . . . but rather by skilled sailors and farmers who arrived in several waves." Implied in their data and in their conclusions (at least as they are reported) are these significant decisions: no cooking fires were set before 300 C.E., and therefore no Hawaiians lived here before that time; and the average annual rate of population growth is correctly calculated at 0.27 percent.[2]

Early in 1989, historian David Stannard stunned commentators who, for the last hundred years or so, have been accepting the all-but-sacrosanct population estimates of 200,000 to 300,000 Hawaiians for 1778.[3] Stannard declared that the number of Hawaiians in 1778 "could have grown to" as high as 800,000 or even a million. He bases his conclusions on: (1) a review of population figures presented in accounts left by early visitors and residents; (2) archaeological features on the main islands, especially those concerned with agriculture, aquaculture, the "carrying power" of certain land areas, and identified house sites; (3) recent revisions in demographical distributions and population statistics for Amerindian societies in North, Central, and South America, all of which seem to have supported much larger numbers of people than have been generally accepted; (4) analogous situations derived from population data for societies in other parts of the world; and (5) the rapid destruction of aboriginal peoples throughout the world in consequence of their exposure to representatives of European civilization.

As before, so again: the question of Hawai'i's population at any time before the 1830s is not yet answered. Controversy will continue to excite the young and bemuse the old—who, in their wisdom, know that some questions can never be answered. The only important datum that scholars can count on is the fact that somehow, from somewhere, in a world not far away but certainly younger than the one we inhabit, the first Hawaiians came to these islands, sailing bravely across the intervening sea.

ぞぞぞぞ

These islands were not entirely lifeless when those first Hawaiians arrived. Nature's means for dispersing creatures of the land—currents of wind and ocean, migratory birds, pieces of driftwood—had carried to them living cells, seeds, spores, and minuscule eggs almost as soon as the lava of which the islands were formed had cooled enough to receive these germs of life. And the ocean was full of creatures of the sea, migrants from waters off the surrounding continents, especially from that fertile source of marine organisms, the straits separating the coasts of Southeast Asia and its innumerable islands.

About 1,900 species of endemic plants (1,729 represented by seed plants and 168 by ferns) and more than 5,000 species of insects and other small endemic land animals had preceded the human colonists and were thriving in places where water was available.[4] Even so, except for a few species of birds (some known today only from fossil remains) and the young fronds or roots of a few kinds of ferns, the islands offered little for hungry people to eat. The colonists would have had to establish here all the plants and animals they depended on for foods, medicines, utensils, and clothing.

These treasures from the homeland, all neatly packaged in leaves, gourds, plaited baskets, pieces of matting, all so carefully watched during the long journey, were carried ashore at the landing place and unwrapped. As prayers to the gods went up, asking their care for the plantings so that the people too might grow, the hopeful pioneers put into Hawai'i's soil coconuts and *kukui* nuts; seeds of mountain apples, of medicinal *noni,* and of gourd vines; corms of taro and tubers of sweet potatoes, yams, and arrowroot; shoots of bananas, breadfruit, *ti,* sugarcane, of '*awa* (the sleep-inducing pepper) and of *wauke* (the paper mulberry) from which *kapa* (the "bark cloth" of Polynesians) is fashioned.

Even before those reverent plantings were made, almost as soon as the voyagers themselves, prostrate on the beach, had heard their priest utter prayers of thanksgiving for the voyage safely ended, they brought ashore the animals whose progeny would give them meat: scrawny pigs, perky little dogs, and lean chickens. Uninvited but inevitable fellow-travelers would have been lice, fleas, and perhaps other such vermin, arriving as parasites on both people and animals. And, inescapable companions of people everywhere in all their migrations, rats and houseflies came with them too.

Unseen, but also introduced, were remembrances of the home left behind: the thoughts, language, customs, and *kapu,* the taboos, of the widespread Polynesian race; the skills and crafts and arts learned from their parents; and, above all, around all, present in every earthly and celestial thing, the immanent gods—those defenses that hopeful souls everywhere must raise against what Freud called "the crushing supremacy of Nature."[5]

These were the four greatest gods: creator Kāne, the father of every thing below and above, who dwelled in the sun; gentle Lono, the giver of peace and of healing, whose abodes were the clouds and the plants of earth called forth by his blessing of rain; aloof and restless Kanaloa, lord of the sea and all it held; and energizing Kū, the source of power in all its manifestations, who often rose up in the livers and minds of men, urging them to war. With him came his consort Hina, the goddess whose feminine attributes complemented the masculine strengths of Kū.

With them would have journeyed most of "the forty lesser gods, and the four hundred, the four thousand, the forty thousand little gods," who moved so easily in and out of the all-embracing spirit world. These lived in mountains and hills, in valleys, caves, and stones; in trees, herbs, ferns, and grasses; in fishes, birds, and beasts of every kind; in springs, streams, swamps, and drops of dew; in mists, clouds, thunder, lightning, winds; and in the wandering planets, the glittering far-off stars.

Always watching, often helpful, usually tolerant, sometimes maleficent, all those gods, great and small, gave a Hawaiian both religion and conscience by decreeing the kapus that their priests told him he must observe. Because he could never escape the surveillance of the gods and of their priests, and because he dared not ignore the promptings from his own 'aumakua, his ancestral spirit guardian, every Hawaiian gave them obedience and respect. If he failed this trust by breaking their laws, they punished him. He paid for his offense in misfortune, loss of property or loved ones or of love itself, in unhappiness, in sickness of body or of spirit. So terrible was their power, so strong was his fear, he believed that if his crime was great he must pay for it with his life: knowing that he was beyond forgiving, he lay down on his sleeping-mat and stayed there until he died.

Every child learned these lessons early in life—from the teachings of parents, from the warnings of priests who spoke for the gods, from the histories of others who were favored or broken by the gods. Whatever they gave to a righteous man the gods could take away if he should lapse into unrighteousness—although, as is the way with deities who are forbearing or preoccupied, "there are times when justice limps."

When, later, they explored their new home, those first Hawaiians became acquainted with two manifestations of divine power they could not have seen in the land of their birth. With a fine sense of relationships, and their realists' humor, they decided that these novel forces must be feminine. The blazing, impulsive, destructive, hot-tempered, and beautiful one who issued so unpredictably from her underground realm they called Pele. The haughty, pallid, silent, cold maiden who never deigned to descend from her lofty mountain citadels they named Poli'ahu.

Precisely because they were realists, they did not scorn the womanly fury they called Pele. As their tales about her reveal, they regarded Pele as their Earth Goddess in her triple manifestations: as Mother, maker of mountains and of islands and of humankind; as Lover-Pursuer-Virago, devourer of men who do not heed her power, no matter how handsome and accomplished they may think they are; and, finally, as Kūkū Wahine, Grandmother, who receives in her wrinkled bosom the bodies of the dead, taking them into her care once more. Among all their great deities, Hawaiians knew Pele best, because they could see her and all her works in the lands she had made for them.

Bare and comfortless though these islands of Hawai'i-loa would have been, and crowded though they were with demanding gods, they were wonderfully safe places in which people could live. They harbored no serious visible enemies, whether human, animal, or vegetable, to endanger the settlers. Only the sea was treacherous, but only occasionally, and Polynesians are accustomed to the moods of Kanaloa. Pele's tantrums presented few problems: being sensible

folk, they avoided her awesome domains, the craters atop Kīlauea
and Mauna Loa, or they simply ran away when she burst out from
one or the other of her fiery lairs, chasing after them in rage.

Only very few of the most intrepid men dared to climb to
Poliʻahu's ghostly realm. They were drawn there not by interest in
her mystifying self, but by search for riches in a few cold dark cav-
erns opening like sores in the mountain's sides: pieces of the hardest
of stones, left like clots of Pele's blood, shed when she labored to
build her snow-sister's house of Mauna Kea. In the highest caves,
more than 13,000 feet above the level of the sea, gasping for breath
in the thin air, trembling with cold and fear, the climbers would
gather up their prizes. Usually they would hurry back to seaside
homes where, warm again and safe, they fashioned from those
obdurate stones the sharp-edged adzes that enabled farmers, woodcutters, and artisans to do their work.

Throughout all the land, in those days, only the gods were jealous,
only the gods could be cruel. They were appeased by prayers and
offerings, their wrath was avoided by obeying the kapus. In those
earliest years people felt no need to be cruel to others. Because they
were so few, so precious, because the islands to which they had come
were so vast and so empty, the companions of Hawaiʻi-loa lived in
peace, with themselves and with their land.

ನ-ನ-ನ-ನ

As the animals and plants they had imported thrived, so did
the people prosper. Before many years passed they and their children
were "spreading like gourd-vines over the plains." From the first settlement new ʻohana, young offshoots, were sent, to farther bays,
more distant valleys, and, in time, to the other islands awaiting them
beyond the narrow straits. Thus did the companions of Hawaiʻi-loa
bring life to the land. And thus, in return, did the gods and the land
give life to the people.

ನ-ನ-ನ-ನ

They claimed the land, taming it to their needs. They were
hardworking, cooperative, ingenious, imaginative, even while they
were being most practical. Stones and woods, bits of shells, teeth,
bones, and tusks, larger leaves, fibers from bark and grasses gave
them tools, clothing, and shelter. They had nothing else to use. They
had no beasts of burden or wheeled carts, no mortar or clay or uten-

sils made from metals. Using only hands, stone adzes, and staves for levers, they built platforms of fitted stones for temples and dwellings, stone-walled terraces for taro patches, stone-lined irrigation ditches, straight level roads and climbing paths often paved with flat stones and pebbles. And shelters made of tree trunks and branches, thatched with plaited leaves or bundles of grasses. And canoes such as they had made at home.

Such industry so impressed their successors that, even in the triumph of conquest, the usurpers did not claim the more durable structures as works of their hands: the conquerors attributed those monuments in stone to "the *menehune*." Vague memories of these menehunes and a very few of their works—such as a short section of an irrigation ditch near Waimea on Kaua'i—survive even now. But the builders themselves have been demeaned: today they have been reduced to obnoxiously cute caricatures of Europe's elves and leprechauns, which look like creatures that might have floated to Hawai'i under a toadstool rejected by Disneyland.

Neither the menehunes' hardiness nor their gods could save them from the invaders who moved in upon them from the south. The first settlers seem to have left behind them, in communities of the Central Pacific, a memory of their discoveries in the northern sea. They may have been nostalgic enough, for a while, to keep in touch with the homeland. In the event, time and distance offered them no protection, and they were subjected to the usual fate of all pioneers. After the passage of several centuries, perhaps as many as a thousand years, a new wave of voyagers came sailing in their double-canoes to the islands of Hawai'i-loa. Genealogies, traditions, customs, kapus, and similarities in language indicate that those invaders departed from a home in or near Tahiti. Probably they moved out from there in response to the same social forces that stimulated the "Great Migrations" that sent other seafarers to the very limits of the Polynesian triangle—Easter Island in the east, New Zealand in the south— and to other places within that vast area.

The newcomers to Hawai'i—certainly their great chiefs and high priests—appear to have been a taller and more warring folk than the menehune. Beyond doubt they were more arrogant: claiming descent from the great gods gave them the conviction that they were chosen to rule. They moved in and took over the islands of Hawai'i (just as, at about the same time, Norsemen moved in upon Britain and the coastal areas of Europe).

The conquerors from Tahiti became the nobles of Hawai'i, the *ali'i*. The menehunes who survived the invaders' entry either submitted and stayed in their homes or retreated to mountain fastnesses and distant islands, such as Kaua'i and Ni'ihau. Those who yielded merged with the *manahune,* the commoners who accompanied the ali'i. Those commoners, known as *maka'āinana,* people who attend the land, were not slaves. But they lived to serve their masters, the ruling chiefs, and the teacher-priests who ruled those lordly ones. As always, upon the backs of commoners was laid the burden.

The conquerors brought new kapus and rituals, new and bloodier demands from Kū. With them fear too entered in: fear of the chiefs and fear of the priests—especially those evil ones who practiced the black arts of sorcery—and fear of death come too soon, in battle, in famine as a consequence of war, in brutal sacrifices in the temples of Kū, the god of war. Upon Hawaiians, as upon societies elsewhere, the ugly pattern was imposed: as people increased in number, their lives diminished in value. No longer precious, life could be squandered—on the altars of Kū, in wars fought at the urging of Kū-kā'ilimoku, Kū-the-Snatcher-of-Lands, who delighted in provoking those games arising out of boredom, those conflicts of greed and assertions of pride without which some chiefs can never be content.

Nevertheless, when all known factors are considered, even though this later Hawaiian society must have been a very docile one, perhaps even a terrorized one, because it was an authentic theocracy managed by priests in the name of the gods, it was also a relatively safe society. Each adult knew his or her place in it, and almost everyone tried carefully to keep to that place. Although the threat of a man's being sacrificed may have been unrelenting, sacrifices were neither numerous nor frequent, as they were in more fanatical religious centers in the Society Islands, or on the blood-drenched altars of Aztec Mexico. And in Hawai'i, until late in the eighteenth century, most wars were little more than border raids, in which few soldiers fought and not many were killed.[6]

The relationships of people to things about them and to each other, and of people to the gods, great or small, were defined by the kapus. As in all societies whose elders are responsible for maintaining law and order under the guise of custom and tradition, those kapus prescribed rules of conduct for almost every thought, deed, and association, enforcing them with threats of punishment if ever a kapu was broken, whether knowingly or unknowingly. The kapus, to use Sartre's term for Europe's equivalent regulations, were forms of "inert violence"—convertible in an instant into exactions of retribution.

Yet, to be fair, most taboos were founded upon respect for order. Order was the gods' first law. In almost every action of his life, even in those which relieved his body's needs, a Hawaiian was required to remember the respect he owed to the *mana,* the spirit power, in himself, in each person around him, and in the *kino lau,* the embodiments, of all the gods in all the places and things they inhabited. In consequence of those ritual sanctions by the group, so universal as to be unquestioned, so thoroughly learned as to be almost involuntary, no one dared to defile land or water or sea, no one caused waste or disarray or ugliness. Land was not blighted, water was not fouled. In return for such respect, the gods gave freely of the fruits of the land and the produce of the sea. And when the gods smiled, the people prospered—and rejoiced.

The rewards of such a life were many: happiness of a sort, if only because no one questioned that this was the only way to live; physical comforts of food and shelter to a considerable degree; the health of cleanliness and good order; a culture surprisingly rich in the material things that the environment provided and the ingenuity of people could adapt. They made the tools that drew foods from land and sea; but they also fashioned the delicately tinted and decorated kapa clothing they wore, the gorgeous feather capes and splendid feather helmets in which they arrayed their chiefs. Their spirits may have been cowed by spying priests and by glowering wide-mouthed images of the gods that sculptors carved and set up in temple precincts; but they also composed merry songs and subtle riddles and remembered in chants their ancestors and their deeds unto the fiftieth generation. Their bodies may have belonged to the chiefs who ruled over them, and through the chiefs to the deities who governed the world; but those bodies also knew the pleasures of love, the excitements of sports and games, the laughter of ribald jesting, the graces of dancing, the solace of rest from toil, the soft embraces of small sons and daughters born of their loins.

Their intellects may have been limited by lack of contact with people from other cultures, but, so wondrous is the human mind, their imaginations leaped over the vast spaces of the encircling sea and they thought the great thoughts of people everywhere, or found stimulus in studying the familiar things of home, recognizing every plant

and animal and type of stone, naming almost every kind of wind and
rain cloud in the air and wave pattern in the sea. A people who used
ten different words meaning "beautiful" could not have been mere
savages. A people who could compose as profound a poem as *The
Water of Kane* and cherish poets who could conceive—and remember, too, without help from writing—the 2,102 lines of *The Kumulipo Chant,* an epic of creation, was not a people to be scorned.

Despite so many restraints, the spirit was still free, in some people
if not in all. They were the questioners, the leaders who managed to
change the way in which they were being forced to live. Not the
authority of the gods did they challenge, but the rule of evil men.
Rebellions and usurpations were not unknown: cruel chiefs, like the
hated Milu of Kohala, who did not take good care of their people,
who thought to rule by force and fear, could be overthrown, vicious
priests could be deposed, and good men could be raised to high
places. The good men, like the High Chief 'Umi, were long remembered, but only the worst of the bad, such as Milu, found places in
the memories of people.

For its time and setting the Hawaiian society was remarkably successful. It was primitive, "neolithic" as anthropologists would say,
only because of its limited material resources. But the things that
Hawaiians made with their simple tools—and with their nimble fingers—and the society they evolved command admiration even now.
It was "savage" only in comparison with the society expected of Uto-
pia, in the way the society of Homer's Greece was savage. And it was
less brutish than were most of its contemporary societies throughout
the world, even those of patronizing Europe, just as it was less brutal
than are most of those that adorn our civilized world today.

It was successful most of all because its people had established a
sensitive and sensible understanding with their environment. They
had no written language, yet they read with wisdom the signs with
which their gods addressed them. Out of respect for the gods,
Hawaiians did not ignore those messages; out of gratitude for their
generosity, Hawaiians did not waste their gifts. They conserved,
replenished, restored. When they plucked a fruit, they planted its
seed to ensure the continuance of its kind. When they cleared a field,
they trampled the uprooted weeds or the ashes from the burned
weeds into the soil of that field, thereby enriching it for the next
planting. During the months from May until September, when shell-
fish release their eggs and fishes spawn their young, Hawaiians put a

kapu on those mother creatures, safeguarding them until their purpose was fulfilled. They learned from the gods the season for planting, the season for gathering in. And, in the brief season which the
gods allot to each living thing, they saw, in common with people in
other places, that for Hawaiians too there is a time to live and a time
to die.

In harmony with the gods who shared with them land and sea and
sky, they observed the kapus. They were a respectful folk. And
because, by their nature, the gods are just, they rewarded this righteous people. Foods and sweet water they gave in plenty and—that
greatest blessing of all, that surest sign of their favoring—children,
many beautiful children. Throughout all the islands, from where the
sun rose at Ha'eha'e on Hawai'i to where it set beyond Lehua, the
gods were kind, the people flourished.

How much of all this pious talk about expressions of respect
for the provident gods and their manifold gifts can we believe in this
age of disrespect for everything? Can we really believe that those
"primitive" Hawaiians, in their "Stone Age culture," actually understood the principles of conservation, perceived the ecological associations among plants, animals, and human beings, when Western societies are only now beginning to realize how important a part these
interdependencies play in the health of Earth and of all the creatures
who live on it? Or are these large claims for Hawaiians' attitudes and
responses merely exercises in creative nostalgia, imagined by sad-
dened writers and embittered rhetoricians, all longing for the good
old days that never really existed—and that, alas, if they did exist,
can never be regained? Europeans too indulged in such wishful
thinking when, caught in the brutalities of the Iron Age, they yearned
for the gentle simplicities of the Golden Age.

In this matter also we cannot be sure about the degree to which
Hawaiians before 1778 practiced those precepts for respecting land,
water, sea, and air, and all the creatures in them. Probably most of
ka po'e kahiko, the people of old, did observe these sensible and
helpful rules. After all, they are recognitions of obligations (or fears)
that are built into the pantheism of all primitive societies, and
Hawaiians most certainly were pantheists. People in Western
societies, as well as in Eastern, accepted these beliefs and followed
their preachments until relatively recently, when, under the blighting

touch of exploitation and industrialization, they rejected them—to their cost. Western societies, in fact, are now "discovering" these principles anew, giving acceptably scientific terms to concepts that pantheists of long ago honored without need for names.

Further evidence to support this conclusion about Hawaiians of old is provided right here, in their islands. Many of these signs of respect were continued far into the twentieth century, especially by farmers and families who lived close to the land or to the sea. (Not all of these people, incidentally, were native Hawaiians.) Furthermore, in a happy proof of the persistence of custom, if not of piety, some of us who learned from our elders to make these offerings of respect still observe some of the ways of old, some of the time.

Upon this insular society, presumably a harmonious one because it had established the relationships with creating deities and neighboring people that ensured continuity of the race—but also a static one because it was almost unchanging and unchangeable—descended the bringers of change.

Naturally, some observers expressed very different opinions, depending on their points of view. The Reverend Sheldon Dibble, while a missionary-teacher at Lahainaluna High School in the 1830s, composed this uncordial description of the people of old:

> The Hawaiians were sorely oppressed, wretchedly destitute, and exceedingly ignorant; stupid to all that is lovely, grand, and awful in the works of God; low, naked, filthy, vile and sensual; covered with every abomination, stained with blood and black with crime. Idolatry also reigned with all its obscenity, frantic rage and horrid exhibitions of bleeding human sacrifices. Then superadd the deadly evils introduced from Christian lands during an intercourse of 40 years, and you will place them in the state in which they were found by the first missionaries who arrived among them.[7]

ぐぐぐぐ

From among the mysteries and theories regarding their past, one incontestable fact about the Hawaiian people does emerge: during most of their history as the northernmost branch of "the widespread Polynesian nation," as Captain Cook called them, they were cut off from frequent contact with people in other parts of the Pacific. Even if the earliest settlers from the Marquesas Islands did make an occasional voyage to the homeland; even if, in their turn, the conquerors from Tahiti did keep in touch with the Society

Islands, such contacts would have been infrequent because of the distances and hardships involved. Probably those return voyages ceased almost as soon as children born in Hawai'i replaced parents who treasured their connections with the islands to the south.

Long before 1778 all voyages between Hawai'i and central Polynesia ended. Not even a memory of the Marquesan home was kept, and Tahiti itself became no more than a legend. "Kahiki" referred to any place beyond the horizon which Hawaiians no longer knew how to find; and Ke-ala-i-kahiki, the Way to Tahiti, served only as the name for the narrow channel between Lāna'i and Kaho'olawe, instead of as a reminder of the best point of departure for the long journey to the southern home. No brave voyagers sailed upon that course, either from the north or from the south. As W. D. Alexander wrote, "there is no further evidence [of voyages to Kahiki] in any of the ancient legends, songs, or genealogies for five hundred years." Hawaiians, knowing only their own islands, thought of Kahiki as "a land of mystery and magic, full of marvels, and inhabited by supernatural beings."[8] "Audacious no more," as Arnold Toynbee sneered, Hawaiians and their fellow Polynesians had become members of an "arrested civilization."[9]

Yet if Hawaiians did not venture away from their islands, and southern Polynesians stayed at home, could strangers from other places have come to these shores before 1778?

On 23 December 1832 a storm-battered fishing boat from Japan, after drifting for almost a year, reached Waialua Bay on O'ahu.[10] Four men, wasted and weak from hunger, thirst, and scurvy, lived through the ordeal, which had claimed five others of the original crew. If that one sturdy vessel survived such a voyage, then quite possibly, before 1832, and before 1778, other derelict vessels could have brought castaways to Hawai'i from the Orient or from islands in the southern and western Pacific.

Fernand Braudel, for example, related "the story of the Japanese junk which sailed from Japan to Acapulco in Mexico in 1610. A gift from the Japanese, it was carrying home Rodrigo Vivero and his fellow castaways." Although Vivero and his crew manned that first ship, "two other junks, both with Japanese crews, later made the same voyage. Such exploits prove that junks were technically quite equal to brave the high seas."[11] They also show that, at least until 1638, when the Tokugawa shogunate forbade Japan's mariners to sail abroad, other Japanese vessels bound to and from Mexico (or to places in Central America) could have visited a Hawaiian island or been wrecked upon its shore. Japanese merchantmen too, before 1638, roamed the South Pacific, licensed to venture from home ports by the Vermilion Seal of the Tokugawa regime.

Chinese vessels, even larger than Japanese and presumably more seaworthy, were not prohibited from sailing wherever their masters chose to go. Expeditions from China, borne aboard great seagoing junks, may have been exploring the Central Pacific during the fifteenth century, continuing the searches begun as early as the sixth century, when "sandalwood junks," seeking the precious wood, traversed the well-known southern routes among the islands of Indonesia.[12] Whether driven by explorers' curiosity or by storms, Chinese ships might have visited the Hawaiian Islands long before Captain Cook's expedition found them in 1778. Ruth Hanner of Honolulu, who has studied hundreds of petroglyphs in Hawai'i, believes that many of them show distinctly Chinese ideographs and motifs, so alien to native Hawaiian inscribings that they could have been engraved only by Chinese or Japanese visitors or castaways.[13]

Even more likely, however, is the possibility that, after 1527, during the 250 years when Spanish galleons sailed between ports in Mexico and the Philippine Islands, one or more of them may have visited the Hawaiian Islands or been wrecked upon their coasts. Dahlgren, Stokes, and other writers have discussed this subject at great length and—basing their conclusions upon the absence of documents, maps, and such tangible evidence from royal archives in Spain and Mexico—decided that Spanish mariners did not discover the Hawaiian Islands. Other writers—foremost among them Dr. A. Mouritz of Honolulu, an indefatigable (and often uncritical) collector of medical curiosa—were equally convinced that Spaniards did discover these islands, but kept their location secret from fear of English privateers and dislike of Dutch merchantmen. In 1963 George Carter declared that, if they did discover Hawai'i or any others of the Polynesian island groups, the Spaniards "deliberately chose to ignore these lands" because they were useless both as "staging areas" and as sources of spices or gold.[14]

Despite the lack of documentary confirmation, the possibility remains that Spanish navigators did find these islands, and that records of their visits were lost, suppressed, or misplaced. A Spanish ship wrecked on a Hawaiian shore could not very well send home documentary proof of its fate. One tradition concerning such a wreck was detailed enough to impress W. D. Alexander, a very skeptical man, when in the late 1880s he wrote his matter-of-fact *History of the Hawaiian People*. During the reign of Keali'ikaloa, eldest son of 'Umi (a celebrated chief who ruled long and well on the island of Hawai'i about 1500 c.e.),

> a foreign vessel was wrecked at Keei, in South Kona, Hawaii . . . only the captain and his sister reached the shore in safety . . . they knelt down on the beach, remaining a long time in that posture, whence the place was called Kulou. . . . The people received them kindly and set food before them. The strangers intermarried with the natives, and became the progenitors of certain well-known families of chiefs, such as that of Kaikioewa, former governor of Kauai [during the reigns of Kamehameha II and Kamehameha III].[15]

Inasmuch as the genealogies of chiefs were supposed to be too sacrosanct for falsification, Kaikioewa's lineage suggests that at least one foreign ancestor arrived from a distant land before 1778. Less reliable is Alexander's identification of the very ship that presented those "well-known families of chiefs" with such exotic forebears. Because "no white people except the Spaniards were navigating the Pacific Ocean at that early period," he concluded that the wrecked vessel was one of a squadron of three ships fitted out by Cortez which departed from Zacatula, Mexico, on 31 October 1527, under the command of Alvarado de Saavedra.[16]

Even so, ships and visitors from any foreign land would have been so rare that they had little effect upon the memories, the genealogies, or the health of Hawaiians. For good or for ill, a complement of new chromosomes might have been introduced into the constitution of a chief or of a commoner as he acquired an extraordinary parent; and, probably to their distress for a time, an inoculum of new microorganisms (as well as a leavening of novel ideas) would have been imparted to the local populace.

ぴぴぴぴぴ

Much more difficult to explain are the "epidemics" which—if they did occur—David Malo mentioned in his *Hawaiian Antiquities:*

> 10. During Waia's reign Hawaii nei was visited by a pestilence, *ma'i ahulau,* which resulted in a great mortality among the people. Only twenty-six persons were left alive, and these were saved and cured by the use of two remedies, *pilikai* [a species of morning glory] and *loloi* [an unknown agent].
> 11. This pestilence was by the ancients called Ikipuahola. . . .

18. After Waia's time another pestilence called *Hai-lepo* invaded the land and caused the death of a large number of the people. Only sixteen recovered, being saved by the use of a medicine . . . composed of some kind of earth *(lepo)*.[17]

Little information of value can be gained from such vague references. The number of survivors can hardly be accepted literally—unless Malo was recounting a tale of an almost legendary past, soon after the first settlers arrived, when the population was so small and so concentrated that it could have been all but annihilated by a single epidemic. The name of Waia, according to Malo, appears very early in the genealogies, soon after Wakea, the Sky Father, and Papa, the Flat-Earth Mother, created the human race. In Malo's time *waia* meant "foul or polluted," and in the opinion of N. B. Emerson, who translated Malo's work into English, "its use here is probably figurative."[18] According to Kamakau,[19] Wai'a was one of the "eight new husbands" Papa took "in revenge" when lustful Wakea "introduced the 'sin' of mating with many women." For this reason alone, Malo's "epidemics" seem to be closer to myth than to history.

More relevant to this book's purpose is the fact that, despite their great knowledge about the past, neither Malo, nor Samuel M. Kamakau, nor John Papa I'i mentioned any epidemics during the later history of Hawai'i's people. Inasmuch as Malo had to reach all the way back to Waia's epoch, to the imagined beginnings of the human race, in order to find a memory of so dramatic an event as a pestilence, we can conclude that the people who lived closer to his time were spared an acquaintance with such terrible—and unforgettable—afflictions.

ぐぐぐぐ

The long isolation from their counterparts in other areas of the Pacific affected every creature that lived on the islands of Hawai'i. Endemic animals and plants, having been established here for much longer times than the human inhabitants, revealed the effects of their separation much more dramatically, at least to biologists, than did the people. In the 5 million years or so since Kaua'i rose above the sea, in the million years and more during which the island of Hawai'i's immense body has been growing upward and outward, the processes of evolution in isolation developed a flora and fauna that are notable for their high degree of endemicity, the relative paucity both of presumed ancestor organisms and of their descendants, the versatility and rapidity with which mutation and speciation have occurred, and the remarkable forms which some of these adaptations to the Hawaiian environment have displayed.

Among animals the best-known examples of such adaptations are those shown by land mollusks, drepanid birds, and a number of insects. In 1948, in his admirable introduction to the series of monographs entitled *The Insects of Hawaii,* E. C. Zimmerman wrote:

> It is estimated that the total number of ancestral species which gave rise to the 3,722 known endemic insects was between 233 and 254. There is reason to believe that future modification of these last numbers may be downward rather than upward. The significant conclusion reached here is the fact that perhaps only 233 to 254 fertilized female insect immigrants could have given rise to the entire endemic insect fauna! (It will be of interest to note here that only 14 original colonizations have given rise to the entire Hawaiian land-bird fauna.) Of all the data that indicate extreme insularity for the Hawaiian Insecta, these seem to be the most striking. How few have been the successful immigrants over the several millions of years available for dispersal and colonization![20]

"The native plants of Hawaii," Zimmerman continued,[21] "form an assemblage which has been referred to as one of the most distinctive floras in the world." Although taxonomists have not yet completed their studies on identifications, derivations, and interrelationships, their estimates for the degree of endemicity of native Hawaiian plants range from 90 to 95 percent.

In a chapter written for Zimmerman's analysis of the Hawaiian biota, botanist F. R. Fosberg stated that "the flora is a small one, typically that of an oceanic island. The total known flora of seed plants . . . is 1,729 species and varieties scattered through 216 genera; that of ferns, 168 species and varieties in 37 genera."[22] Fosberg considered that these 1,729 species of spermatophytes (or seed-bearing plants) were derived from 272 "original immigrants," and that the 168 species of pteridophytes (or ferns) were derived from 135 immigrant ancestors.[23]

In both groups, the majority of immigrants came from the Indo-Pacific and the Austral regions. For the seed plants, "an average of one successful arrival and establishment every 20,000 to 30,000 years would account for the flora."[24] This flora "is exactly the type that might be expected to be descended from a random aggregation of chance waifs carried overseas by a combination of factors such as storms, currents and birds."[25] Of plant adaptations to the Hawaiian habitat, best known are "the shrubby violets, the arborescent lobelias, the peculiar composites,"[26] and the noble leguminous tree, *Acacia koa,* which, until long after Cook's expedition visited these islands, grew nowhere else in the world.

Although both Zimmerman and Fosberg stressed that their figures are tentative, their general conclusions are beyond question: they affirm the isolation, both geographical and temporal, of the Hawaiian Islands and all the creatures that lived upon them in 1778. Moreover, by implication, the small number of cosmopolitan or nonendemic plants and animals represented here is further evidence that the human population did not maintain a prolonged contact with their homelands south of the equator. If they had done so, at least a few more of the animals and plants found in those southern islands would have been introduced to Hawai'i, either by intention or by accident.

The effects of long isolation on the aboriginal Hawaiians themselves have not been so clearly defined, if only because people are not studied so easily as are plants and animals. The fact that most Hawaiians were dead long before the modern techniques of anthropology, demography, epidemiology, genetics, immunology, medicine, microbiology, and pathology could be directed to studying them adds to the difficulty. Under the circumstances, the best that can be done now is to make some inferences and deductions about the Hawaiian people based on the present state of knowledge in these disciplines.

This heady game of hindsight is a dangerous one. It is made all the more precarious when several unknown factors, as well as a clutch of treacherous variables, must be employed in establishing the premises of an argument. To begin with, we cannot know with certainty The Truth about health and sickness and causes of death among Hawai'i's people before 1778—or, for that matter, at any time before the middle of the twentieth century, by when at last the methodologies of the medical sciences (and those of their practitioners) were sufficiently improved to give reliable meaning to biostatistics. Today we can only guess about the roles these factors played in the history of native Hawaiians. The following essay presents some guesses—discreetly offered, in the tradition of science, as hypotheses—about what might have been the state of public and individual health among the people of old. These hypotheses may not present The Truth. Yet, too, they may not be false. They do help to explain the tragic history of Hawai'i's native people in the calamitous time after 1778.

In that climactic year, the one immediately following the last they were to know as members of their isolated primitive society, between 200,000 and 300,000 natives are thought to have lived upon the eight habitable islands of Hawai'i. (In 1989, however, Stannard declared that the native population in 1778 was much higher, "between 800,000 and a million."[27])

In that fateful year of 1778, explorers from a greater society "discovered" these islands, and thereby brought to their inhabitants many of the wonders and most of the evils of Western civilization. For more than a century after that critical year, the evils of civilization outnumbered and overwhelmed its benefits. The impact on Hawaiians was disastrous: their society was shattered, and as it died Death came for its people too, in many guises, which they could neither recognize nor combat. By 1900 only 29,799 native "pure-blood" Hawaiians remained alive, and the islands their ancestors had found and settled were no longer theirs to own. Today, no one knows how many pure-blooded Hawaiians are living in the state of Hawai'i. Even the most generous estimate can manage to grant no more than 5,000. The melodramatic title that Stannard gave his book about this tragedy—*Before the Horror*—is intended to shock.

ぺぺぺぺ

The endemic flora and fauna of Hawai'i have been as badly affected by foreign influences as were its indigenous people. Introduction of grazing animals, forage grasses, ornamental plants along with alien insects, mollusks, nematodes, and microbes attached to them or present in soil around their roots, and, more recently, the use of machines, insecticides, and herbicides in agriculture and engineering, have utterly destroyed native plants and animals on millions of acres of Hawai'i's land. Many indigenous species are extinct. Most of the survivors live in jeopardy. In no other place in the world have so many species of endemic plants and animals become extinct in so short a time.[28]

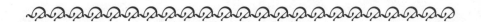

Two

Two Unprovable Hypotheses

Anyone who studies the history of Hawai'i cannot doubt that, since 1778, infectious diseases introduced by foreigners have claimed more Hawaiian lives than all other causes of death combined. Reasons for the Hawaiians' susceptibility to these infections can be inferred from the few facts that are known about themselves and about their environment. These facts, interpreted in the light of present knowledge in relevant medical sciences, lead to two major hypotheses.

HYPOTHESIS I
A significant proportion of the native population may
have been so inbred as to be genetically predisposed to suffer to
an extraordinary degree from the contagious diseases of civilization
when these were introduced in 1778 and thereafter.

Argument: If we assume that only a small number of voyagers came to live permanently in Hawai'i, first from the Marquesas Islands and later from Tahiti or its neighbors, and if we assume that their number was not markedly increased by subsequent immigrants, visitors, or castaways from any source, then we must conclude that the entire population of aboriginal Hawaiians were descendants of that limited number of ancestors. In other words, the Hawaiian colony of the Polynesian nation was derived from a very small gene pool. Moreover, if, as some anthropologists believe, the *entire* Polynesian race itself was descended from "a small . . . extremely small . . . founding group," then of course the Hawaiian offshoot of that Polynesian stock would have been even more narrowly delimited in the genetic sense.[1]

Of necessity, this initial colony of Hawaiians was enlarged

by interbreeding of progeny who very soon would have produced closely related children. Interbreeding may not have been actually incestuous to begin with but, within a very few generations at the most, matings between consanguineous individuals would have been unavoidable. The likelihood of such unions would have been increased if, in the earliest centuries, when the population was still sparse and localized, matings were arranged between related males and females who lived in the same small area, because people had not yet dispersed to distant places.

According to the most generous calculations—starting with as many as a hundred pioneers, half of whom would have been women able to bear children; an average of four children for each woman during her lifetime; an equal representation of males and females in each successive generation; the most favorable circumstances for raising children to maturity; and a generation time of 20 years—in theory those colonists could have produced 3,200 descendants during the first hundred years after they arrived in Hawai'i. In reality, because no human population is ever that fortunate in the ability of its members to survive and to reproduce without loss of offspring, the actual number of living Hawaiians at the end of their first century probably would have been closer to 1,600—or less. Naturally, anthropologists who employ other methods for measuring population growth (not to mention the help of speedy computers) will arrive at different estimates. Their differences simply emphasize the fact that all such figures are merely guesses which have no value except to the diligent savants who propose them.

The fact that, even after 1778, Hawaiians—especially nobles, the ali'i—did not proscribe matings between siblings, cousins, and other consanguineous persons, suggests that from the beginning taboos against interbreeding were not decreed or enforced. (Casual couplings among experimenting youths before "marriage" would have complicated genetic heritages even more.) In truth, the idea of increasing the mana of ali'i offspring by mating brothers with sisters, or fathers with daughters, uncles with nieces, and so on, would have encouraged inbreeding. Commoners, not so constrained by respect for bloodlines, probably had greater freedom in the choice of mates.

If these assumptions are accepted, then in the course of centuries, by the process known as "gene drift," potential weaknesses or strengths in the ancestral gene pool would have been enhanced among interrelated descendants. Weaknesses of hereditary nature in people of all societies are manifested in many ways. Some have been known for a relatively long time, such as hemophilia, color blindness, harelip, and other obvious physical ailments or traits. More subtle defects, recognized only relatively recently, are diabetes, phenylketonuria, acatalasemia, agammaglobulinemia, and cystic fibrosis. More such defects are being detected with dismaying frequency.

When they are challenged by factors in the physical or social environment, most individuals who show such signs of abnormality are eliminated either by nature's attrition or by the attentions of society. Hawaiians, in common with other Polynesians, were accused by foreigners of being ruthless in eliminating monstrous or sickly infants, and by such a practice may have eradicated most if not all of the obvious failures of inbreeding. Less conspicuous failures, such as the metabolic deficiencies, may not have been destroyed deliberately, but individuals so afflicted would have languished and died for want of adequate medical care. Such corrections of errors in biology, whether achieved by nature or by social sanctions, probably explain why Captain Cook and his companions observed only a few cases of sickness, idiocy, and congenital defects among Hawaiians they saw on Kaua'i and Hawai'i. But those few cases indicated that not all defective people were eliminated mercilessly.

Lieutenant James King's entry in his journal, written in 1779 as the British expedition sailed away from the Sandwich Islands for the last time, summed up the explorers' observations about diseases in four short paragraphs:

The Venereal is certainly now the Worst, & we are divided in our opinions whether they had it before or no. They did not appear to me to have any Name for it, & at last calld it sometimes —— [burning]. The next in fatality to this is the disorder arising from their debaucherys in the excess of the Kava. In these People the Skin looks as if parchd by the Weather. It is of a blackish appearance, but in its excess, it is mixt with a whiter Cast, & Scales peal of the Skin; the Eyes are red, inflamd, & very sore, the body is Ememecat'd [emaciated] & infirm, & it makes them very stupid.

Boils are very general, & we supposed those foul humors to arise from too much Salt which they eat with flesh & fish.

We saw here more deform'd people than in all the other [Southern] Islands put together, some had prominences before & behind, or were what we call humpd backd; one young man, had neither feet or hands; We saw two dwarfs, one was an old man 4 feet two Inches, perfectly well made, the other was a fat chubby woman, & many of their lower class of people were ill made. They brought to us a blind man to be cur'd; & a squinting sight was pretty common. An old woman at Neeneehow was wrong in her senses, & a man at Owhyhee still more so. & we could not but be surprised, that these two personages, had a very particular regard paid to them.

Old men are often to be seen. . . .[2]

Two paleopathologists in the twentieth century have presented evidence that seems to contradict Lieutenant King's observations about the number of deformed people he saw in Hawai'i. Warner F. Bowers,[3] who examined "864 pre-European contact burials from the sand dunes at Mokapu, Oahu," looking for "pathological and functional changes," did not even mention genetic defects in his report. Ivar J. Larsen,[4] who studied more than 500 skeletons from the same burial site, found "no suggestive genetically induced skeletal defects." Even so, the obvious question arises: can we extend to the whole aboriginal Hawaiian population the conclusions drawn from so small a sample of skeletons, all of which came from the same small district?

When nothing in the Hawaiians' almost unchanging physical environment challenged them, they—or, better, their genes—were not forced to adapt to change or challenge. If a genetic weakness was not challenged, it could persist and be compounded by further inbreeding of couples who shared the hidden trait. Thus, a person with a masked or latent defect could live normally, even healthily, and might have survived to an advanced age without showing any sign of the hidden trait.

Although not all geneticists are convinced that gene drift occurs today to a significant extent among human beings, the phenomenon does occur among populations of plants, animals, and microorganisms. It might plausibly have occurred among a human population as isolated and as limited in numbers of progenitors as was the Hawaiian race. Although we have no evidence other than Lieutenant King's account that such genetic weaknesses did occur among Hawaiians before 1778, we should reckon with the possibility that they might have been present. They certainly are not lacking among "pure-blood" and "mixed-blood" Hawaiians of today.

A trait such as agammaglobulinemia—the incapacity to synthesize adequate amounts and kinds of gamma globulin, from which are derived most of the antibodies that protect a person against invading microorganisms—need not have been an important deficiency either to individuals or to families during the centuries of isolation, when microbes that cause major epidemic diseases were not present in the islands. But it would have been revealed as a lethal deficiency, with almost explosive speed, when that isolation ended and the defective members of the population were challenged at last by *epidemics* of new diseases against which they could produce no early defense. A masked defect of this kind would explain why whole families were destroyed by foreign diseases, and why other families, presumably not so attainted, managed to survive.

Similarly, even today certain individuals in isolated tribes cannot produce sufficient amounts of HLAs—human lymphocyte antigens —to protect them against infectious organisms. Some Eskimos and Amerindians have been shown to suffer from this genetic deficiency. Some Hawaiians, not yet studied for this trait, undoubtedly will be found to be deficient in HLAs.[5] In addition, "many of the HLA-linked diseases are related to malfunctions of regulation" in the physiology of tissue cells.[6]

But then perhaps this whole exercise in suppositions is erected on misconceptions retained from older times, before modern forms of treatment were made available to "isolated and primitive people." In the late 1960s, a joint U.S.–Venezuelan scientific expedition in the rain forests of the Orinoco–Amazon river basin "observed the effects of a full-scale measles epidemic on isolated and primitive tribes who were probably encountering the disease for the first time." Sick Indians in one tribe who received "proper care" showed a mortality rate of 4 percent. Sick Indians in another tribe who received no such care had a mortality rate of 17 percent. Proper care, administered by the expedition's physicians, meant "fluids, aspirin, antibiotics, and cooling measures." The scientists concluded that "there is no basis for the widely held belief that American Indians have a racial susceptibility to measles." Another team of investigators decided that "they have no genetic susceptibility to tuberculosis."[7]

In other words, proper treatment rather than genes (or primitive circumstances) is the important factor that determines whether a sick person recovers or dies from an infectious disease. This is good news indeed to poor or primitive peoples in the world today—if only they can arrange to receive "proper care."

Not all consequences of inbreeding are necessarily harmful, as centuries of experience with hybridizing plants and domestic animals have shown. Among human beings, too, potential strengths can be enhanced—sometimes—when siblings or close relatives are mated. In several accounts about Hawaiians, an aliʻi who was the issue of a nīʻaupiʻo marriage (meaning, literally, "bent midrib of the coconut leaflet," figuratively, "of the same stalk") between brother and sister or uncle and niece, was noted for a splendid body and a superior intelligence. Admittedly, however, we have no idea how many failures were born to such unions, or how many of those apparent successes carried within them latent weaknesses that were not recognized while they lived. One of the causes of the lamentable barrenness of Hawaiians, both chiefs and commoners, both male and female, during the nineteenth century may have been genetic defects resulting from inbreeding. And perhaps a hereditary deficiency of this kind was responsible for the peculiar familial distribution of leprosy, when that terrible disease made its assault on the Hawaiian people in the decades after 1830.

HYPOTHESIS II

Hawaiians before 1778 were not acquainted with
the major infectious diseases that afflicted populations in
other parts of the world.

Argument: Hawaiians were not germless, of course. As do people everywhere and at all times, they harbored a normal microflora and microfauna upon the skin and upon membranes lining the gastrointestinal tract and other apertures and orifices. For all people everywhere, as microbiologists have learned, the gastrointestinal microflora especially is essential to their normal growth, development, and nutrition when they are young. And, let us recognize, some of the germs we harbor can help us to die when we are old or weakened by other troubles.

But—except perhaps immediately after those rare occasions when castaways or visitors might possibly have come among them—Hawaiians as a whole were spared the ravages of the great epidemic pestilences that compounded the miseries of so many peoples in the rest of the world. The most serious of these diseases were bubonic plague, cholera, typhoid fever and the other enteric fevers, the several kinds of dysenteries, tuberculosis, leprosy, typhus fever, yellow fever, poliomyelitis, smallpox, measles, influenza, malaria, yaws, rabies, and, above all, the several venereal diseases (or the sexually transmitted diseases, as they are called today). Furthermore, Hawaiians as individuals would have been singularly free of the serious acute or chronic infections that afflicted people elsewhere—and that, after 1778, devastated Hawaiians as soon as the causative agents of those diseases were introduced among them.

This second hypothesis does not mean that Hawaiians were absolutely free of all infections. No man, even one on an island, is ever spared some hurt from the "normal" microorganisms he harbors: always, among those parasites which live with him and upon him, usually to his advantage as well as theirs, are some opportunistic ingrates that turn against the body that feeds them if ever they are given the chance to do so. That chance is offered them in a variety of ways, not all of which are known as yet, but which are summed up in the catchphrase "when the resistance of the host is lowered"—as it is from "insults" presented by malnutrition, acute or chronic fatigue, any degree of physical injury, organic dysfunctions, psychological traumata, old age, and the terminal weaknesses of dying.

Paleopathologists, in examining the bones and teeth of several hundred Hawaiians who died before 1778, found signs of a variety of infectious processes. They indicated, among people less than forty years of age, a low incidence of dental caries, sinusitis, mastoiditis, arthritis, osteomyelitis subsequent to wounds, and chronic ulcerations of the skin.[8] H. G. Chappel, a dentist who studied the teeth in 161 skulls, noted:

> Pyorrhea seems to have been remarkably prevalent . . . far more so than caries of the teeth. . . . Of those over 40, more than half showed the disease in an advanced stage. . . . Alveolar abscess, pyorrhea, osteomyelitis, antral disease, and tumors [in bones] prove that the ancient Hawaiians had to contend with the same diseases that are found in mouths today.[9]

The same microorganisms that left signs of their activity in the very bones and teeth of their victims could also have caused ulcerations and abscesses in the softer tissues, such as gums, flesh, and viscera, as well as the agonies of puerperal sepsis and the pains of rheumatic fever. Such infections would have been confined to individuals, however, and were not passed to numbers of people on an epidemic scale.

If members of the colonizing expeditions from central Polynesia did bring any virulent microorganisms with them from the homeland, those germs—assuming that they resembled pathogens of today, as we have every reason to believe they did—soon became adapted to their hosts and thereby lost their ability to harm either the immigrants or their descendants. "Given enough time," wrote René Dubos, "a state of peaceful coexistence eventually becomes established between any host and any parasite. . . . Throughout nature, infection without disease is the rule rather than the exception."[10]

Among pathogenic microorganisms important in the eighteenth century, one possible exception to this generalization is *Treponema pertenue,* the spirochete that causes yaws. It is so persistent and so contagious a troublemaker (and yet, paradoxically, so mild a pathogen) that once it is introduced into a population it is ineradicable, unless all of its victims are treated with modern chemotherapeutic drugs, such as organic compounds of arsenic or antibiotics like penicillin.

If individuals seriously ill with infectious diseases were allowed to accompany the migrating colonists, they would have died of hardships during the voyage to Hawai'i or soon after arriving in the harsh new land to which they had come. When they died, their pathogens would have perished with them. Moreover, in the small and dispersed settlements that would have been established during the first century or so, opportunities for healthy human carriers of germs to pass virulent microbes from one place to susceptible recipients in another location would have been so severely limited that, in effect, transmission did not occur. Therefore, in one way or another, either by gradual loss of virulence or by actual extermination, serious pathogens would have disappeared from the isolated Hawaiian population.

Recent research by microbiologists, immunologists, and epidemiologists supports these conclusions. Loss of virulence by species of bacteria, rickettsias, and viruses—with the notable exception of the retrovirus that causes AIDS—occurs with surprising rapidity. In the case of a person who is taken ill with an infection (and who is not treated with antimicrobial medications), recovery is actually dependent upon his body's immunological triumph over the invading microbes. During the short interval of sickness followed by convalescence, the patient becomes adapted to his invader—and the invader, in turn, if it is not completely eliminated, becomes adapted to its host, with a demonstrable loss of virulence. It may even survive in the host, for a long time, apparently without ill effect, until years later it strikes again after regaining a measure of virulence.

In some die-hard pathogens, however, a variation in virulence seems to occur: a microbe that has "lost its virulence" in one host can regain it in another host—or even, after a time, in the same host. Usually virulence is regained when the avirulent microbe is passed rapidly among members of a population of nonimmune hosts. Such rapid transmission to susceptible victims, combined with nutritional components they helpfully provide, will favor the revival of virulence. But some pathogens are so fiendishly adaptable and changeable that they can regain virulence while they are still parasitizing the body of the same host—who can never shake off the infection. The organisms that cause undulant fever, the recurrent fevers, and AIDS are notable for this degree of adaptability.

Changes in virulence of a microbe may be either genotypic (that is, effected by mutations in the genetic composition of the pathogen which are passed on to its descendants) or phenotypic (that is, effected by alterations in their metabolic functions, which are controlled by environmental rather than by genetic mechanisms).[11]

This interplay of adaptations in an individual also happens in a whole population of human beings who are continually exposed to cases of infectious diseases and to apparently healthy carriers who harbor virulent pathogens. Sooner or later an epidemic arises, caused by pathogens let loose on a populace. The epidemic runs its course and subsides, as hosts and pathogens become adapted each to the other, and arrive at last at a sort of truce.

P. L. Panum's observations in 1846–1850 upon the speed with which measles, common colds, and other contagions—introduced by sailors aboard trading ships calling at port towns in the isolated Faeroe Islands north of Scotland—waxed, waned, and disappeared in the resident population were among the earliest of many reports on the mutual adaptability of human beings and their pathogens.[12] The medical experiences of Hawaiians after 1778, whenever their shores and ports were visited by foreign sailors, were similar to those of the Faeroe Islanders—except that Hawaiians, having been isolated for centuries rather than months, suffered much more severely from the alien germs unwittingly introduced by those alien visitors.

The difficulty with which even a virulent strain of a microbe is able to cause an epidemic is also well established. The conjunction of factors which must be attained before an epidemic can develop is so seldom achieved that even in large cities filled with people such outbreaks are astonishingly, mercifully, rare. Moreover, the bio-chemical interrelationships between potential pathogen and possible victim are so complex that only a few of them are known as yet.

At the present time, epidemiologists agree that the process by which an epidemic does arise depends on these six factors, at least:

1. The presence of a source of the fully virulent microorganism (in actual cases, convalescents, apparently healthy carriers, animal reservoirs, and, for some pathogens, in insect hosts which act as transmitting agents)
2. The release from the source of infection of a large number of viable cells or units of the infectious microbe
3. The survival of sufficient numbers of cells or units of the infectious agent between the time they leave the host source and the time they enter the body of the new host
4. The presence in an exposed population of a relatively high propor-tion of susceptible individuals
5. The frequency of contacts, either direct or indirect, between those susceptible individuals and the pathogens released by the host sources: the more contacts that are achieved, the faster will the pathogens be spread, and the sooner will the epidemic develop
6. The success with which the transmitted microbes can invade, estab-lish themselves, and multiply in the tissues of the new host

For example, the highly contagious viruses which cause mumps, chicken pox, measles, German measles, influenza, hepatitis, and poliomyelitis are always present in some individuals of the populace in a large city. Until recently, smallpox too would have been included in this list. But early in the 1980s a determined program conducted by WHO throughout the last remaining foci of the disease succeeded in eliminating the virus that causes smallpox. For the first time in his-tory the human race has been freed of a major pathogen. But let us not be smug because of this singular conquest. Nature—or Nemesis, or Fate, or Providence, whatever we want to call it—always a few steps ahead of us, is still creating brand-new pathogens to fill the places of the ones we think we have subdued.

Yet epidemics of diseases occur only when the six prerequisite cir-cumstances just mentioned (and possibly others still unknown) are fulfilled. Usually the new susceptible population is furnished by the crop of children born in a community during the interval since the last epidemic of a specific disease occurred. And opportunity for rapid distribution of the viruses is provided when those children are sent from sheltered homes to kindergartens, day-care centers, and schools. For these reasons, epidemics of measles in temperate zones "tend to appear in two- to three-year cycles," and epidemics of German measles occur at intervals of one or two years, usually during winter and spring. In Hawai'i, however, according to reports from the State Department of Health, epidemics of German measles arise at intervals of about four years.[13]

Hawai'i's tourist industry proves each year that epidemics are not easily started. In 1989 alone, more than 6.6 million tourists came to visit these islands, once upon a time the most isolated landfalls on earth. Those hordes of transients would overwhelm the resident population of about 1.1 million, if most of the newcomers did not prefer to frequent the fleshpots of Waikīkī. Nonetheless, despite this ceaseless flood of bodies and germs, no serious epidemics of major infectious diseases have occurred for many years—with one significant exception. A few minor "outbreaks" of food poisoning (caused by the latest prevailing serotypes of salmonellas) are noticed by public health officials (who are well aware that only relatively few of those cases are ever reported). No doubt a small number of tourists catch the local variety of Mexico's "turistas." Most certainly, in a fine show of reciprocity, lots of locals catch from flitting transients the viruses that cause common colds, "intestinal flu," or the latest in circulating strains of the influenza virus. But none of these minor interferences with the well-being of our stay-at-home islanders is really serious. We get sick for a few days, soon we get well again, and very few of us are so uncooperative as to die from any of these quite ordinary clinical experiences.

When we consider that, among those 6 million visitors, at least a few bodies could so easily be carrying within them so many of the world's more fearsome microorganisms, we should be both amazed and grateful that none of these potential killers has caused sickness and death on a scale that is new to Hawai'i. But the pathogens seem to have been held in check: none of them exerts any statistically significant effect on our general well-being or on our morbidity and mortality rates. So far.

Why are we so lucky? The answer to this question lies in our remembering those six factors that must be satisfied before an epidemic can begin. The likeliest explanation for our being spared is the kind of protection that Hawaiians after 1778 could not call upon in their own bodies: islanders today are already immune to most of the important disease-producing microbes that go careering around the world. They have met them before (or close relatives of them) in sicknesses they have survived or in representatives of them in the vaccines they have received. Because of those previous exposures, they have built up antibodies to the threatening microbes, and therefore are relatively safe from them.

Only one of the dangerous "foreign diseases" has moved in to stay. This is AIDS, caused by a retrovirus. Because this protean virus is so determinedly different from all others of the pathogens that human beings have met before, it is the most terrible scourge to be let loose among human beings in the history of mankind. As best our health officials can tell, AIDS arrived in Hawai'i either in the very late 1970s or in the early 1980s. This epidemic has not "run its course," in the considerate way that most imported plagues have done, leaving their hosts either removed by quick death or safely immunized and therefore protected by the exposure. This one, researchers tell us, is not kind. Dr. Robert Gallo, who led the American team that discovered this virus, calls it "unforgiving." It does not grant the boon of immunity—or that of quick death.

Even worse. In these Years of Grace, no vaccine, no antiserum, no specific medication to arrest the virus's depredations is available. We can only hope that they will be found soon.

ဆဲ-ဆဲ-ဆဲ-ဆဲ

Any agent, whether it is physical, chemical, biological, or sociological, that breaks the links in the chain of events that must precede an epidemic will prevent such an outcome. Recognition of this principle is the basis for most of the measures employed at present in preventive medicine and public health. The fact that, at the very least, physical and social circumstances among aboriginal Hawaiians interfered with that sequence of events is the basis for the hypothesis that those people of old were unacquainted with the major infectious diseases that prevailed in the rest of the world. Evidence to support this opinion is indirect, but it is provided by so much information drawn from so many disciplines and observers that the sum of their contributions is persuasive.

Immunological: The most overwhelming evidence is found in the terrible vulnerability of the Hawaiian people themselves, in the rapidity with which they sickened and died when, after January 1778, they were exposed to foreigners and their germs. During the decades that followed, in a pitiless processional of death, most of the contagious diseases of civilization were introduced. And all of these

—even sicknesses like the common cold, or measles, mumps, and chicken pox (which Westerners dismissed as mere "diseases of children")—were unrelenting in the toll they exacted from Hawaiians. Such weakness in a people apparently stalwart and vigorous puzzled the few foreigners who bothered to think about their plight; gave moralists cause to assert that Hawaiians were "decadent," "debased," and even "debauched"; and demoralized the race that provided its victims.

Both foreigners and natives offered many "explanations" for this weakness, some naive, a few ingenious, many derogatory, but none even near to being correct. No one before the late 1880s—when Pasteur, Koch, and a few of their contemporaries established the sciences of microbiology and immunology—could have begun to understand its nature. Today, with our knowledge of the principles of immunity, we are forced to conclude that—most certainly because they had been isolated for so long in space and in time, and possibly because of the genetic constitution of whole families among the inbred population—Hawaiians were so vulnerable because they lacked protective antibodies with which to combat microorganisms they could not have encountered before foreigners introduced them.

Medical: Despite a considerable competence in the diagnosis of injuries and other physical disabilities which native physicians had developed, and despite their use of a varied materia medica for the treatment of those physical ailments, both the native physicians and the general populace were utterly unacquainted with the signs and symptoms of acute communicable diseases when these were introduced. Moreover, Hawaiians had neither medicines nor regimens with which to treat patients afflicted with these contagions. Native physicians were perceptive enough, however, to recognize immediately that, in "the venereal distemper," Captain Cook's sailors had presented the people of Hawai'i with something new in the way of sickness.

Lieutenant King, very much concerned about the effects that the venereal diseases were showing among Hawaiians, noted on 1 March 1779, when the British expedition returned to Waimea, Kaua'i:

One man, without my putting questions to him . . . told us that we had left a disorder amongst their women, which had killed several of them, as well as men. He himself was infected with the Venereal disease, & described in feeling terms the havock it had made, & its pains,

&tc—I was never more thoroughly satisfied of a doubtful point than from this Circumstance, that we were the authors of the disease in this place.[14]

Native physicians tried to find medicines for treating these venereal infections, as well as any other ailments they would have recognized as being new to Hawaiians. Unfortunately, their experience and their resources were so limited—as indeed were the medications available to all physicians anywhere in the world at the time—that they were doomed to fail.

Sociological: The inexperience of native physicians, *kāhuna lapa'au,* when confronted with infectious diseases was reflected in the behavior of the whole populace. They lacked not only the protection of antibodies: they lacked almost every one of those cultural and psychological preparations for coping with infectious diseases which identify a society that is accustomed to them. They lacked awareness of the signs and symptoms of epidemic sicknesses, the good sense to take even the most elementary care of their suffering persons, the charity to help relatives and neighbors when they fell ill, or, conversely, the sense to avoid sources of infection when these appeared in a community. Like Tahitians and other Polynesians, Hawaiians too could be unreasoning, feckless, helpless, often hysterical, sometimes brutal. Their behavior—until Christian missionaries taught them the virtue of charity and their own despair plunged them into apathy—revealed a people to whom epidemic diseases were new and mystifying—and terrifying.

Linguistic: Although Hawaiians had developed a large and versatile vocabulary, including many terms showing their knowledge of the material world (as well as the concerns of the intellect and the spirit), they did not have words to identify specific infectious diseases or their varied symptoms. After 1778 new terms were devised as the need for them arose. In some instances, a disease practically named itself to a people with a facility in wordplay. Thus, *ka ma'i 'ōku'u,* "the squatting sickness," was a natural descriptive epithet for an intestinal infection characterized by a severe dysentery. In other instances the new diseases received names that were translations or transliterations from English. Smallpox, for example, was known as *ka ma'i pu'upu'u li'ili'i,* "the sickness of small bumps," or simply "kamolapoki."

Even more instructive is the fact that certain words used throughout islands in the South Pacific for diseases known to Polynesians living there were not included in the vocabulary of Hawaiians. *Kona,* or *tona,* in the dialects of southern and central Polynesia, referred to yaws, and later, after Europeans introduced the disease, to syphilis (because the early lesions of the two infections are similar in appearance). In Hawai'i *kona* had a number of meanings (as do many Hawaiian words), but none referred to a disease of any kind. Similarly, *feefee,* or *fefe,* the Tahitian word for filariasis, that other unmistakable malady which was endemic among some southern Polynesians when European explorers discovered them, was not used in Hawai'i. The medical meanings of these two words disappeared from Hawaiian consciousness because the diseases they signified did not occur in Hawai'i. The absence of mosquitoes explains why filariasis was unknown here. (Indeed, it still is absent, although the mosquitoes have arrived.) The absence of yaws is not so easily explained. Hawaiians may have ended all contact with the southern homelands before that contagion was introduced there; or, if they did bring the disease with them to Hawai'i, carriers and lesions soon died out, taking with them the very memory of its name.

No one knows how or when yaws or filariasis (and the mosquito vectors of filariasis) were introduced into central Polynesia. Recent studies by entomologists and epidemiologists suggest that both mosquitoes and diseases reached those central islands relatively late in history, after Hawaiians had ended their voyages to and from Tahiti. Thus, P. A. Buxton wrote in 1928: "We presume that yaws has prevailed in most parts of Melanesia and Polynesia since long before the coming of the white man to these islands. . . . It seems possible that some of the more remote islands were free of yaws till the coming of European shipping, and that the disease was spread to those places by traders, blackbirders, and missionaries."[15]

Although Great Britain's Captain Samuel Wallis, who is credited with having discovered Tahiti in 1767, did not mention the presence of either yaws or filariasis among the island's people, Captain Cook's accounts of his first visit there, in 1769, and his second, in 1773, leave no doubt that both diseases were well established among Tahitians.

Leon Rosen believes that "an examination of early data from the Marquesas Islands indicates that neither elephantiasis [filariasis] nor [*Aedes*] *scutellaris* mosquitos [vectors of the microfilariae of *Wuchereria bancrofti,* the organism causing filariasis] existed in that area until relatively recent times. . . . It is not until 1884 that one finds reference to elephantiasis in this area." And that reference, he adds, was "certainly an instance in which the etiology of the elephantiasis might be obscure."[16]

Traditional: Even when a people possesses a written language, its histories and traditions do not necessarily tell the truth about its past. Traditions especially are likely to be collections of myths and fables, distorted memories, superstitions, delusions, boastings, equivocations, and outright lies—inventions of conceit rather than records of fact. How trustworthy, then, are the traditions and histories of Hawai'i's people, who did not develop a written language but relied on erring memory to preserve the chronicles of their past? Unfortunately, as anyone can prove to himself at any time, even well-trained memories are neither infallible nor omniscient: "Of all liars, the smoothest and most convincing is memory" (as someone has said).

In Hawai'i, as elsewhere, traditions are not reliable sources of facts. Nonetheless, they can serve as indicators of the interests, experiences, and preoccupations of the society that created them. Of native Hawaiians, only four—David Malo, Samuel M. Kamakau, John Papa I'i, and Kepelino—wrote extensive accounts that might be considered to present histories of times past. But because they learned to write long after their ancestral society had been sundered by foreign influences, these earnest men had to rely on fallacious memories and variable "traditions" for the materials they put in their chronicles. Their "fragments of history," as I'i was humble enough to call his own contributions, must be read with a very questioning mind.

The fact that Malo and I'i wrote very little about epidemics and diseases in the decades just before 1778 *might* mean that the genealogists, tellers-of-tales, and priest-historians who were responsible for preserving the experiences of their society had few occasions of such a dramatic kind to remember. Kamakau claimed as much when, in 1870, he wrote: "Foreigners had not yet come from other lands; there were no fatal diseases *(luku)*, no epidemics *(ahulau)*, no contagious diseases *(ma'i lele)*, no diseases that eat away the body *(ma'i 'a'ai)*, no venereal diseases *(ma'i pala a me ke kaokao)*."[17]

Kamakau hangs us upon another horn of the historians' dilemma: by 1870 he was an embittered man, a self-appointed proclaimer of doom, a professional Hawaiian with many an ax to grind. Hacking at foreigners for causing all the troubles that had befallen Hawaiians was almost the only consolation to natives who still survived, and

Kamakau certainly led his people in playing this national game. In this particular statement, at least, he is not above suspicion.

Observations of Foreign Visitors: These accounts, interpreted in the light of their times, are the best sources of information, but even they are regrettably inadequate.

As explorers, Captain James Cook and his fellow scientists aboard HMS *Resolution* and HMS *Discovery* were instructed by "the Commissioners for executing the Office of the Lord High Admiral of Great Britain & Ireland &c" to make all the multitudinous observations that members of an expedition sent into unknown quarters of the world were expected to perform—and more.

Believing that they were the first Europeans to "discover" the Sandwich Islands, Cook and his associates were doubly interested in comparing "the Indians" living here with their relatives in the South Pacific. Captain Cook himself—generous, enlightened, observant, far in advance of contemporary naval officers in his regard for the health and well-being of Britain's seamen—was very much concerned about the effects that his companions would have upon a populace not previously exposed to Europeans.

Some of his officers reported every manifestation of sickness or physical disability they encountered among the Hawaiians. They found very little to record, as the quotation from Lieutenant King has shown—aside from the venereal diseases, which they believed had been transmitted to Hawaiians by members of their own expedition, and the puzzling assortment of symptoms (which they mistook for signs of leprosy) that were exhibited by chiefs who were addicted to the narcotizing *'awa,* the intoxicating juice extracted from roots and stems of *Piper methysticum.*

We must allow for the probability that most diseased and crippled Hawaiians were not present among the crowds of healthy folk who gathered from miles around to see "the floating islands" and the god-like visitors they bore. Sick and disabled natives need not have been hidden away. (Some explorers suspected they were secreted in caves on Easter Island.) Simple inability to walk from their homes to Waimea Bay on Kaua'i or to Kealakekua Bay on Hawai'i could account for their absence. Yet when the visiting British themselves explored the countryside beyond Waimea and Kealakekua, collecting specimens of plants and birds, observing the habits, customs, and appearance of the people, they could have had opportunity to see unhealthy natives among the well. The few cripples and deformed individuals they did remark suggest that the incidence of diseases of any kind was very low. So does the fact that, after consorting with natives, eating quantities of their foodstuffs, and drinking their water (which, by modern standards, could well have been polluted both chemically and microbiologically), no member of the expedition contracted an infectious disease from Hawaiians, except for "the venereal," given to the natives by Britons in the first place.

Whether the low incidence of physical disabilities was a natural consequence of Hawai'i's isolation, or was an artificial consequence of the natives' practice of killing defective infants, is a question that cannot be answered. The presence of a very few hunchbacks, cripples, insane persons, and even one man born without hands and feet proves that infanticide was by no means ruthless or universal.

On the other hand, the observations made by another group of early explorers were very different from those recorded by Captain Cook and his company. Captain the Count Jean-François Galaup de La Pérouse and several members of his expedition aboard France's ships *Boussole* and *Astrolabe* landed on the southwest coast of Maui, at the place we now call La Pérouse Bay, on 30 May 1786.

La Pérouse's own account of the visit is polished, urbane, elegantly philosophical:

> About 120 persons, men and women, waited for us on the shore. . . . The women showed by the most expressive gestures, that there was no mark of kindness which they were not disposed to confer upon us . . . but they were little seductive. Their features had no delicacy, and their dress permitted us to observe, in most of them, traces of the ravages occasioned by the venereal disease. As no women had come on board in the canoes, I was disposed to think, that they attributed to the Europeans those evils of which they bore the marks; but I soon perceived that this remembrance, supposing it is real, had not left in their minds the smallest resentment.
>
> I shall here take the liberty to examine, whether the modern navigators are the true authors of these evils, and this crime, with which they reproach themselves in their narratives, be not more apparent than real. To give my conjectures the greater weight, I shall support them by the observations of M. Rollin, a very enlightened man, and surgeon of my ship. He visited in the island several inhabitants attacked by this disease, and observed appearances, the gradual development of which would have required in Europe 12 or 15 years. He likewise saw children of 7 to 8 years of age, in whom it prevailed, and who could only have contracted it during the period of gestation. I must further

observe, that Captain Cook, on his first arrival at the Sandwich Islands, landed only at Atooi and Oneehow; and that nine months after, on his return from the north, he found that the inhabitants of Mowee, who came on board, were almost all affected with it. As Mowee is 60 leagues to the windward of Atooi this progress seems to me to be too rapid not to afford some doubts on the subject.[18]

The Dissertation on the Inhabitants of Easter Island and the Island of Mowee, by M. Rollin, M.D., Surgeon of the frigate *La Boussole,* describing what he and his fellow physicians saw during that incredible day in that ghastly place is absolutely confounding—and exceedingly damaging to my second hypothesis. Here, complete, is the section of the *Dissertation* that refers to the diseases that he identified among Maui's residents and their animals:

The beauty of the climate, and the fertility of the soil, might render the inhabitants extremely happy, if the leprosy and venereal disease prevailed among them less generally, and with less virulence. These scourges, the most humiliating and most destructive with which the human race are afflicted, display themselves among these islanders by the following symptoms: buboes, and scars which result from their suppurating, warts, spreading ulcers, with caries of the bones, nodes, exostosis, fistula, tumors of the lachrymal and salival ducts, scrofulous swellings, inveterate ophthalmia, ichorous ulcerations of the tunica conjunctiva, atrophy of the eyes, blindness, inflamed prurient herpetic eruptions, indolent swellings of the extremities; and among children, scald head, or malignant tinea, from which exudes a fetid and acrid matter. I remarked, that the greater part of these unhappy victims of sensuality, when arrived at the age of nine or ten, were feeble and languid, exhausted by marasmus, and affected with the rickets.

The indolent swellings of the extremities, which we observed among the natives of Mowee, and which Anderson, surgeon on Captain Cook's ship, remarked also among most of the inhabitants of the South Sea Islands, is nothing more than a symptom of an advanced state of elephantiasis [that is, Elephantiasis Graecorum or leprosy], as I assured myself, as far as was possible, by examining a great number of lepers in the hospitals of Madeira and Manilla.

In this period of the disease, the skin has already lost its sensibility; and if the activity of the virus be not checked by proper treatment and regimen, the swollen parts soon lose entirely both their irritability and sensibility, the skin becomes scaly, and phlyctenae are formed, filled with fetid and corrosive matter, which will occasion, without extreme care, gangrenous or carcinomatous ulcers. The nature or quality of the food may concur with the heat of the climate to nourish and propagate this endemic disease of the adipous membrane; for the hogs even, the flesh of which forms the chief part of the food of the inhabitants of Mowee, are many of them extremely measly. I examined several, and their skins were scabby, full of pimples, and entirely destitute of hair. On opening these animals, I found the caul regularly so sprinkled with tubercles, and the viscera so full of them, that, in the least delicate stomach, the sight could not but have produced a nausea. Among the diseases with which these islanders are so deplorably afflicted, there are some that seem to be produced by the venereal virus in all its activity but it appears for the most part under a degenerated form, or combined with psora or itch.

The shortness of our stay (a few hours), and other circumstances, did not permit me to acquire any information respecting the mode of treatment employed by the natives for the cure of these disorders; but to judge from their inactive suffering, and the progress of their infirmities, I am induced to think, that they are acquainted with no means of alleviating the misery of their condition.[19]

What can be said of this report? It is so much in opposition to the observations made by Cook, his officers, and his ships' surgeons only eight and seven years before, as well as to those made by all visitors who came after M. Rollin, at least during the next forty years, that we can scarcely believe he was describing a community of Hawaiians.

As earlier and later observers made very clear, Hawaiians living in all other communities, from Kaua'i to Hawai'i, were not that dreadfully diseased, that universally revolting. Those other foreigners, in fact, extolled the cleanliness of the natives, the beauty of the young women, and the vigor of the young men. If even a small proportion of Hawaiians from any place had been as afflicted and as repulsive as were those the French explorers saw on Maui, the grand romantical stories about the many charms of Hawai'i's people would not have been started and could never have been perpetuated far into the nineteenth century.

Surely M. Rollin's report cannot be accepted literally as applying to all the people of Maui specifically, or to all Hawaiians in general. In the first place, no physician then or now, by mere visual appraisal alone, while strolling for a few hours among a pressing crowd of curious people, could possibly make—correctly—the number and variety of diagnoses that M. Rollin recorded so casually, even if he was aided by his colleagues. What reliance would we place today on the diagnoses of even the world's most expert doctor if, as he sauntered among the many tourists and the very few Hawaiians crowding the sands of Waikīkī Beach, this presumptuous man declared: "Ah, yes. This one has tuberculosis of the lungs. And that one has syphilis. And that one over there suffers from gonorrhea. Whereas this one has worms, and his neighbor shows all the signs of leprosy"? Could we not, through all this patter, detect a pretentious charlatan? A deceiver, a *kahuna ho'opunipuni,* Hawaiians of old would have called him. A *kahuna a ka 'alawa maka,* one who "sees at a glance" the nature of any affliction.[20]

In the second place, several of the diseases Rollin claimed to have recognized (as well as others he did not mention) share a number of symptoms, especially those conditions involving the skin and underlying tissues. Even today an expert dermatologist (perhaps because he knows so much), trusting to his eyes alone, would have great trouble in arriving at a diagnosis for a patient with skin lesions resembling those of leprosy. He must rule out several other conditions which can mimic leprosy—such as syphilis, tuberculosis, yaws, leishmaniasis, the lesions caused by certain species of fungi and yeasts, "eczemas" caused by a variety of microorganisms as well as by allergies, not to mention other disorders attributable to hormonal dysfunctions, autoimmune responses, cancerous growths, vitamin deficiencies, and infestations with scabies mites, body lice, and certain kinds of worms.

Furthermore, in order to establish a diagnosis, a modern dermatologist would have to call on a number of laboratory tests designed either to confirm the presence of the causative organism of the disease, in the case of true infections and infestations, or to eliminate the possibility of its presence in those conditions that are not contagions.

Physicians have learned much since Rollin's day, when the roles of so many different microorganisms, allergens, chemicals, vitamins, and hormones, in health and in disease, were not yet known, and before laboratory techniques to aid in diagnosis were established. Dr. Rollin, we must remember, did not have the benefit of this accumulated knowledge, which exacts caution from the diagnostician of today.

Nevertheless, M. Rollin and his associates were not blind. During those few hours ashore they saw horrors enough to make them hasten from that awful beach as soon as some of the ships' casks had been filled with water from the solitary spring. In fairness, we must assume that M. Rollin himself was neither fool nor charlatan. How, then, can we account for that assemblage of diseased and loathsome people and animals?

At least three explanations are possible. The first and easiest would be to accept Rollin's statements as being correct in all particulars and implications. Yet to do so contradicts the observations not only of all other early visitors to Hawai'i, both before and after La Pérouse's landing, but also—and even more important, as this book is meant to discuss—the testimony offered in the destruction of the Hawaiian race in the years after 1778.

A second explanation would suppose that the shore, if not the whole district around La Pérouse Bay, was a lazaret to which all the diseased people of Maui had been banished, just as, after 1866, Hawai'i's lepers were segregated at Kalaupapa on Moloka'i. This supposition is highly improbable, inasmuch as nothing like such a settlement, set aside exclusively for diseased people, is known elsewhere in Hawai'i or in Polynesia. Even so, Hawaiians were intelligent enough—and possibly ailing enough—to develop a medical profession that has been considered to be superior to that encountered in other places in Polynesia. And some chiefs and priests were humane enough to establish a number of *pu'uhonua,* places of refuge, on each island, in which people who had broken a law or who were fleeing from wars, political stresses, or the wrath of punitive chiefs and priests could find sanctuary. A place of refuge comparable to a hospice for diseased and disabled folk would have been a logical extension of the concern offered to healthy unfortunates. W. D. Alexander mentioned one such pu'uhonua on O'ahu: "The heiau of Waolani in Nuuanu was sacred to fugitives and the sick."[21] If such segregated communities did exist, they would explain why Captain Cook and his associates did not see as many diseased natives as La Pérouse and Rollin saw.

If the people at La Pérouse Bay were indeed victims of advanced as well as congenital syphilis (not to mention leprosy and a few other contagions), the question of its origin becomes all the more pertinent. Only one answer to this question is possible: they must have received the disease from foreigners before 1778. Who, then, were those foreigners?

As has been discussed in an earlier essay, the most probable visi-

tors would have been travelers aboard Spanish galleons, on their
voyages between Mexico and the Philippine Islands. Less likely visitors, but possible ones, would have been Chinese or Japanese mariners or fishermen. Natives from any other islands east of the Asian
continent must also be reckoned with. All these voyagers could have
come to Hawai'i in the same unplanned way that brought drifting
Japanese fishermen toward Hawaiian shores on several occasions
after 1800. Wherever they might have come from, all would have
carried their germs with them.

All these unprovable possibilities still leave us with the great unan-
swerable mystery: why were those miserable people at La Pérouse
Bay the only ones in all Hawai'i to show the signs and symptoms of
advanced syphilis and leprosy—and only M. Rollin knows what
else?

A third explanation seems to be the most natural and the least
strained: because of its location on the hot, dry, almost waterless leeward coast of Maui—one of the most inhospitable places in all
Hawai'i even today—that whole area at La Pérouse Bay must have
been inhabited by a dirty, unwashed, unkempt, undernourished, and
brutish set of miserable people who showed in their bodies the perpetual squalor in which they lived. A general infestation with scabies
mites, affecting both people and animals, complicated in many
instances by fungus infections of the skin and by scurvy and other
vitamin deficiencies, could have presented the astonished Frenchmen
with the whole array of hideous symptoms that M. Rollin reported.
In addition, the older people could have contracted both syphilis and
gonorrhea during the eight years since Britain's sailors presented the
women of Ni'ihau and Kaua'i with those mementos of their call. And
the "tubercles" Rollin noticed in those mangy measly hogs could have
been lesions caused by the cysticerci of parasitic tapeworms of swine,
or possibly with germs other than the tubercle bacilli, such as Johne's
bacillus, *Mycobacterium paratuberculosis,* which in swine provokes
lesions similar to those of tuberculosis but which do not infect
human beings.[22]

As a matter of record, Rollin himself suspected that scabies—"the
itch" as he called it—might be contributing to the morbid symptoms
he saw. He blamed "the venereal virus in all its activity" for some of
"the diseases with which these islanders are so deplorably afflicted,"
but he also conceded that "it appears for the most part under a
degenerated form, or combined with psora or itch."[23] And here this

attempt to explain M. Rollin's controversial *Dissertation* must end —in bewilderment and uncertainty.

Pathological: Paleopathology is a relatively new discipline. Its judgments are dependent upon the acumen of pathologists, the reliability of the laboratory techniques they may employ, and the state of preservation of the bones or mummies they are able to examine.

Of the many infectious diseases that beset human beings, only a few leave lasting traces in their victims' bones. The fainter of these markings, which are little more than superficial erosions, may disappear while the bones lie buried, especially when they are consigned to wet earth or sand. False traces may be inscribed after burial—by the action of enzymes or other chemical agents secreted from roots, worms, flesh-eating insects, and assorted saprophytic microorganisms, or by the action of numerous kinds of reagents derived from the surrounding soil or from the decomposing body itself. Obviously, to decipher the meanings hidden in such a delicate calligraphy is extremely difficult; and a diagnosis based on such a reading is likely to be almost as much an act of divination as was a Chinese scapulomancer's prediction of a client's fate gained from his reading of the pattern of cracks that appeared on the dried shoulder bone of an ox when he touched it with a red-hot poker.[24]

A few kinds of infections, however, do affect bones in such a manner that structural changes, often evident during life and persisting after death, are so characteristic as to be pathognomonic. Foremost among these infections are tuberculosis, leprosy, syphilis, yaws, arthritis, and osteomyelitis of any etiology. Equally reliable signs of less serious diseases are cavities in teeth and changes in the surfaces of the bones enclosing the cranial sinuses.

Bones of Hawaiians who lived and died before 1778 are not easily found. Most of them disintegrate too rapidly while buried in Hawai'i's damp earth. Others that may have resisted decay are sealed in hidden burial caves or in graves now covered by many square miles of asphalt or concrete. Until recently, the skeletons (or portions of them) from only about 1,000 autochthonous Hawaiians, preserved in the Bernice Pauahi Bishop Museum, have been studied for signs of disease.

Warner F. Bowers, who looked for "pathological and functional changes . . . in 864 pre-European contact Polynesian burials from the sand dunes at Mokapu, Oahu," found no indications of tuberculosis, leprosy, or syphilis in those relics. He did find about eight cases of osteomyelitis following chronic infections of leg bones, nasal sinuses, and mastoid bones, and "six instances of subperiosteal new bone formation along the shaft of the lower tibia." Those shin bones came from three men and three women who were between twenty-five and forty years of age when they died. "From the location, these [formations of new bone] probably resulted from trauma or the inflammation of an overlying skin ulceration. This is inferred because the lower shin area is the most common site of chronic skin ulcers. Again, by inference these may have resulted from yaws."[25]

Bowers' inference about yaws may be consistent with theory, but it is not supported by epidemiological evidence or by history. In fact, from 1778 until the present time not a single case of yaws has ever been observed among island-born residents (and almost never among immigrants). This is proof that *Treponema pertenue,* the organism causing yaws, was not present among Hawaiians before 1778. A disease as extremely contagious and as persistent as is yaws—and, before modern chemotherapy became available, as ineradicable— could not have attacked only a very small fraction of the aboriginal population and then obligingly disappeared.

The skeletons Bowers examined, however, all of which came from a single burial ground at Mōkapu, O'ahu, represented only a very small sampling of the indigenous population. To draw from that small number great generalizations about the absence of diseases can be as foolish as is the insistence that yaws was epidemic among the people of old because six leg bones show formations suggesting responses to infection with *Treponema pertenue.*

In the early 1960s Ivar J. Larsen,[26] an orthopedic physician, examined bones from more than 500 skeletons that had been recovered from sand dunes at Mōkapu, O'ahu. (Given the source, more than likely at least some of those bones had been examined by Bowers in the 1920s.) Larsen saw "no changes suggestive of syphilis in the long bones, teeth, or skulls . . . and no extremity arthropathy . . . suggesting gonorrheal infection." Moreover, in a polite refutation of Bowers' claim, Larsen added, "bone lesions to justify the diagnosis of yaws were not seen." He found no signs of poliomyelitis, muscle dysplasia, ricketts, scurvy, or osteomalacia, and "no suggestive genetically induced skeletal defects." The only evidences of microbial disease that he did find came from cases of septic arthritis and bone infections.

In other words, the studies of Bowers, Larsen, and others indicate that Hawaiians who lived and died before 1778—*and* whose bodies were buried at Mōkapu—had not yet been exposed to the important epidemic diseases that leave proof of their presence in bones. But, as might be expected, individuals among those Hawaiians did suffer from noncontagious infections caused by opportunists among the microorganisms they harbored.

At the present time, then, paleopathology offers no strong dispute to the hypothesis that aboriginal Hawaiians were free of the major infectious diseases. In 1969, however, G. H. S. Chung et al. published a report indicating that they had found some congenital defects in such remains, the most frequent being clubfoot.[27] Blaisdell declared that clubfoot "persists in the highest frequency among modern Hawaiians compared to other ethnic groups in Hawai'i."[28]

Nutritional: Nutritionists who have evaluated the foodstuffs eaten by native Hawaiians, as well as paleopathologists who have examined their bones and teeth, agree that the kinds and amounts of foods available in normal times provided them with calories, organic components (including essential amino acids, vitamins, and other growth factors), and minerals sufficient to build sound healthy bodies and to maintain them in good condition.[29] The diet may have been "simple and monotonous," as Carey D. Miller said, "but, except for food shortages, temporary or prolonged, was one of relatively high nutritive value."[30]

Neither Bowers nor Larsen found those malformations of bones that are consequences of vitamin deficiencies, such as scurvy and ricketts. H. G. Chappel, who studied the teeth in 161 skulls, stated that "the well-formed teeth and high grade of enamel is proof that the food taken into the body during the time when the teeth were forming was sufficient both in quality and quantity." He believed that "the excellent quality" of the teeth disproved the statement "frequently heard in Honolulu" (in the 1920s, when he made his examinations) that "Hawaiian soil is so poor in lime salts that the vegetables do not furnish a sufficient amount of calcium to make good bones and teeth."[31]

We can assume, then, that except for periods of famine—attributable either to troops of marauding enemies during times of warfare or to spells of drought—native Hawaiians ate well enough and often enough to keep them in good nutritional health. This being so, their physiological condition would have helped to protect them, most of the time, from the attack of opportunists among the microorganisms they harbored normally upon and within themselves.

Zoological: Inasmuch as many of the insect vectors for viral, rickettsial, and protozoan pathogens were not present in Hawai'i until long after 1778, we can safely say that the diseases transmitted by these vectors could not have troubled native Hawaiians. The absence of specific animal hosts for those or other pathogenic microorganisms—and the absence of the intermediary animal hosts required by certain species of flukes and flatworms—extends the list of diseases which could not have been present in ancient Hawai'i.

Mosquitoes were not introduced until 1826, when (according to resident foreigners who marked the occasion all too well), the whaling ship *Wellington* brought them from San Blas, Mexico, to Lahaina, Maui. Mosquito larvae were dumped ashore by *Wellington*'s sailors as they rinsed water casks before filling them from Lahaina's stream.[32] The pestiferous interloper from San Blas— "enemy of all repose and ruffler of even tempers" as terrible-tempered Herman Melville complained in *Typee*—would be identified eventually as *Culex quinquefasciatus,* and is still the only species of the genus present in Hawai'i.[33] In other parts of the world it is an important vector of the several organisms that cause filariasis and certain types of virus encephalitis in human beings, heartworm in dogs, malaria in birds, and fowlpox. Even though this mosquito is established now on all the Hawaiian Islands, it has not yet been related to any cases of filariasis or viral encephalitides among island residents.

Two other species, *Aedes (Stegomyia) aegyptii* and *A. S. albopictus* complete the surprisingly meager representation of mosquitoes in these islands. They are vectors of the viruses that cause yellow fever and dengue fever. Although they were not recognized in Hawai'i until about 1895, one or the other of these mosquito species must have been present on O'ahu at least as early as 1852. During the summer of that year residents of Honolulu experienced for the first time an epidemic of dengue fever, which they called "Boohoo Fever," because people sick with it had "an uncontrollable disposition to cry."[34] Descriptive epithets like "Boohoo Fever," "Breakbone Fever," and others have been used for hundreds of years by foreigners living in Asian countries to describe the symptoms in places where dengue is endemic.

Yellow fever has never occurred in Hawai'i, although a "scare" excited Honolulu's residents in 1912. Outbreaks of dengue fever have been infrequent; the last epidemic, a long one, happened in 1943, when American combat pilots returning from the western Pacific's war zones brought the virus back with them to Waikīkī, from which it spread among residents on much of southern O'ahu.

For some reason, *Anopheles* mosquitoes have not yet been established in Hawai'i, possibly because a sufficient number of larvae—or, in this age of airplane travel, an adequate number of adult forms—have not been released in an area where they can survive and proliferate. This kindness of Nature, for which careless humans can receive no credit, means that the several species of malaria plasmodia that may be present in visitors, immigrants, or residents who have traveled abroad in malarial regions cannot yet be transmitted to islanders who stay at home.

While lice and fleas arrived together with the first Polynesian colonists and their animals, the most important diseases they transmit—typhus fever and bubonic plague—could not have affected aboriginal Hawaiians. Bubonic plague was introduced from the Orient only in 1899—and with a most unforgettable effect. Old World typhus, caused by *Rickettsia prowazekii,* has never been reported among residents. The milder endemic typhus or New World typhus, caused by *R. typhi,* is encountered occasionally in humans and is thought to be transmitted from wild rodents by means of fleas parasitic upon household pets, such as dogs and cats. "Scrub typhus," or tsutsugamushi fever, has never been reported from island residents, even though since World War II its causative agent, *R. tsutsugamushi,* has been imported often enough in American military personnel who have served in Asian countries before being returned to stations (or hospitals) in Hawai'i. Here, too, the insect vectors of *R. tsutsugamushi,* several species of acarine mites belonging to the genus *Trombicula,* have not yet arrived in the islands. The other rickettsial diseases have not been established here, although "Q fever" appeared briefly in Honolulu during the 1950s.

Nothing is known about the incidence of parasitic roundworms, flukes, and tapeworms in aboriginal Hawaiians although, as Windsor Cutting wrote, "parasites probably were introduced into Hawaii with the first colonization by man."[35] Because of their observance of the taboos for disposing of body wastes, most of the people of old probably were not infested with hookworms, pinworms, ascarids, and other roundworms that are passed more or less directly from human hosts to human recipients. Their swine (and they themselves) may have suffered from trichinosis, caused by *Trichinella spiralis,* but no evidence about the presence of this disease before 1778 has been found.

The rat lungworm, *Angiostrongylus cantonensis,* which causes eosinophilic meningoencephalitis in people who have eaten its intermediate hosts in the raw state (such as garden slugs, African snails, freshwater prawns, land crabs, and perhaps salad greens sheltering small garden slugs or land planarians), almost certainly was not present before 1778. The first human case in Hawai'i was recognized only in 1961. All evidence indicates that this nematode arrived in Hawai'i (indeed, in all Polynesia) only very recently.[36]

On the other hand, a few native Hawaiians may have contracted infestations with a variety of cestode tapeworms (such as *Taenia solium, Hymenolepis nana,* and *Dipylidium caninum*) from their domesticated pigs and dogs and from wild rats—provided those animals were infested to begin with. The horrendously "measly" pigs M. Rollin saw at La Pérouse Bay support this suspicion, but do not prove it.

The major diseases of humans caused by trematodes, or flukes, could not possibly have troubled indigenous Hawaiians. Those infestations peculiar to the Orient—such as schistosomiasis, clonorchiasis (or opisthorchiasis), and paragonimiasis—were absent because either the flukes themselves or the mollusks that serve as their intermediate hosts were not present. None of these diseases has occurred as yet among island-born residents who remain in Hawai'i. The few cases diagnosed in Hawai'i have been limited to islanders who were born in the Orient (or have visited places there), to American military personnel who have served in Oriental countries, and to Japanese soldiers interned on O'ahu as POWs during World War II.

The liver fluke associated with cattle, *Fasciola gigantica,* also was absent, because cows were not introduced until 1793. The heterophyid fluke, *Stellantchasmus falcatus,* for which snails and mullet serve as intermediary hosts, could have been present before 1778, but would not have caused serious or epidemic disease. Even today it is found only infrequently in human hosts in Hawai'i.

Arthropod ectoparasites upon both people and animals (such as lice, fleas, and scabies mites) would have been inescapable and very difficult to control. Fleas and lice, large enough to be seen, were observed by Captain Cook's associates, but the minuscule mites of scabies escaped their notice. William Bayly, astronomer with the British expedition, seems to have been more aware of head lice than were his shipmates, who did not bother to comment upon such constant companions of their times. Bayly thought that Hawaiians who cut their hair short did so "in order to destroy the lice which they have in great multitudes among it."[37]

Fleas and lice are big enough to be removed from the human body with fingers, forceps, combs, and other grooming devices. Scabies mites, *Sarcoptes scabei,* are too small to be seen easily, and therefore are removed only with difficulty. They are controlled most effectively by being killed in place, with steam baths and hot mud baths (such as many a European spa offered for the easing of people who suffered from "the itch"), or by anointing the entire body, from head to foot, with unguents containing some form of sulfur or a modern chemical sarcopticide. Even though their Fire Goddess Pele emitted quantities of sulfur from many steam vents at Kīlauea, Hawaiians did not know about using the golden-yellow crystals for treating the itch. In consequence, those who were so unfortunate as to catch the infestation were forced to endure it as best they could until, finally, after 1820, American missionaries told them about the value of sulfur salves and fumigants.

The varied lesions that can develop around female mites burrowing in the human skin are astounding and horrifying: they range all the way from mere reddened swellings, through pustules, weeping ulcerations complicated by secondary infections with bacteria, fungi, or other microorganisms, to exuberant crenellated proliferations of tissue that resemble lepromata or cancers run amok. This diversity of effects is represented unforgettably in the hand-colored illustrations of lesions caused by scabies mites that were prepared by D. C. Danielssen and W. Boeck for their pioneer work on leprosy, *Om Spedalsked,* published in Christiania, Norway, in 1847.

As Danielssen and Boeck intended to show, these many different responses to the infesting mites can be mistaken by uninformed people for lesions of serious infections such as are seen in cases of erysipelas, tuberculosis, leprosy, syphilis, tertiary yaws, and leishmaniasis. The damage done by scabies mites alone could account for the repulsive appearance of the natives at La Pérouse Bay—and that of their animals—which so dismayed the visiting French mariners that day in 1786.

These many references by no means complete the account of pathogenic microorganisms that may have affected native Hawaiians since 1778. Some of these microbes have been implicated very recently by epidemiologists, while others are only now being recognized as pathogens. Examples are the protozoa that cause giardiasis and the several kinds of amoebic dysentery; cases of these in Hawai'i are rarely reported. Other pathogens are the leptospiras causing icterohaemorrhagic fevers and the chlamydias involved in "chronic fatigue syndrome" (misnamed "yuppie disease") and certain sexually transmitted diseases. Beyond doubt other pathogens, still extremely difficult to detect, are present among islanders—or will be imported in the future.

Environmental: Located, as they are, in a region of the earth that is neither entirely tropical nor yet definitely temperate, the islands of Hawai'i enjoy a climate such as fabulists in the Middle Ages granted only to the Isles of the Blest. With "Airs, Waters, Places," as the Hippocratic writings called these features in the environment, few indigenous Hawaiians could have found any reason to complain.

Along coastal lowlands and in green valleys, where most of the populace lived in scattered family farms or in "dispersed communities" (as anthropologists prefer to call them), no extremes in temperature occurred such as discomfort inhabitants of temperate or equatorial zones. Rains won from Lono's clouds by the high mountains gave quantities of pure water to windward districts on the major islands. The people there drew the Water of Kāne from streams, irrigation ditches, springs, and, in a few places along leeward coasts, from shallow wells.

Hurricanes rarely vented their fury upon islands so well tempered by expanses of ocean, and strong winds or gales were infrequent. Even earthquakes were usually gentle; and the archipelago's active volcanoes offered spectacles to be looked upon in awe rather than terrors to be fled. No venomous reptiles, no beasts of prey, lurked in fields and forests. In this protected realm the only hazards Hawaiians dreaded were the sharks in the sea, cruel men, and unpredictable gods.

Although they did not understand this, because they knew no other land to compare with theirs, Hawaiians of old were granted the most salubrious environment on earth in which to dwell. It was so benign, so unchanging, that they thought not at all of their good fortune, and they found no need to coin a word meaning weather. They

were not subjected, therefore, to the stresses of intense cold or ener-
vating heat that affect human metabolism in less favored countries,
in consequence of which people there are made more susceptible to
infections with microorganisms derived from themselves or from
neighbors.

Nor were Hawaiians so numerous that their islands could
not accommodate them comfortably. Because they did not live in
crowded, filthy, noisy cities—and because in their respect for the
land, the water, and the air that the great gods had given them, they
did not pollute their dwelling places with excrement and litter, with
stenches and clamor—they were spared most of the social stresses
which (as we today are learning all too brutally) are the consequences
of crowding and pollution. And yet, in being spared the assaults of
hurtful weather, crowding, and contamination, Hawaiians were fortunate and favored for only so long as they remained insulated from
the rest of the world's people: the very kindness of their environment
proved in time to be almost as great an unkindness as was their isolation. Without the many attritions of a more demanding environment
to cull the weak from the strong, too many of the weak survived, to
become the victims of foreigners' germs and foreign pollutions.

As the good gods in their power had ordained, and as the people
knew only too well (because the priests who were the gods' intermediaries never let them forget), Hawaiians were subjected to many
other psychological stresses and tensions which must have made
them miserable in subtle ways before foreigners arrived with their
new kinds of troubles.

In 1858, the Reverend John F. Pogue, moralizing in the manner of
Christian missionaries, reminded his readers:

> Life was Extremely dangerous under the chiefs during [the ancient
> times]. It is justified to call it—"bloody times *(wa koko)*" because men
> were killed mercilessly and without justification; their chiefs had no
> compassion upon them. Their bodies were placed on the same altars as
> the sacrifice-hogs . . . until rotting set in.[38]

Not one to let a good message go to waste for want of support in
fact, Pogue may have been indulging here in pulpit hyperbole. In any
event, the idea of psychological stress that he meant to emphasize is
clear.

Beyond all doubt, psychological traumata of almost intolerable
intensity and variety afflicted most Hawaiians after foreigners with

their strange artifacts and alien values disrupted the indigenous society. Those new psychological stresses, as well as the new kinds of microbes, most certainly played important parts in the long dying of the Hawaiian race.

Experiences of Other Isolated Societies: Hawaiians were not the only people who suffered the onslaughts of diseases new to them. The same tribulations that were thrust upon them have been inflicted so often upon so many peoples, both before and after 1778, that the experience must be recognized as being both inevitable and inexorable. Always, when a weak society is confronted by a strong one, the weaker must yield to the stronger. This is one of History's few axioms, for it is but an expression in human terms of one of Nature's most ruthless laws. The law applies to all aspects of a failing society —from the tools its members use to the heaven they envision—but it is revealed most strikingly in the number of deaths it exacts from the people who are subdued, whether by weapons, or ideas, or diseases. The history of the human race is full of melancholy illustrations of this rule. Nowhere is it more clearly demonstrated than among the people of Oceania, and nowhere is its proof better documented than for the islands of Hawai'i. "The white man's civilization," wrote Robert Louis Stevenson, mourning the dying of the Polynesians whom he so much admired, "was scarcely less fatal than the white man's bullet."[39]

Whether the emissaries of the stronger society come as invaders or as friends, their effect on the weaker is the same. Spain's greedy conquistadores and zealous padres brought destruction and death to the Aztecs of Mexico and the Incas of Peru even more with the germs of smallpox, measles, syphilis, gonorrhea, and tuberculosis those warriors carried in their bodies than with muskets, cannon, pikes, and swords. North America's white settlers wiped out Indian friends as well as foes more with fevers, however unplanned, than with firearms and firewater.[40]

Today primitive tribes in Papua New Guinea's high mountain fastnesses and in South America's dark jungles are being devastated by the diseases of civilization before they have even seen a civilized man. Even when they come with the best of intentions, representatives of civilization, regardless of color, are unmitigated dangers, if unwitting ones, to primitive peoples. Explorers, traders, trappers, and missionaries have been much more effective as sowers of diseases than as sharers of knowledge or savers of souls.

On occasion, by one of those ironies that Tragedy can arrange, a member of the threatened society is himself the bringer of death to his own people:

On January 12, 1875, soon after Fiji was placed under our Colonial Government [Dr. William Squire reported to the Epidemiological Society of London], the chief Thakombau arrived at Levuka in HMS *Dido,* on his return from Sydney. While there he or some of his party had measles. On January 6, during the voyage home, one of his sons and a native attendant fell ill with measles. They were treated in a house built for them on the ship's deck, and made so good a recovery that no obstacle was raised to their landing on the 12th. Two or three days after landing, another son of the chief returning with him was seized. . . . At this time visitors from all parts thronged the house when he was sick. On January 24–25 there was a great assemblage of native chiefs, some from the more distant parts of the large island. A strong force of native constabulary attended. Any new case of measles in the native village had not at this time attracted notice. On February 12 a despatch from Mr. Layard announced measles to be epidemic among the natives, and that nearly one hundred of the native constables were down with it. . . .

Excessive mortality resulted from terror at the mysterious seizure, and the want of commonest aids during illness; there were none to offer drink during the fever, nor food on its subsidence. Thousands were carried off for want of nourishment and care, as well as by dysentery and congestion of the lungs; the worst dangers from overcrowding were incurred in the small houses, and the worst dangers from cold by the sufferers rushing to the water, where they could continue immersed.[41]

That is how measles came for the first time to the people of Fiji. It spread from Levuka to all the larger islands of the group, and in four months killed more than 20,000 people—"one-fourth to one-fifth" of the entire native population.

All island communities, wherever they lie, are subjected to this kind of microbiological warfare. Panum perceived how the people isolated in the Faeroe Islands responded to the flow and ebb of germs, arriving with sailors aboard merchant ships, receding as the resident islanders either died or recovered from the most recent wave of sicknesses—until the next time around. This book attempts to show, on a larger scale, how the people in the Hawaiian Islands, these "Crossroads of the Pacific" as mariners used to call them, responded to the microbial invasions they were forced to contend with.

For island populations such assaults can never end. Always, as long as visitors come and go, dangers too will come. Most of them will subside, in time, but now that AIDS has come to Hawai'i at least one threat will not soon go away.

In fact, in these days of restless traveling about the world, the islanders do not have to wait any more for strangers from other lands to descend, trailing their germs behind them. Islanders, too, send tourists out into the big world. And, not surprisingly, when they come home again they too may come bearing alien germs.

Thus, on 29 January 1989, two young officers, members of the U.S. Army Reserves, returned to Honolulu after participating in a joint Japan–U.S. training exercise in Hokkaido. Within a few days both men became ill with rubella, or German measles. Before their ailment was diagnosed, they transmitted the rubella virus to five susceptible adults. So began an authentic epidemic, a minor one to be sure, of little importance to the adults affected. But the virus represented a serious threat to the really vulnerable people in the community—pregnant women and the fetuses they carried. Fortunately, public health measures to interrupt the cycle by which pathogens are distributed—isolation of actual cases, passive and active immunization of susceptible contacts—contained the epidemic, preventing it from becoming a greater hazard.[42]

Physicians and public health officials were much better informed and prepared in 1989 than Fiji's medical authorities could have been in 1875—or Hawai'i's at any time before the 1980s. In the future, however, perhaps Hawai'i will play another and more positive role in matters concerning epidemic diseases—a role better than the passive and accepting one it has assumed for the past 200 years. In February 1989, Dr. C. Everett Koop, at that time Surgeon General of the U.S. Public Health Service, visited Honolulu, in part to commemorate the hundredth anniversary of the Public Health Service as a commissioned corps. While here, he "met with a group of visiting Pacific island health officers . . . to discuss issues affecting island nations." During the meeting Dr. Koop said: "Hawai'i will play a major role in the future of health research as the bridge between the United States and other countries in the Pacific Basin."[43]

Such speeches, full of grand promises, are the stuff of which *shibai,* sham, is made. Residents of these islands have heard equivalent prophecies, about all possible subjects, for 200 years and more. Whether or not Hawai'i's politicians, physicians, and health planners will ever allow their state to achieve that helpful role remains to be seen. But at least the Surgeon General tried to point them in the right direction.

ಲ್-ಲ್-ಲ್-ಲ್

Although no one today can be certain about any of the aspects of personal and public health in Hawai'i before 1778, information drawn from many sources (and interpreted according to the logic of several biomedical disciplines) permits these deductions to be made:

• Because of their extreme geographic isolation, Hawaiians were spared any experience with the major infectious diseases that afflicted the populations of Asia, Europe, Africa, the Americas, and even those of central Polynesia.

• Because they were not germ-free, individual Hawaiians, like people everywhere, did experience sporadic, idiopathic infections and infestations caused by organisms present in their own normal microbiota or in those of their domestic animals.

• If they brought any pathogenic microorganisms with them in their migrations from central Polynesia, those pathogens either died out during the centuries after contact with the homeland ceased, or they became so adapted to their hosts as to be relatively harmless.

• Implied, but beyond proving, is the possibility that centuries of inbreeding among a progeny descended from a very small number of ancestors may have produced a population in which, by the process known as gene drift, many members of whole families would have been made vulnerable to infection with virulent microorganisms when these were introduced in and after 1778.

• While in theory Hawaiians before 1778 might have maintained certain microorganisms that can cause one or more serious epidemic diseases indigenous to themselves, this possibility is not supported by evidence from any source.

• The possibility that they were as acquainted with major epidemic infectious diseases as were the people of Europe, Asia, and the Americas is incompatible with observations made by the British discoverers of Hawai'i, as well as with the history of Hawaiians since 1778.

• Protected by distance, favored by environment, Hawaiians were healthy, if not happy, until their isolation came to an end in that fateful fatal year of 1778.

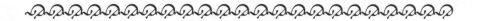

THREE

The Native Medical Profession

In Hawai'i, too, the "people of old" suffered from sicknesses of body and of spirit. They, too, out of their need, sought help from physicians and priests, from healers, quacks, sorcerers, and gods. In the stratified Hawaiian society, with its several castes and many subcastes recognized according to lineage, duties, or training, physicians were called *kāhuna lapaʻau,* experts in medicine. The medical profession itself was known as *ʻoihana lapaʻau.*[1]

Because kāhuna lapaʻau served as priests as well as physicians, usually they were associated with temples of healing, *heiau hoʻōla.* Each of the major islands supported at least one heiau hoʻōla which was noted for the excellence of its teachers and the efficacy of treatments they prescribed for their patients. Such a temple of healing was famed Hono-a-Kāne in Kaʻū on Hawaiʻi. Another was Pākākā heiau of the priests of Lono in the village of Kou on Oʻahu. This heiau stood on the point jutting into the bay of Māmala, near the little inlet on the southern shore of Oʻahu that in time would be called Honolulu.[2] The heiau would have stood about where Aloha Tower rises now.

Still another was Ke Aīwa heiau at 'Aiea on Oʻahu. The very name, Ke Aīwa, "the mystery," referred to the power of a kahuna lapaʻau as it was expressed in his skill in the diagnosis and treatment of illness. The word *aīwa,* in its turn, was derived from an older form, *aīwaīwa,* meaning "the mysterious, the incomprehensible." Implicit in both terms was the question, asked in awe: "Who can explain the mystery and power of their medicines?"[3] And Kapuaīwa, "mysterious kapu," referring to this power acquired through his divine lineage, was one of the sacred names given to the child who later became King Kamehameha V.

During the most ancient times, a heiau hoʻōla and its attendant priest-physicians were dedicated to one of the four greatest gods, Kāne, Kū, Lono, or Kanaloa, in his different manifestations, or to the Moon Goddess Hina, wife of Kū. As the people multiplied, so did the number of kāhuna lapaʻau increase. As methods of diagnosis and treatment became more diversified, new temples of healing were founded and lesser gods also were regarded as patron deities. David Malo, one of the first Hawaiians to write about his people's past, named three of these: "Those who practised medicine prayed to Maʻi-ola. Kapualakaʻi and Kau-ka-hoʻo-la-maʻi were female deities worshipped by women and practitioners of medicine."[4] Ultimately, several heiau hoʻōla were established on each of the major islands in order to serve residents from nearby districts as well as patients who came from afar.

In 1951, at ceremonies "rededicating" Ke Aīwa heiau after it had been partly restored, Sir Peter Buck, at that time director of the Bernice Pauahi Bishop Museum, said:

> In Polynesia the advancement of medical science was confined by superstitions. The Hawaiians formed an exception. They broke out of the chains of superstitions and sought remedies for human ills in other fields. The temple of healing is unique in Hawaii. The Hawaiians came to know the therapeutic uses of certain plants. They organized a profession of herbalists who had to be trained and pass rigid tests before they were recognized by the people.[5]

Sir Peter was applying the European definition of herbalist to all kāhuna lapaʻau. Moreover, in giving such high praise to Hawaiʻi's native physicians, he seems to have overlooked those of other Polynesian societies.

In many respects, heiau hoʻōla were similar to temples of healing founded in the Mediterranean area by priest-physicians such as the disciples of Aesculapius. In Hawaiʻi, as in Greece or Egypt, such hallowed precincts included the temple itself, where an image of the protecting deity might be exhibited and where his mana was believed to be present, as well as auxiliary structures in which priest-physicians together with apprentices lived, studied, and stored their utensils and medicines.

Stringent kapus regulated every thought and action of kāhuna lapaʻau and their disciples. The mysterious powers derived from the presiding god and from the priests who were dedicated to his service were believed to be so great that all evil spirits were held at bay. An ordinary man would not dare to enter the heiau before he was purified at its gate by aspersion with *wai ea,* a holy water containing salt and turmeric.

Unlike Aesculapian temples, however, heiau hoʻōla ordinarily did not serve as hospitals or dispensaries. Generally a kahuna lapaʻau attended an ailing person in the patient's own home, although on occasion a chief of high rank might be accommodated in a temporary house built for him within the temple area or just outside its entrance.

Some of the medicinal herbs favored by physicians of the temple might be cultivated in the adjacent gardens. Mary Kawena Pukui remembered that, when she was a child in Kaʻū, her family "had about a half-acre in medicinal herbs and plants."[6] In most instances, however, plants were sought in their natural habitats, as were the animal and mineral components employed in therapy.

Apprentices were boys and youths of good character, carefully selected, as are medical students today, according to their abilities and motivation. Although usually sons of kahunas, or of chiefs, were chosen as apprentices, worthy commoners were not denied the opportunity to become physicians. Apparently the profession was exclusively masculine. Women were forbidden entrance to heiau hoʻōla, even great chiefesses, even the wives and daughters of the physician-priests who served the god within. And, for those ancient times, no mention is preserved of a woman kahuna lapaʻau or, indeed, of a woman kahuna of any kind.

After many years of training by a master teacher, a successful apprentice became a practicing kahuna lapaʻau. According to his interests, he could remain at the temple as an assistant to his master, or he could join the staff of another heiau hoʻōla, or he could establish a private practice by settling among the people in some place remote from a temple of healing. More than likely an ambitious physician, or one who conceived a different approach to diagnosis and treatment, could found a new heiau hoʻōla.

No account of kāhuna lapaʻau has ever discussed the nature of the training by which a good physician prepared himself spiritually for the demands of his profession. In other words, how did he develop the mysterious ability to communicate with the spirit world, to receive messages from gods great or small, from spirit ancestors and other invisible forces?

Writers of a century ago could reveal very little about this psychological aspect of a physician's training because, not being initiates themselves, they could not know what it entailed—and probably were baffled by it as well. More than likely, assuming that an effective kahuna lapaʻau can be compared with an effective psychic of our time, or with a proper Siberian shaman, Tibetan lama, or Hindu guru, he developed himself through continual exercises in spiritual discipline, having acquired the fundamental techniques from his teachers in the heiau hoʻōla in which he had been trained. This preparation of his psychic abilities would have been absolutely necessary because, without the capacity to receive and sustain the power emanating from those spirit forces, his own mana would have been inordinately strained—or, even worse, burned out, with consequent suffering for himself and no help at all for his patient.

Samuel M. Kamakau did imply this meaning: "If the *kahuna* was an upright person he could be guided properly by true revelations of his spirit guides; the secret things of his ancestors would be revealed to him, and all the hallowed things about which he did not know." An upright kahuna was "commanded" through apparitions, visions, phantoms, shadowy forms, and "by visual knowledge . . . through seeing and talking with an *akua* who had assumed human form." In short, to use the language of today's psychics, he became clairvoyant, clairaudient, a "seer," a "sensitive." An upright *kahuna ʻaumakua* was recognized "in the purity of his person and of his deeds, and his true piety. Then the *akua* would help him by revealing the cause of the trouble, the wrongdoings the patient had committed, and what offerings the patient must give to pay for his wrongs."[7]

The belief that a genuine kahuna lapaʻau could communicate with entities in the spirit world, and therefore needed to develop his own spiritual powers to a high level in order to receive revelations from akua, ʻaumakua, and other such guides, establishes another link between Hawaiians and the cultures of their origin in Southeast Asia. Anthropologists, ethnobotanists, and zoologists have long since demonstrated this connection of Hawaiʻi to Asia in their several sciences, as have linguists and students of mythology and religion. To these relationships the kahuna lapaʻau should be added: to some extent he is a more modest version of Asia's shaman-priest-prophet-physician. Far removed in space and time from his Asian counterparts, of course, and undoubtedly differing from them in the rituals and the materia medica he could use, the kahuna lapaʻau still put his faith, and his need, in the deities and the powers of the spirit world, just as his ancestors did long ago, before ever they sailed forth from Asia across the Great Sea.

Concepts of Sickness

As has been said in the preceding essay, present evidence indicates that in the centuries between the time the first colonists from central Polynesia settled in the Hawaiian Islands and the discovery of these islands by Captain James Cook's expedition in 1778, the Hawaiian people suffered from no epidemic infectious diseases. Kamakau, most learned of early native historians, held the same opinion:

> In very ancient times, many people observed the rules of the art of healing, but in later times most of them abandoned medical practices because there was not much sickness within the race. Foreigners had not yet come from other lands; there were no fatal diseases, no epidemics, no contagious diseases, no diseases that eat away the body, no venereal diseases.[8]

This is not to say that the people of old were not acquainted with sickness and disease. If only because they were human they knew well enough the signs of illness, the meaning of pain. But most of their ailments were consequences of physical injury—of bones broken in accidents or in battles; of cuts, bruises, and festering wounds inflicted by work, play, or warfare; of the miseries of childbirth and the ravagings of childbed fever—or of the usual organic dysfunctions and the deteriorations of aging from which people in all societies suffer.

Their worst afflictions came from the very real cruelty of other people and the imagined cruelty of their gods: in a theocracy in which great gods and lesser gods lurked everywhere, each one jealous for the respect due to him and his kapus, in which clever priests and proud chiefs maintained their power by enforcing those kapus, the incidence of psychogenic ailments must have been very high. The ease with which a Hawaiian could lie down on his mat and die, when he was persuaded that an implacable god or a malign sorcerer demanded his life in forfeit, indicates that fear was more powerful than hope. Anxiety and terror, which make their claims upon people even today, and manifest their effects in so many sicknesses of psyche and body, must have been even more potent causes of illness among members of a society as dominated by gods and priests as was that of Hawai'i.

In common with other Polynesians and other primitive peoples throughout the world, Hawaiians believed that health, prosperity, and happiness were the rewards of piety, expressed in reverence for the gods; of conformity, expressed in respect for the kapus as these were announced by chiefs and priests; and of rectitude, expressed in their relationships with family and neighbors. Sickness, poverty, misfortune, the unhappinesses of failure, were punishments imposed directly or indirectly by the gods for having broken their kapus. A man prospered when his mana, his spirit power given him by the gods, was not burdened with guilt or depleted by offenses against the kapus. But when his mana was weakened for any cause—whether by his own act; or by the decree of an affronted god; or by the malice of an ancestor spirit, an 'aumakua; or by the machinations of a sorcerer —he suffered. Sickness could be caused by "failure to obey the mandate of an 'aumakua (i.e., in the naming of a child), or from unintended or intentional offense to an 'aumakua (e.g., by eating an animal which was the totem of the sick one's family), speaking maliciously about a relative or an 'aumakua, promising something and failing to fulfill the obligation."[9]

To Hawaiians, as to most primitive peoples, thoughts, too, and therefore the words with which thoughts were uttered, were charged with mana. "Words bind," they believed, "and words make free." "Ua hewa ka waha," a man said, when he recognized that he had offended: "The mouth has committed an error." And the evil effects which befell him in consequence of that error were called na hua 'olelo, "the fruits of speech."[10] E. S. C. Handy, in his Polynesian Religion, gave this translation of the lament uttered by a fallen chief, "whose mana had failed him":

> What is my great offense, O god?
> I have eaten standing, perhaps, or without giving thanks,
> Or these, my people, have eaten wrongfully.
> Yes, that is the offense, O Kāne-of-the-water-of-life.
> O spare; O let me live, thy devotée,
> Look not with indifference upon me.
>
> I call upon thee, O answer thou me,
> O thou god of my body who art in Heaven.

O Kāne, let the lightning flash, let the thunder roar,
Let the earth shake.

I am saved; my god has looked upon me,
I am being washed, I have escaped the danger.[11]

During the long centuries of isolation, Hawai'i's priest-physicians developed several modes of diagnosis and treatment for ailments. Physicians trained according to the different schools of thought were able to treat injuries to bones and muscles, or disturbances of mana, quite satisfactorily. Samuel M. Kamakau, writing in 1866–1870 about *ka po'e kahiko,* the people of old, assigned physicians to eight major categories, according to their specializations:

1. *Kahuna ho'ohāpai keiki* and *kahuna ho'ohānau keiki* (who induced pregnancy and delivered babies)
2. *Kahuna pa'ao'ao* and *kahuna 'ea* (who diagnosed and treated childhood ailments)
3. *Kahuna 'ō'ō* (who kept closed the fontanel and who practiced lancing)
4. *Kahuna hāhā* (who diagnosed internal ailments by palpation)
5. *Kahuna ka 'alawa maka* and *kahuna 'ike lihilihi* (who diagnosed ailments by insight or close observation)
6. *Kahuna 'anā'anā* and *kahuna kuni* (sorcerers who used magic in treatment, either for good or for evil)
7. *Kahuna ho'opi'opi'o* (who used counteracting sorcery)
8. *Kahuna makani* (who treated the spirits of illness)[12]

Kamakau also called them *kāhuna 'aumakua* because, in their attempts to identify sicknesses and proper methods for treating them, all physicians, regardless of specialization, invoked the aid of *'aumakua,* spirit-guardians, or of *akua,* gods.[13]

A physician who administered medicines of any kind was also called a *kahuna lapa'au lā'au. (Lā'au* means "tree, plant, wood," and a number of other things more or less related to vegetable sources, even though some medications were derived from animals or minerals.) Other kinds of specialists may have practiced some form of medicine, but Kamakau did not name them. Neither did David Malo, when he wrote his *Hawaiian Antiquities* in 1836–1839, nor John Papa I'i, when, in the late 1860s, he wrote his *Fragments of Hawaiian History* about the period from 1800 to 1854.

A manuscript in the Bishop Museum adds details that Kamakau, Malo, and I'i did not mention:

1. The chiefs had a separate kahuna or kahunas.
2. The multitudes had separate kahunas.
3. The *Maka-i-o-Uli* order of kahunas [was] separate: they were the medical kahunas.
4. The kahunas of the travelers were separate.
5. The kahunas who wore dried *ti* leaf coverings (mountaineers) were separate.[14]

Surgeons were not named separately in Kamakau's classification, even though certain operations were performed frequently, such as circumcision (or, more correctly, subincision) and lancing of boils or other superficial abscesses, while others were seldom attempted, such as the rather more difficult trepanning of a cracked skull. Presumably these surgical interventions were performed by kāhuna 'ō'ō. Hawaiian surgeons, in any event, seem not to have been as proficient as those of Tonga and Samoa.

Activities too menial for the august members of the medical profession to perform were passed on to apprentices or to lowly assistants, such as midwives, *pale keiki,* and nurses, *kahu ma'i.* Either males or females could serve in these lesser roles.

Pukui confirmed Kamakau's descriptions for kāhuna lapa'au and their functions in the days of old.[15] But, as we shall see later, she indicated that, for the decades after foreigners and their influences came to these islands, kāhuna lapa'au and their methods changed considerably to meet the needs of those new and different times. She did add, however, an engaging (and revealing) explanation for the roles that their major gods played in Hawaiians' concepts of medicine:

> Lóno, Kū, and Hina, and to some extent Kāne, would remain through generations the constantly invoked gods of medicine. Lono, because he caused all plants to grow, reigned supreme. . . . Kū and Hina continued to symbolize the balance embodied in well-being. For Kū was maleness; Hina was female. Kū was erect; Hina supine; Kū was east, the morning; Hina was west and the evening; Kū was the external factor, Hina the internal. Kū was the right side and right hand; Hina, the left. Thus, what could be more life-restoring than plants, gathered ritually with right and left hand, kept separate for external or internal use, or blended, Kū-with-Hina, for poultice or potion?[16]

Nowhere else in all Hawaiian accounts of kāhuna lapa'au and their practices can we find a clearer statement of the relationship between Hawaiian beliefs and the oriental concept of Yang and Yin.

Jungian analyst Rita Knipe, in her perceptive book *The Water of Life, A Jungian Journey Through Hawaiian Myth,* extended this thought to a higher and universal level:

> The lunar aspect of healing is not expressed solely by [Hina] the moon goddess, but by Hina and Kū in conjunction. . . . [In] the Kū and Hina godhead of duality, with its implied union of male and female, a third reality is constellated . . . which may be considered the archetype of healing or of health. Kū-with-Hina, like the yang-with-yin symbol of Chinese Tao, symbolizes the balance embodied within the conjunction of opposites, with resultant harmony and health.[17]

Because Hawaiians did not create a written form of their language, and therefore were unable to keep records of their history, very little is known about the nature of their ailments and the state of their medical art before 1800. When natives did learn to write, in the syllabary which American missionaries devised for them between 1820 and 1827, some of them wrote a great deal, upon every conceivable subject, and with a zest for which today's antiquarians can be grateful. Even so, whatever they wrote must be read with extreme caution because by the time they were able to put their thoughts on paper, their society had been exposed for more than fifty years to foreign practices and ideas. Whether or not a native was aware of this, his thoughts were no longer his own to express, but were forever tainted by foreign influences. And, phenomenal though his memory may have been, however much he may have honored his people's traditions, these too were exceedingly unreliable sources of information for historians of his time or today.

Accounts written by foreigners are equally suspect because of the innate biases of those haoles (as all foreigners were called in those days), as well as their ignorance of native customs, language, and psychology. In consequence, almost everything written about Hawai'i and its people before the year 2000 *(sic)* must be read with considerable skepticism, especially when it concerns native practices of which haoles disapproved and about which natives were defensive. To most haoles the natives' religion, social relationships, sexual mores, diseases, medicines, other remedies, and "medicine men" were subjects for disapproval if not outright condemnation.

Small wonder, then, that most Hawaiians quickly learned to dissemble, or to remain silent, when an inquisitive anthropologist-type haole approached them with prying questions, poised pencil, and

opened notebook. Small wonder, too, that a staunch native, proud
of his heritage and wanting to protect it, did not put into writing his
knowledge of certain respected matters. The ones who hastened to
take up *peni* and *pepa* were half-haole already, alas, full of vainglory
and eager to vaunt themselves with the new-learned *palapala*. Often,
too, they were full converts to the new Christian religion, all too willing to share their naive ruminations with the American missionaries
who had taught them this gratifying pastime of writing. In either
case, the very fact that they were educated and influenced by foreign
teachers made them unreliable reporters and interpreters of the way
things actually were in the days of old. A close reading of the works
of David Malo and Samuel M. Kamakau, who were introduced to
the joys of writing by the Reverend Sheldon Dibble, their teacher at
Lahainaluna High School, reveals how quickly the Yankee missionaries' theology and morality were inculcated in those most assiduous
pupils.

Fortunately for the purpose of this appraisal, a great number of
manuscripts written in Hawaiian by kāhuna lapaʻau during the latter
half of the nineteenth century have survived. Some of these papers
are preserved in the Bernice Pauahi Bishop Museum, in the Kalākaua, Liliʻuokalani, Kalanianaʻole, Kamakau, Henriques, Poepoe,
and Lono Maguire Collections, while others are deposited in the
Archives of Hawaiʻi. Most of these manuscripts have been translated
into English by Mary Kawena Pukui or her predecessors at the
Bishop Museum. Supplementing those slighter works are later trea-
tises written by Akana, Akina, and Kaʻaiakamanu (1922), Green
and Beckwith (1926), Handy, Pukui, and Livermore (1934), Pukui
(1942), and by Handy and Pukui (1958).

As might be expected, the monograph entitled *Outline of Hawaiian Physical Therapeutics,* prepared by Handy, Pukui, and Livermore, is the most authoritative of these studies, and will continue to
be so. Nonetheless, after most of the translated manuscripts and all
of the published accounts have been read, some further conclusions
can be drawn that will serve to amplify their classic report.

In *Polynesian Religion,* published in 1927, Handy summarizes
native concepts about cause, diagnosis, and cure of sickness in these
biased terms of white men:

Physical malady and death were believed to be the result of psychic
causes or conditions, rather than physical; and hence the chief means

chosen to combat illness were psychic. Broadly speaking, the evils that were thought to destroy a man may be classified as of two kinds: demons that acted of their own accord or at a god's or necromancer's behest, causing illness, sometimes by entering the body; and curses of black magic that acted directly on the psychic nature. When a man fell sick, first it was necessary to discern the nature of the trouble. The causes of illness being psychic, diagnosis was necessarily by psychic means, these being mainly of two kinds, through revelation by familiar spirits speaking through a human medium, and by clairvoyance. If the trouble was caused by an angered god or spirit, then expiation or placation was required, and gifts or sacrifices were presented and other measures taken to mollify the angry psychic being. When it was a case of a demon in the sick body, various modes of exorcism were resorted to, including the recitation of potent spells, the application of heat, the use of evil-smelling herbs. Spells of black magic were capable to being counteracted by a powerful magician, who attempted usually to cause the trouble to revert upon its sender, or a curse might be removed if the witch who had laid it could be bought off or otherwise persuaded to relieve the victim. Finally there were various types of spells and rites designed to restore health and life to the sick body, and practices resorted to for the purpose of bringing back into its body the soul that was believed to have left it.[18]

Kamakau expressed the same philosophy from a more naive (and native) point of view:

The god was the foundation [of medicine], and secondly came prayers. Third, came schooling in the kinds of diseases; fourth, in the kinds of remedies; fifth, in the art of killing; and sixth, in the art of saving. . . . It was [the god] who knew without error the treatment; it was he who pointed out the nature of the ailment and the things that pertained to this or that disease in man.[19]

Erwin H. Ackerknecht, a European physician of the twentieth century who studied the medical systems among many societies throughout the world, both ancient and recent, wrote in terms that related Hawaiians to the universal experience:

Illness, like death or an accident, is generally not regarded by the primitive as a natural event. It is the consequence of supernatural actions or forces. Even a cold may be explained by such causes. Mystical object-intrusion, loss of the soul or one of the souls, spirit intrusion, breach of taboo, or witchcraft are the most common causes of illness.[20]

Diagnosis

Although a kahuna lapaʻau used the techniques of diagnosis emphasized at the temple of healing he had attended, more than likely all
physicians followed this general procedure described by Kamakau:

> If the illness was a very serious one, one that a *kahuna* could not com-
> prehend, and it was beyond the knowledge of the *kahuna* who treated
> for it, then it was due to the *ʻaumakua*. It was very difficult to dodge
> the "smoke" of the *ʻaumakua*. And they "entertained" introduced dis-
> eases.
>
> It was not well to treat [with medicine] a person whose illness had
> been sent by the *ʻaumakua* lest the force *(mana)* of the medicine cause
> his death. If the *kahuna* was an upright person he would be guided
> properly by true revelations of his spirit guides; the secret things of his
> ancestors would be revealed to him, and all the hallowed things about
> which he did not know. In order to rightly guide the *kahuna*, and for
> him to know the proper sacrifices and offerings and suitable pres-
> criptions to use in treatment, he was commanded through [appari-
> tions, visions, phantoms, shadowy forms, and by visual knowledge],
> through seeing and talking with an *akua* [god] who had assumed
> human form. So it was in ancient times, and so it is now [that is, in
> 1867–1870, when Kamakau was writing his newspaper articles about
> the past].
>
> The [signs of] uprightness of a *kahuna ʻaumakua* were: the purity of
> his person and of his deeds, and his true piety. The *akua* [god] would
> help him by revealing the cause of the trouble, the wrongdoings the
> patient had committed, and what offerings the patient must give to pay
> for his wrongs. *Kahuna ʻaumakua* who did not keep their bodies clean
> and did not obey the laws of the land as well as those of the *akua* were
> likely to be led wrongly by their "angel watchmen," and their work
> [would] be made erroneous. Evil spirits would aid them, and their
> work would be wrong.[21]

Yet, because kahunas were also reasoning men as well as intermediaries between gods and suffering mortals, some physicians attempted
to supplement divine assistance with observations and treatments of
their own.

Kāhuna Hāhā

Foremost among such diagnosticians was the *kahuna hāhā*. He
"belonged to the order of Lono—that is Lonopuha. It was a very

ancient order of medical kahunas."[22] *Hoʻohāhā* means "to feel," and the function of a kahuna hāhā "was to 'feel' for the disease, to locate it, and to prescribe for it." He uttered the ritual prayers as well, and never forgot his dependence upon the gods, but at least he looked at his patient, examined him, and relied on physical evidence more than did the other kinds of kāhuna lapaʻau.

He learned the art of diagnosis first from "the table of pebbles," *ka papa ʻiliʻili:*

> This was an arrangement of pebbles in the form of a man, from head to foot. . . . There are one hundred to one thousand diseases that snuff out the life of a man, and a *kahuna haha* must know everything about the body of a man, from the soles of the feet to the crown of the head. . . . Those who had studied until they were well grounded in knowledge and skill could predict when a man would die, and a death so forecast could be averted if the man listened to advice. . . .
>
> By the time the instruction with the *ʻiliʻili* . . . was finished, [an apprentice] knew thoroughly the symptoms and the "rules" . . . for treatment of the diseases. . . . Then the teacher would bring in a man who had many disorders and would call the pupils one by one to go and "feel" . . . for the diseases. If the diagnosis . . . was the same as that of the teacher, then the teacher knew that the pupil had knowledge of *haha*.[23]

Kāhuna Hoʻohāpai Keiki and Kāhuna Hoʻohānau Keiki

These specialists can be likened to modern gynecologists and obstetricians in the services they provided, if not in the knowledge they possessed. They claimed to be able to induce pregnancy "among barren women who had ceased bearing,"[24] as well as in women who had not yet borne children.

Physicians from "the orders of Ku, Lono, or Kane" relied upon prayers and offerings to those great gods. "The plant-using *kahunas* of Ku and Hina" employed supplications, sacrifices, potions, and decoctions. "A child obtained thus, through entreaty or prediction, was entirely different from one born from natural pregnancy. He was not obtained from humans, but from the *mana* of the gods."[25]

Confident of his powers (although we can wonder with what accuracy he made these predictions), "the *kahuna* could foretell whether the child would be a boy or a girl, depending upon which sign he saw first when he went outside," presumably from the house of the woman for whom he invoked divine intervention. If, for example, he saw an *'ō'ō,* a pointed digging stick (which to him, untroubled by Freudian complexes, would have been merely a tool used only by men, not a phallic symbol), the child would be a boy. If he saw an *i'e kuku,* a mallet used only in women's work of making kapa, the child would be a girl.

Ka po'e kahiko, the people of old, "used to pray ritually . . . that the race might increase, and flourish, and sprout from the parent stock." In consequence of these rituals, expressed in prayers, offerings, and observances of the kapus, "thriving seedlings *ka po'e kahiko* bore; great gourds filled with seeds they were. But today [in the 1860s] they are poison gourds, bitter to the taste."[26]

Even so, "when there were too many births, the women were given a concoction to stop births."[27] The context of this statement implies that this kind of intervention was given to individual women who became pregnant too often, and was not used as a means of controlling the population of a district (as it would have been in crowded Tahiti or other islands in central Polynesia). Nonetheless, the practice of contraception and abortion (not to mention infanticide) seems to have occurred in Hawai'i both before and after 1778, even when Hawaiians were dying faster than they were being born. Today, when effective contraceptive and abortifacient agents would be of great value for population control in our overcrowded world, no one has been able to ascertain the nature of the "concoctions" which Hawaiian gynecologists administered in order to "stop births." If, indeed, Hawaiian kahunas did use certain plant or animal components with full knowledge of their efficacy, the secrets have been kept very well.

Handy, Pukui, and Livermore, on the other hand, were much more circumspect in discussing these matters than was Kamakau. After asserting that "Hawaiian women apparently were unacquainted with any contraceptive medicinal agents," they mentioned "physical and ceremonial measures resorted to after the birth of a first child, believed to be effective in preventing subsequent conceptions. . . . And in the recipes at hand there are several which purport to induce embryonic abortion."[28] Being very proper Victorians, however, they carefully refrained from identifying in their report either the recipes or the ingredients. The information may very well be found in their notebooks, if these are still preserved in the Bishop Museum.

A kahuna ho'ohānau keiki was much more than a midwife; not

only did he assist at the birth of a child, he also gave prenatal care and psychological support to an expectant mother. A midwife *(pale keiki)*, either male or female, may well have been the kahuna's helper in the more routine tasks associated with delivery of a child. The obstetrician prepared the mother-to-be by giving her, "after the seventh or eighth month a potion of the *ho'opahe'e* (that which makes slippery) to drink frequently." This ho'opahe'e was a mixture of water with a "slippery" sap obtained from any one of several kinds of plants, such as "the *māmaki* tree, or *kikawaiō* fern, or *pālau* yam, or *hau* tree," each of which produces a viscous material rich in mucins and other complex polysaccharides or polypeptides. Kamakau stated that this "slippery" concoction was supposed to relieve the mother of pain only if her child was born prematurely;[29] but Handy et al. believed that all mothers were given such a "lubricant" when labor pains set in.[30]

Some kāhuna ho'ohanau keiki and midwives—"but they are few and far between," said Kamakau—"would assume the birth pains." Most of them "give potions and plants to help delivery, but do not transfer the pain to others."[31] Some physicians in primitive societies (and a few sympathetic husbands in modern ones) are credited with the ability to transfer or assume the birth pains, thereby relieving a woman in labor.

From our modern point of view, the functions of native obstetricians and the treatments they prescribed are relatively simple and comprehensible, no doubt because for most Hawaiian women in times of old—especially after they had borne their first offspring—birth was a natural, uncomplicated experience.

Kāhuna Pa'ao'ao and Kāhuna 'Ea

With these specialists, the "pediatricians" and "internists" of their time, the inquirer is led into a realm of utmost confusion, far different from the ordered problems associated with pregnancy and parturition. This confusion arises because today no one can be quite sure what was meant by those collective nouns, pa'ao'ao and 'ea.

Dorothy Barrère, who edited the translations of Kamakau's works, tried valorously to reduce to terms resembling the jargon of modern physicians the jumble of signs and symptoms associated with those conditions according to the jargon of the old kahunas. "In general," she concludes, "pa'ao'ao was a classification for malfunctionings of the body, and 'ea is a classification for diseases now recognized as infections."[32] This neat dichotomy is helpful "in general," but, on evidence provided by Kamakau and other native writers, it is an oversimplification which does not accommodate a number of exceptions to the rule. Nor does it account for other writers' attempts to define the terms. Elsewhere in Kamakau, for example, Barrère also translated pa'ao'ao as "predispositions"; Pukui and Elbert, in their Dictionary as "latent childhood diseases"; Pukui, as "a comprehensive name for many organic ailments, such as habitual constipation, inactive liver or kidneys, weak lungs, etc."[33] In that same work, Pukui defined 'ea as "a general name for several kinds of sickness, including soft bones, bad breath, coated tongue, inability to gain weight, and so on."

The reasons for these discrepancies are understandable: they can be attributed primarily to the difficulties of making correct diagnoses for certain kinds of diseases. These difficulties, to be sure, confronted not only Hawaiian kahuna lapa'au but also physicians in every country the world around during those "unscientific" times. And even today modern physicians, with all their "scientific training" and whole batteries of laboratory techniques to aid them, are not always able to establish a correct diagnosis for some illnesses which affect some of their patients. In any country many cases of disease are not correctly diagnosed until after autopsy; and, for a few cases of obscurest etiology, a diagnosis is never made. A disadvantaged kahuna lapa'au can hardly be blamed, then, if he missed a diagnosis or because he did not employ the terminology of pathology or the techniques of laboratory sciences now in use.

Kamakau himself was not a physician, and, despite his vast knowledge of many subjects, he may have been as confused as are we who read him when in 1870 he wrote:

> Such pa'ao'ao ["predispositions"] as 'opu lauoho ("hair stomach"), ha'alele makua ("parent deserter"), papa ki'i ("bound bowels"), mapele manawa ("soft [depressed] fontanel"), and many others, if not treated in childhood would develop in maturity into severe ailments—ninole (emaciation), hoki'i (tuberculosis), nae (consumption), hano (swelling of the abdomen). There are many ailments that result from pa'ao'ao and wai 'opua ("cloudy secretions").[34]

Such a mixing of the signs and symptoms of sicknesses with the names of actual diseases, both infectious and noninfectious, offers a clue to the meanings of the kahuna's terms: in contrast with the concept of the (more or less) specific etiology of a disease held by physicians today (and with the corollary opinion that signs and symptoms are the *effects* rather than the causes of a disease), the kahuna's terms are both naive and erroneous.

Confusion is much compounded when we read further in Kamakau:

> The signs and symptoms in a newborn infant that reveal the presence and kind of pa'ao'ao are: first, the cuttlefish, *muhe'e;* second, the cuttlefish with the swaying head, *muhe'e pulewa;* third, the red cuttlefish, *muhe'e makoko;* fourth, the white cuttlefish, *muhe'e kea;* fifth, the multi-colored cuttlefish, *muhe'e lehua;* and sixth, the flattened cuttlefish, *muhe'e papaki'i.*[35]

Barrère's footnote to explain this bit of recondite word-play called upon a footnote from an effort Martha Beckwith had made earlier to give meaning to this obscurity: "The cuttlefish markings which determine a child's future health were real blotches on the infant's abdomen supposed to resemble the shapes of cuttlefish. The disease was diagnosed by studying these markings. They were especially prominent on the fifth day."[36]

A kahuna 'ea faced even more difficult problems, because two kinds of 'ea were recognized, and each of these was divided into two sub-groups:

> The *'ea huna,* "hidden" [latent] *'ea,* or *'ea mahani,* "vanishing" [evanescent] *'ea;* and the *'ea ho'ike,* "revealed" [manifest] *'ea,* or *'ea waka,* "flaming" [acute] *'ea.* The *'ea ho'ike,* or *'ea wawaka,* can be seen by the untrained eye and can be removed in childhood. The *'ea huna* does not show itself in childhood, but if nothing is done about it then, in maturity it shows itself by . . .[37]

At this point Kamakau presented the native names for a number of "serious ailments that children and youth get; they are passed down from the grandparents to the parents, and from the parents to the children." These names, Barrère's translations, and plausible diagnoses suggested by Frank Tabrah, M.D., are easier to read in the form of a list than in a compacted paragraph:[38]

pala	"yellow rot"	gonorrhea
ka'oka'o	"red rot"	syphilis
'ala'ala	"scrofulous sores"	tuberculous adenitis

puhi ka'oka'o	"red puffiness"	secondary syphilis
kua puhi	"burst back"	boils or abscesses
kua 'o iwi	"back pierced by bone"	inanition
kua nanaka	"back split open"	confluent lesions on back
po'o hua'i	"erupted head"	
ihu 'ole	"no nose"	syphilitic saddle nose or damage from leprosy
maka 'ole	"no eyes"	blindness
po'o pilau	"stinking head"	impetigo or eczema
po'o lehu	"ashy [scaly] head"	
umauma naha	"cracked chest"	inanition, starvation

Kamakau continued:

> *'Ea* is the condition that "played host" to the introduced diseases . . .
> *kaokao* (syphilis), *pala* (gonorrhea), and *pu'upu'u hebera pake* (leprosy). So declared a certain *kahuna pa'ao'ao* and *kahuna 'ea* in 1821.
> Kama was his name, and he was skilled in treating *pa'ao'ao* and *'ea* in
> young people and adults. He diagnosed by critical observations, by
> insight, and by "feel" (palpation). He would choose the age when persons should be treated with medicines for *pa'ao'ao*, as well as the
> proper medicines for *'ea huna*, or *'ea mahani*. When the persons took
> the proper medicines—at the age the *kahuna* had chosen—they would
> not get a "sudden" illness (*ma'i ulia;* such as a stroke) or an introduced
> disease.
>   As *'ea* used to kill one man with its "poison" . . . so now the race is
> being killed by *'ea,* through its playing host to "poisonous" introduced
> diseases—[gonorrhea, syphilis, leprosy, and smallpox].[39]

Nowhere can be found better evidence of the reasoning by which
kāhuna lapa'au arrived at their diagnoses—or of their bafflement
when confronted with the need to diagnose a bewildering array of
ailments, some of which were infectious, some functional, others
congenital, still others were new to them as well as to their patients.
And nowhere can we find better proof of the responsibility—and
courage—with which kāhuna lapa'au tried to diagnose and treat
those ailments. Nothing stopped them, not even the failure of their
medications, not even the discouraging fact that, after 1778, more of
their patients must have died than ever were saved, either by their
prescriptions or by their prayers.

Other Kinds of Kāhuna Lapaʻau

The several other classes of specialists—especially those who practiced sorcery, whether for good effect or for evil—although interesting in themselves, do not come within the scope of this study, because they were not primarily concerned with the diagnosis and treatment of diseases which might have been infectious. No doubt they played important parts in the medical profession, but those roles would have been psychological, or religious, rather than as curers of ailments caused by microbes.

The kahuna ʻanāʻanā, "the witch-doctor who prays people to death" as foreigners invariably misconstrue him, has received more attention from them than have all the other native physicians combined. Ready-made for haole imaginations to cast as the fanatical villain—but never as the sympathetic healer—he has appeared in travelers' tales and lurid novels, impossible pantomimes and ridiculous films, ever since word of his existence was carried back to Europe by the discoverers of Polynesia's ensorcelled isles. Even today, for most people the word *kahuna* means "sorcerer," but not priest, certainly not physician. Yet, strange to say, the kahuna ʻanāʻanā has never been the subject of a sober study, which would place him correctly in proper context with respect to his colleagues—both ancient and modern—in medicine and in psychology. Studies of his counterparts in other primitive societies suggest that the kahuna ʻanāʻanā in Hawaiʻi may not have been all bad: "The black magician, far from being antisocial, may just enforce the tribal lore by his threats and maintains the public order without coercion."[40]

Kamakau's eighth category for native physicians, kāhuna makani, has given considerable trouble to many translators. The word *makani* has several meanings, "wind," "gas," "ghost," and "spirit" among them. Pukui and Barrère, in the approved version of Kamakau published in 1964, eased out of their uncertainty by defining a kahuna makani as one "who treated the spirits of illness." Pukui and Elbert in their *Dictionary* define kahuna makani as "a priest possessed by the spirit called makani."

K, a younger Hawaiian man, holds a very different opinion—and a much more satisfying one for people living in this New Age. K's definition is derived from his own training as the son and grandson of kāhuna lapaʻau. He believes that a kahuna makani (to use terms familiar to us today which were not available to Pukui and Barrère in the 1950s) was a psychic, a seer, a clairvoyant, who was able to communicate with 'aumākua in the spirit world. (The 'aumākua could be the physician's own spirit guides or those of the patient.) K's account, cast in modern terms (the analogues are mine, because he is not so mechanistic) makes the relationship between kahuna and 'aumakua seem either entirely plausible—or entirely fantastic. According to K, a sort of dossier, a "file of information" about every Hawaiian, living or dead, in past, present, or future, is established in that very sacred place, Waipi'o Valley on the island of Hawai'i. (This concentration of spirit forces there is, of course, the primary reason why Hawaiians have always considered Waipi'o Valley to be so sacred.) The kahuna makani's psychic powers enable him to make contact with the 'aumā-kua who maintain this "retrieval and information system," and to learn from them the causes of the patient's distress. E. S. C. Handy, whose rather patronizing opinions about kāhuna lapa'au's methods of diagnosis and treatment were presented in his work entitled *Polynesian Religion*,[41] would have been amazed to learn how closely his description coincides with the belief expressed by K.[42]

Therapy

As every Hawaiian knew, whatever the gods had given him they could also take away. To avoid the loss of the gods' favor, a sensible person practiced a form of prophylactic placation by obeying the many kapus and by making those offerings and sacrifices which were decreed by the priests who interpreted the wishes of the gods.

When, by some act of omission or commission, whether intentional or unwitting, a man became ill, he understood immediately that he had incurred the displeasure of at least one of those jealous deities. This was the first rule in the shifting, uncertain relationship between capricious gods and hapless mortal. Knowing this rule, the sick person turned to a priest-physician for help. The prime function of the kahuna lapa'au was to ascertain which of the gods had been affronted and how the victim of that god's displeasure could best appease the angered deity. If, despite every device of physician and patient, the god could not be identified or persuaded to relent, the sick man felt that he was doomed.

The priest-physician, then, was diviner, confessor, interpreter, intercessor, counselor, and exorcist, before ever he administered a medicine. Healing the sick spirit, by restoring the depleted mana of an ailing patient, was the first step in therapy. When that was well begun, cure of the body would follow—if the god so willed.

In these respects, certainly, Hawaiian kāhuna lapaʻau were no different from physicians in other primitive societies throughout the world. Ackerknecht summed up their services in an aphorism: "Primitive medicine is magic medicine." In his opinion, medicine men were successful because their remedies affected the mind (or psyche) of a patient, rather than his body. "Primitive medicine is but a part of the magical system. . . . The medicine man [possesses] an aura of secular and clerical power." In other words, he offered psychotherapy, and this in turn often helped the body to recover its health. And psychotherapy was effective because, as Charcot declared in the early years of psychology, "the best inspirer of hope is the best physician."[43]

Engagement and Regimens

When he accepted a case, a kahuna lapaʻau strove with all the power of his own mana for the very life of the patient. He did not assume this responsibility without asking the advice of his personal ʻaumakua and the god of his heiau hoʻōla: "The foundation of the knowledge and skill of the kahuna lapaʻau was the god," as Kamakau insists. "It was he who knew without error the treatment; it was he who pointed out the nature of the ailment and the things that pertained to this or that disease of man."[44]

If advice from the spirit world was not received promptly, the kahuna withheld his decision until it did come to him—often in dreams, sometimes in other portents, which prayer and fasting prepared him to receive and experience helped him to interpret. "Wait, I will sleep," he said, "and if I have a good dream tonight I will treat you."[45]

Both physician and patient knew that together they were engaged in a very serious rite. As partners in this attempt to regain the favor of the displeased deity, they hoped that the mana of the priest could induce the mana of the gods which were present in the medicines he administered to enter into the body of the sick man. Medicines were accessories to the cure; they were not regarded as being the sole agents by which health would be restored to the ailing body.[46] In some instances—such as with the ripened fruit of noni (Morinda citrifolia), which to certain people smells like a very mature Limburger cheese and to others like vomit—the mana resident in a remedy was supposed to be reinforced by "its disgusting smell and taste."[47]

The commingled mana from these several medicines would strengthen the patient's own languishing mana to the point where the evil forces that the offended god had sent to make him ill would be routed from his body. Only when they had been exorcised, by prayer as well as by medicines, was the sick person able to regain his health.

Recently another explanation has been offered for the restoration of an ailing person's depleted mana. It proposes that the patient heals himself, because his mana already exists within him. This mana, even if it is depleted, just needs to be "strengthened" or "evoked," by the patient, not by the physician.[48] This "newer" theory is derived from principles of holistic medicine that have been revived and emphasized since the 1960s. Such ideas have been invoked before, by physicians and faith healers the world around, since at least the time of the Egyptians. To people who accept this approach, the physician or "healer" is essentially an accessory, an encourager, perhaps even a disciplinary force, but he is not really indispensable to recovery.

Once he had assumed responsibility for treating a sick person, the kahuna lapaʻau took complete command over the patient, his family, and the servants who attended him. Chiefs as well as commoners submitted to his discipline; everyone and everything in the household were placed under a kapu. According to his specialization (and the school in which he had been trained), a kahuna lapaʻau could use only prayer in treating a case, or prayer together with physical therapy or medication. "Purely physical aspects of treatment," Handy reported, "include crude surgery, trepanning, massage, sweating or baking, bathing, purgation, and the administration externally or internally of drugs made from herbs."[49]

The Course of Treatment

For "the plant-using *kahuna* of Kū and Hina," and for specialists in children's diseases, kāhuna paʻaoʻao and kāhuna ʻea,

> the procuring of a remedy was much work. . . . Some other classes [of kāhuna] had a few medicines—as much as could be put into the flap of a *malo* [loincloth]. Others had their remedies "at their fingertips" . . . using words to explain what kind of diseases the patient had, what kind of medicine to use, and how to treat the patient.

Such kahunas, especially the sorcerers who used ʻanāʻanā [black magic] and kuni [magic using fire], had "a healing jaw, *he ā ola*": they achieved their effects with prayers alone.[50]

In order to be sure that his messages reached their goal, the kahuna forbade his patient to eat certain kinds of foods. Such items as *lipe'e-pe'e* seaweed and *he'e,* or squid, for example, were interdicted because "pe'e meant to hide away and *he'e* to flee, hence the gods would hide the information sought after and cause it to flee."[51]

Some kahunas would not do "anything of importance" for a patient on certain nights of the moon, because the very names of those nights would be ill-omened. Thus, the *'ole* nights were inauspicious because *'ole* means "no" or "not." So was the night of Muku, which means "cut off short." Māhealani, the night of the full moon, was not propitious, unless "the *kahuna* desired to know where *(māhea)* a certain thing was hidden." On the other hand, nights named for the great gods, Kāne, Kū, Lono, and Kanaloa, were good times for initiating treatment. So also was the night of Hoaka, "casting a shadow," when "the gods could be persuaded to come and 'reveal their presence by casting their shadows' on the *kahuna.*"[52] Kahunas, evidently, were as infatuated with words as are poets, and as ready to use them as are professors.

When at last, by all the means he could command, the kahuna had received messages from a spirit guardian or from the great gods, and by these had understood the cause of his patient's illness, and when all other signs were favorable, he began the actual course of treatment. Always prayers were said. Here is the prayer of Halulu and Pu'ueke, "two learned men whose knowledge is as deep as the ocean":

O, Kū, listen,
Listen in the night,
While there is silent darkness in the heavens,
heal the patient.
Here are the diseases, the *papakū* and the *haikala,*
O Kū,
Take to the cloudless sky where the sooty tern flies,
The groaning, the weakness, the weakness of the eyes,
The sharp pains, the unfelt pain, the pain like being beaten with staves,
The severe sweeping pain,
The greenish bile, the white phlegm,
The vomiting of substance the color of *kukui* leaves,
bile,
The *papakū* of Hauola.
Healed by you, O Kāne and Lonoleimakani,

Take away the swelling,
Hold back the life of the patient,
So that his canoe may again float in the sea.
Amen, it is freed.[53]

Pukui and Elbert define *papakū* as "a disease with severe constipation, or accompanied by vomiting, back-pains, belching, red eyes,"
and *haikala* as "severe cramps, said to have often proved fatal."

Usually the patient was placed on a strict diet. Often, but by no
means always, medicines, *lāʻau*, would be prescribed. The nature of
the medicine, and the route by which it was administered, varied
with many factors. No part of the body, no aperture or orifice, no
palpable muscle or organ or perceivable membrane, was denied the
attention of some physicians. Distinguished persons, naturally, required more elaborate rituals and procedures. Sometimes, as in the
case of a very great chief, an entire community was required to par-
ticipate.

In general, for a patient of ordinary means and a commoner's status, the procedure went something like this: Under the supervision of
the chosen kahuna, the patient and his family were prepared psychologically by means of the ceremony of *hoʻoponopono*, "to make
right." This was "a spiritual cleaning; a forgiving of one another in
the family; a confession of sin and so on, so that there would be no
obstruction of the *kahuna's* work from within [the patient or his fam-
ily]. He might then devote himself to the work of appeasing the
offended *ʻaumakua,* or return the evil influence [*hoʻihoʻi*] to its
source."[54] This *hoʻomalu,* or period of quiet, which followed the ceremony of hoʻoponopono, must continue throughout the whole time
of treatment, without "quarreling, pleasure-seeking, and idle-gos-
sip." More than just incidentally, "pleasure-seeking" included sexual
indulgences by anyone concerned for the recovery of the patient.
Such continence was imposed not because the sexual act itself was
considered to be disrespectful, but because participants in such indulgences exposed themselves to possible risk: the loss of mana and
attendant pollution.

In essence, this "time of confession," as once it was called, this
"group therapy" as it might be considered today, impressed upon the
patient and his family the need to remove all psychological obstacles
to recovery. When this cleansing was achieved, "the medicine to be
given would go 'straight to the mark, *i kaukāhi ka laʻau.*' "[55] While

the patient was being made ready in this manner, the kahuna would prepare himself, spiritually and physically, for communing with gods or ʻaumākua, in order to receive clues, instructions, and other "revelations from the night, *na hōʻike a ka pō.*"[56]

During this critical time, while presumably the ailing man continued to suffer physically if not psychologically, the patient and his family, as well as the kahuna, were alert to receive communications from the spirit world in signs and portents mundane as well as psychic. Dreams and visions were the usual means by which psychic messages were conveyed, but extraordinary events and unexpected visitors in the material world could be helpful also. The age, sex, and relationship of a visitor, the articles carried, or the first words uttered by that guest—all could be interpreted as being messages from spirit guardians responding to the patient's need.[57]

The massing of all these psychic forces for his benefit, drawn from the conjoined mana of his physician, family, friends, and guardian spirits, must have been the single most important factor in the relationship between a patient and his doctor. "How can the forces of evil resist?" the sick man would have asked. "How can my ʻaumākua deny me their help?" In trying to "set things aright" in the affairs of the spirit before beginning an attempt to assuage the miseries of the body, Hawaiian physicians showed their knowledge of human nature as well as their faith in divine clemency. By concerning themselves "with the whole man in his total environment," as Dubos has written,[58] they not only learned all they needed to know about their patients, but also gave those patients a tremendous psychological advantage. In this respect, if in no other, kahunas practiced the very best kind of medicine: they healed with heartening art, rather than with cold impersonal science. Today's word for this ideal medical treatment is "holistic."

In *Charmides,* Plato long ago expressed the essence of this art, which is known to all good physicians:

> The reason why the cure of so many diseases is unknown to the physicians of Hellas is because they are ignorant of the whole which ought to be studied also; for the part can never be well unless the whole is well . . . for this is the great error of our day, that the physicians separate soul from body.

This, indeed, is the great error of our day. Unhappily for those of us who live in these frenetic times, with besieged physicians, computer-ized analyses, and assembly-line "processing" of bewildered and cowed patients crowded into dingy clinics, the relationship between a sick Hawaiian of old and his healer is something for us to envy if only because today it is almost impossible to achieve.

Opening Medicine

A kahuna who employed medications usually started therapy with an "opening medicine." Often this was an "opening" in more than one sense of the word, inasmuch as cathartics seem to have been favored initial drugs. These ranged in efficacy from mild teas brewed from *moa (Psilotum nudum)* or certain other plants, through a variety of potions of intermediate activity, such as were provided by *kukui* nuts *(Aleurites moluccana)*, to a truly heroic type of clystering, using *waikī*, a purgative concocted from kukui sap and the flesh of the bitter gourd, *ipu 'awa'awa (Lagenaria sicereria)*, which only very strong men could endure.[59] "Sometimes it killed, but those who survived enjoyed vigorous health afterward, up to extreme old age."[60]

Dr. Thomas Holman, a member of the pioneer company of American missionaries sent to the Sandwich Islands in 1819, wrote the earliest declaration of haole horror over the effects of kahunas' therapy:

> The medicine they give seems to be more for the purpose of driving ahhooah [akua] out of the person, than of healing the disease. . . . [Medicines] are composed principally of cathartics, and those of the most drastic kind. I have known several instances of death from their operation. The cathartic offset frequently continues for several days, and oftentimes terminates in inflammation and death.[61]

Collecting Herbs for Medicines

When through the preparation of ho'oponopono the peace of ho'omalu was attained, the time had come for gathering the herbs which the physician intended to administer to his patient. Whatever the medicine was to be, its components were collected and prepared according to the strictest of rituals. "A person close to the patient" or a young apprentice to the kahuna was chosen to perform this important task.

Before departing upon his errand he was told what plants to seek, where to find them, and, above all, the prayers he would address to deities in the plants as he plucked the portions of them the kahuna lapa'au lā'au wished to use. Respect for the plants was mandatory, because they were *kino lau*, physical manifestations, of the gods whose mana was incorporated within them:

> If the *kahuna* ordered the gathering of *popolo* leaves [*Solanum americanum,* which later *kāhuna lapaʻau* would acknowledge as the "foundation of Hawaiian pharmacy"][62] the person directed to gather the leaves was taught a prayer addressed to Ka La, the sun, for the *popolo* was an embodiment of Kane as the sun.

The manner of gathering the medicinal herbs was strictly decreed, as formalized as a temple rite. Unless the kahuna lapaʻau himself had been instructed by ʻaumākua to gather herbs at night (in which event they were plucked at midnight, "the hour of deep silence"), the physician's emissary performed his duties at sunrise. "It was not good to go and urinate, to have a bowel movement, to glance backward, to meet anyone, to be called back, to hear a bird. Silence was the one good thing in getting medicine."[63]

Facing the rising sun, the gatherer uttered the prayer he had been taught, revealing with it the name of the patient who needed the medicine. Then, standing with his back to the sea, his face toward the mountains,

> with his right hand [which was guarded by the male deities, *akua kane*] he would pluck leaves from the right side of the plant, addressing Ku, a male god. With his left hand [which was guarded by female deities, *akua wahine*] he plucked leaves from the left side of the bush, addressing Hina, wife of Ku.
>
> Leaves plucked with the right hand were used for internal medicines, those plucked with the left, for exterior medication.
>
> Only enough leaves were gathered for one day's treatment.[64]

While the officiating priest-physician uttered the canonical prayers required for each step in the procedure, his apprentice prepared the medicine in the presence of the patient. Because "the life-giving rays of Kāne" must enter into the mixture, all compounding of medicines was done in the bright light of day.

Administering the Medicines

Generally, doses of the medicine were "prescribed in fives, to be taken five times in succession (whether in a single day, morning and night for two and a half days, or for five days in succession), or in multiples of five. Thus, a tonic might be prescribed for 'five times five' days in succession."[65]

Handy was unable to obtain a satisfactory explanation for "the symbolism of these numbers," which, he noted, strongly resembles "Chinese medical practice based on Taoism." From statements made by David Malo, Handy believed that the symbolism entered into Hawaiian medicine long before Chinese immigrants settled in Hawai'i.[66] In 1989 the interval is just as likely to be three days as five, for reasons equally unknown. Perhaps deference to the Christian trinity is involved. A simple adaptation to the pace of modern living is equally plausible. "One present day Hawaiian," according to the writers of *Nānā i ke Kumu*,[67] believes that "the ritual of five" was "aimed at keeping the treatment going a little bit longer than necessary, to make sure it is continued long enough."

Seldom was a kahuna lapa'au lā'au content to use only a single ingredient in his prescriptions. As Kamakau observed, "there remain many other medicines, from the sea to the mountains—as many as there are diseases in man."[68] Compounding of two to six or more ingredients was common, and the formulas for preparing them were jealously guarded and carefully followed. Here are three examples of relatively simple preparations that used lā'au, that is, components derived from plants; they are taken from Handy et al.:

I. For suppressed urine *(mimi pa'a):*
ingredients: (1) arrow root, five small tubers; (2) sugar cane, a long stalk; (3) coconut fibers.
compounding: grate 1; strain through 3; pound or chew 2, and mix with juice of 1.
treatment: drink this five times in one day, praying before drinking.
pani [closure]: cook and eat a whole rolled-up taro leaf *(lu'au).*

II. For *'ea huna,* or hidden sickness, in a child:
ingredients: (1) *pili* grass; (2) coconut.
compounding: burn 1 to ashes; roast the meat of 2 and extract juice; mix 1 and 2.
treatment: rub this on the tongue and on roof of mouth.
pani [closure]: cook and eat one *'a'ama* crab.

III. For general weakness and wasting away of body:
ingredients: (1) *'ala'alawainui pehu,* stems, one hatful; (2) tree fern *(hapu'u),* one young shoot; (3) *hala,* eight shoots; (4) *'ohi'a,* two pieces of bark the size of palm of hand; (5) white sugar cane *(ko),* three segments; (6) *noni,* two fully matured fruits.
compounding: pound together 1, 2, 3, 4, 5, and 6; strain and clean juice; boil; cool.

treatment: drink all of this, then eat two *iho-lena* bananas, then drink water. Take morning and evening for five consecutive days. *pani* [closure]: eat white-fleshed fish, broiled on charcoal, a *kukui* nut, and a young taro leaf thoroughly cooked. End the treatment by drinking boiled sea water as a laxative.[69]

A remedy for treating gonorrhea used the tips of the aerial roots of the *hala* (*Pandanus odoratissimus* or other species), pounded to a pulp with salt. This viscous preparation, strained well in order to remove the coarser remnants of the hala root, was drunk by the suffering patient.[70] The efficacy of this prescription is not known, but the kahunas' reasons for choosing hala roots are obvious: nothing else provided by the land resembles a tumescent penis as much as does the aerial root of a *Pandanus* tree (which the matter-of-fact Hawaiians called *ule*, penis). Moreover, word-magic entered into this therapy, inasmuch as *hala* means "sin, error, offense," while *ho'ohala* means both "to cause to sin" and "to cause to miss, to dodge, to turn aside."

These recipes may appear to be naive, but in their time they were not very different from the remedies employed by contemporary physicians in China or in Europe and America. In eighteenth-century England, for example, Mrs. Palmer's compilation of recipes for a great variety of medicines recommended one of them, "Lady North-cliffe's snail water," for treating "consumption, convulsions, palseys, vapours, etc." It was prepared according to this formula:

> One peck of garden snails and two quarts of earthworms, [mixed] with two handfuls each of Angelica and Celandine, three handfuls of Wood Sorrel, Agrimony, Betony, and new Dock roots, three large handfuls of inner bark of Barberry, and three and a half handfuls Rosemary tops and flowers, one and a half handfuls of Bearsfoot, one handful of Rue, one ounce of Fenugreek, one ounce of Turmeric, and half pound Hartshorn shavings, one half ounce Saffron, three ounces Cloves, three gallons strong ale, and one quart canary wine, all distilled in an alembic.

In England of the Tudors, "oyle of red dogge" was lauded by Alexis of Piedmont as a cure for many ailments. This required "a red-haired dog, strangled for the purpose, and boiled in ale; St. John's wort, wild marshmallows, wall worts, and saffron were added." And, as late as 1737, Pomet was recommending "use of the left hind hoof of an elk as a cure for epilepsy."[71] We of the twentieth century should not sneer at this remedy. Until 1938, when at last phenytoin (Dilantin) appeared in our pharmacopeia, we had nothing better for the treatment of epilepsy.

Some Chinese remedies could be even more unappetizing. This one was employed well into the twentieth century by Chinese immigrants in Hawai'i, "to reduce fever and to stop vomiting in young children":

> [Take] two cockroaches (the large variety with wings). Remove wings, head, legs, and intestines. Wash the shells clean and place in a bowl having a rough bottom. Grind fine with elephant's tusk, scraping a little of the ivory into the bowl. (This [tusk] is medicinal and can be purchased at a Chinese drug store.) Add about two teaspoonfulls of boiling water and feed a teaspoonful to the baby, or two if necessary.[72]

In the unlikely event that the worried Chinese mother who wished to prepare this concoction could not find those big winged cockroaches, she could substitute earthworms—dug up "from under a banana tree only"—or garden snails.

Not all European or Oriental prescriptions were as unsavory or as complex as these, of course: many an English or American housewife made simples and elixirs and cataplasms with ingredients which were more pleasant both to collect and to apply. Physicians used, among other things, cassia, senna, flax seed, rhubarb, jalap, theriac, larkspur, foxglove, aconite, and poppy juice, many of which are still employed in medication.

These extensive examples of folk remedies from other peoples are presented in order to show that Hawai'i's kahunas were not the only physicians who chose herbs according to their names or shapes or who trusted to their content of magical mana with little knowledge of their physiological effects. Indeed, by comparison, kāhuna lapa'au seem to have been much more restrained than were Lady Northcliffe and other herbalists in Europe who—whether out of determination or desperation—threw almost everything but recognized deadly poisons into their capacious alembicks.

In contrast, the remedies used by physicians belonging to several tribes of Indians in eastern North America were much simpler than those used by Europeans. In this respect, although not in actual content, they resembled those employed by Hawai'i's native physicians.[73] So, also, did their methods of diagnosis rely upon communication with the spirit world. Apparently, physicians in primitive societies were content with simple remedies, while those of more advanced societies resorted to remedies of greater complexity—perhaps because they had learned from bitter experience that simple medications were not powerful enough to safeguard patients against their more numerous afflictions.

When all else failed—or when medicines were not indicated—a kahuna lapaʻau could turn to "the universal remedy," as Kamakau calls it: seawater. Either this was drunk by the patient, "for cleaning purposes," or, after it had been converted into a species of holy water by addition of turmeric *(Curcuma domestica)* and prayer, it was sprinkled on persons or premises in a rite of purification that was almost universal. "No evil spirit belonging to others would remain in a house so sprinkled."[74]

Closing Medicine (the Pani)

Treatment was always concluded with the *pani,* or closure. This was a morsel of food, usually taken from a creature of the sea, chosen for its relations to the suspected cause of illness or to ingredients employed as medicines. According to Handy et al.,[75] "the prescription of the *pani* . . . appears to be determined by the interrelationships of marine forms of life with those on land, as described in the Kumulipo Chant of Creation." All plants from the land were matched with "opposites" found in the sea. Thus, if the *ʻalaʻala wai nui* (a succulent herb belonging to the genus *Peperomia*) was used as a medicine, its pani would be *ʻaʻalaʻula* (a branching, velvety-green succulent seaweed with similar morphology, *Codium edule*). "Very often [the pani] consisted of the *kapu kai* (ceremonial sea-bathing), and the eating of the *kala* seaweed or *kala* fish, or any other thing with the word *kala* (forgiving, or freeing) in its name."[76]

In many cases, of course, treatment was not successful: "the sick person did not recover, but died, and his wealth was gone." A succession of failures caused people to doubt the powers of a kahuna, "and that man became disgraced."[77] Even so, strong faith could be rewarded:

> When a man fell ill, and his eyes were clouded as if entangled in cobwebs, and death had been predicted for him, and none could save him from death, then if he recovered it was "a life from the *ʻaumakua*." Many lives were known to have been thus saved. . . . The *ʻaumakua* and the ancestral deities absolved men from their sins. They were the healers.[78]

Then, too, many Hawaiians of old seem to have been able to choose the time to die. This enviable ability to decide for "self-willed death" was recognized by all: "Na kānaka ʻokuʻu wale aku no i kau ʻuhane," they said during the reign of Kamehameha III: "The people dismissed freely their souls and died."[79] The person who made that decision may have been ill, or full of grief, or weary of life, or simply made aware by ʻaumākua that the time had come to depart. Once the choice was made, death came within a few days, easily, manageably, with dignity. If recent tales can be believed, a few sensitive Hawaiians are still choosing this way to die.[80]

Tests and Safeguards

Neither kāhuna lapaʻau nor foreigners gave any indication that native physicians had developed a method for testing medicines in order to avoid poisoning their patients. A few species of endemic plants are said to be quite toxic; and legends grew up about certain extremely poisonous plants which were employed by sorcerers but not by physicians. Nonetheless, fear of poisonous herbs did not deter some physicians. The several kinds of ʻākia (Wikstroemia spp.), which contain substances that do paralyze fish in tidal pools, were employed by physicians in treatment of asthma or costiveness, apparently without ill effect upon the people who received them.[81]

On the other hand, Kamakau remembered the cautious experimentation of Palaha,

> the first priest who taught the use of the enema, through observing how stagnant streams are cleared of rubbish and stench by a freshet. He tried the enema first on his dog with success. Then he tried it on his sick father, the enema below and the cathartic above. At his father's command Palaha cut open his body when he died to observe the cause of his illness.[82]

Although kāhuna lapaʻau may have performed preliminary tests upon domestic animals, or possibly even upon human subjects selected from slaves, criminals, and captives, more than likely they did not bother to do so. Palaha's sick father is the only known instance of a human subject used intentionally in the gathering of evidence. No doubt astute kahunas had long since noticed what happened to people or to animals that ate toxic plants. Ackerknecht declared that medicine men in primitive societies choose their remedies "by instinct, or perhaps by magic."[83] And quite probably all primitive physicians, elsewhere as in Hawai'i, learn something about the effects of the medications by observing the reactions of patients who take them. Among people as fatalistic as were Hawaiians, harmful as well as helpful effects of treatment would have been attributed to gods, not to physicians or their medicines. Accusations of malpractice would have been the least of a kahuna's worries in those good old days.

This thoroughly empirical method of using as sources of medicines the alien plants and animals introduced into the islands after 1778 seems to have been continued unquestioned throughout the nineteenth century. Fortunately for both kahuna and patients, most of the introduced plants were not harmful. No doubt the few that are toxic, such as oleanders, certain milkweeds, and castor beans, claimed a modest number of victims before more observant kahunas learned to avoid them.

Offerings to Gods and Payments to Priests

The incorporeal gods expected nothing for themselves from a sick person save his return to piety from the excursion into error which had drawn upon him their wrath in the first place. What the gods had taken away they could restore—and for this revision in their attitude toward him, a person beseeched them with prayers and mollified them with proofs of penitence. The best possible proof was the change in attitude toward the gods and their kapus which the ceremony of ho'oponopono helped the patient to attain. When once again he respected the gods and walked in the ways of righteousness, the gods were appeased and his mana was made whole.

But, as everyone knew, the priests who were the intercessors between gods and people were themselves creatures made of flesh, blood, bone, and appetites. Like the folk they attended, they too must eat, must be clothed, must be thanked for their ministrations. Kāhuna lapa'au did not hesitate to make their wants known. They were sustained by "sacrifices and offerings to the gods," to use the euphemism devised by priests in all societies, and by more business-like fees charged for services rendered.

Payments were decided according to a "sliding scale," based on the seriousness of the ailment from which a patient suffered and on his ability to pay. In general, wealthy chiefs were charged higher fees than poor commoners; but a very sick commoner paid more for physicking than did a chief who suffered only a minor indisposition. Nevertheless, both chiefs and commoners, out of hope or out of pride, often made much more lavish "offerings" than were required by priests. And some kahunas, alas, were very greedy, at least in the opinion of their denigrators:

> It was characteristic of ancient *kahunas* to desire wealth of the patient. . . . The *kahuna* would go to the patient's house, looked at him, and said, "Have you no black pig, no red fish? If you have not, you shall die." The patient was frightened. The *kahuna* was fond of pig and they would kill many pigs for treating the one sickness, four, five, or more to be cooked for the one sickness. The *kahuna* said the pig would please the *kumu pa'a* [family god]. If no pig was offered one could not feel better.[84]

Kamakau is more generous toward kāhuna lapa'au than the Reverend Pogue had been:

> Sacrifices and offerings to the *'aumakua* were not all the same. For minor punishments . . . such as illness suffered by a member of the family, a small fire [for a cooked offering] was made morning and evening for five times, and then a final offering [*pani*] of a few *lu'au* leaves or an egg . . . and the illness would be ended. If it was a serious illness, one that confined the sufferer to the house, then the final offering was an *'awa* plant and a pig.
>
> This was a customary thing to do, and was the work of the family; it could not be done by outsiders or strangers because their voices and appeals would not be heeded by the *'aumakua*. . . .
>
> The chiefs made offerings to the *'aumakua* in proportion to the wrongs committed against the god. Sacrifices alone were not the atonement. . . . The first thing to do was to build the *moku hale* [a house apart, for receiving the offerings. When this house was finished and sanctified], offerings were placed on the offerings-rack. *Kahiki, popo'ulu,* and *iho-lena,* . . . [fine] *kapas* were given in sacrifice to the god. The god would heed the offerings . . . and death and troubles became as nothing.[85]

As was only to be expected, in matters of recompense sorcerer-kahunas were "the most notorious." That was because

> they demanded a great price of the patient in the way of sacrifices and offerings. However, the foods provided by the patient and his relatives were for their consumption, and not for that of the *kahuna* and his relatives; but if, through *aloha,* the patient's family wished it, the *kahuna* and his relatives would eat of them too.[86]

On the other hand, Kamakau continued on the same page, "the poor did not often make a feast; very few could afford one." They made "humble offerings . . . for the little misfortunes that came to a person of small account. . . . Sometimes such small offerings were acceptable if the *akua* had compassion upon the giver."

Animals offered either in sacrifices or in payment were not used as means for auguries, as they were in ancient Greece and Rome. Sensible Hawaiians, priests and petitioners alike, merely ate them. In some communities, where presumably the demand was great, the kahunas' families raised "sacred" chickens for patients to purchase. These pampered creatures, sanctified by prayer, bathed regularly, fed on coconut milk and sweet potatoes, did not run wild, like common chickens, but were confined to houses fitted with elevated roosts made of bamboo. Their droppings, caught upon banana leaves spread afresh each morning, were buried with the same care that was accorded the dejecta of people.[87]

A whole pig—or, sometimes, several pigs—would be the most acceptable offering "to please the god." On other occasions, different kinds of fish would be specified. "The patient ate part of the fish, the priest took out first the eye and gave it to him [with] a piece of the tail, and the rest of the fish he could not eat. This was the way some *kahunas* practised."[88]

From the information now available—some of which has been provided by foreigners, most of which is presented in accounts written by kāhuna lapaʻau later in the nineteenth century and by other Hawaiians, such as Samuel Kamakau and John Papa Iʻi—several conclusions can be drawn.

First: The rationale of Hawaiian medicine, with respect to both diagnosis and treatment of physical ailments, was based on *symptoms* rather than on causes (as is the rationale of modern medicine in Western countries). The reason for this approach is understandable, inasmuch as the usual causes of diseases—such as microorganisms, organic dysfunctions, genetic defects, and nutritional deficiencies—were not yet recognized, even to physicians in Europe and America. Because human beings exhibit only a few symptoms for any disease, whatever its nature may be, a confusion about cause, and often about treatment, is still a major problem for physicians today. A skilled diagnostician, as some modern physicians will admit, is the one who makes the right guess in more than 50 percent of his cases. How much more baffling the problems of diagnosis must have been for physicians in all societies before the end of the nineteenth century. The whole complex process of arriving at a correct diagnosis was made all the more difficult for physicians, in any society, because of the lack of definitive laboratory techniques such as have been introduced and developed only in the twentieth century.

Second: The extreme geographical isolation of Hawai'i made its people unacquainted with any other way of living—and thinking—than their own. Because they were denied any opportunity to share the experiences and the accumulating wisdom of other societies, Hawaiians had nothing with which to compare the social system they had developed in the centuries of their isolation. They had nothing but intelligence to lighten their ignorance, and only respect for the gods (and fear of the gods' surrogates on earth) to restrain their egotism.

Nonetheless, after comparing the medical art evolved by Western physicians with that practiced by kāhuna lapa'au, one is impressed with the fact that, except for surgical techniques, the therapeutic regimens used by foreigners were not much better than those used by kahunas. Both were based upon guesswork, custom, and hope; both employed botanicals and minerals of uncertain content and unpredictable effect; and both relied heavily upon purges for catharsis of the bowels and upon trust in the physician (or in the patient's god) for easing of his spirit. Both systems, in other words, were little more than accretions of superstitions and magic, compounded with liberal dosages of hope, and only rarely fortified with an inquirer's intelligence. That attribute, if ever it was employed, was expended on diagnosis rather than treatment. In some respects, Western medicine was even more benighted than was the native: Hawaiians were spared the debilitations of needless bloodletting and leeching, the savageries of surgery without anesthesia, the torments of cauterization of severed flesh with red-hot irons or boiling pitch, the brutality of being chained to a stake or thrust into Bedlam when they were mad.

Yet, because they were so certitudinous, foreign physicians living in Hawai'i invariably condemned their native counterparts. Even a man as sympathetic toward Hawaiians as Dr. Gerrit P. Judd was just as dogmatic as any "benighted" kahuna and much more intolerant. And, of course, he was as blind to the deficiencies of haole medicine as he accused kahunas of being blind to the weaknesses of theirs. The one great advantage he had, in common with other foreign physicians, was a broader experience with patients, diseases, and medicaments from countries beyond Hawai'i. This kind of experience, reinforced by the corpus of knowledge in medicine accumulated since before the time of Hippocrates, enabled most foreign physicians to see that the symptoms of a sickness were the *consequences* of a disease, not its causes. This was a discovery that Hawaiian physicians, in their isolation, had not managed to attain.

Third: The ailments which aboriginal Hawaiians suffered were distinguished by their physicians according to the symptoms presented and, on this basis, were assigned to several categories. Of these the pa'ao'ao and the 'ea seem to have been the most important. Judging from the terms used to describe them, most of these ailments appear to have been caused by organic dysfunctions, physical injuries, congenital defects, or psychological stress. Although microorganisms harbored by the people undoubtedly caused some kinds of infections, kāhuna lapa'au did not identify the more subtle forms such as those which affected the internal organs. External infections were recognized: boils, ulcerations of the skin, dermatomycoses, and the complications following wounds from childbirth, warfare, or accidents in work or play.

Fourth: Techniques of diagnosis for obvious ailments were relatively straightforward; those for obscure ailments were essentially divinations, whose methods were rigidly prescribed and formalized. Techniques of treatment were chosen according to directions that a kahuna lapa'au "received" either from his own akua and 'aumakua or from those of his patient.

Fifth: The limited number of categories for diseases—and of kahuna-specialists to treat them—is further evidence to support the hypothesis that no major infectious diseases affected Hawaiians before 1778. While this shortage of evidence for epidemic diseases might be attributed more to deficiencies in methods of diagnosis than to actual absence of those contagions, it is difficult to believe that generations of "experts in healing"—not all of whom would have been unobservant and unthinking—could have overlooked the dramatic signs and symptoms of severe epidemic infections had they been present.

Sixth: An astonishing number of different plants, animals, and minerals were employed by kāhuna lapa'au lā'au for treating ailments classified as pa'ao'ao and 'ea diseases. Probably the assorted prescriptions and treatments were varied—and variable—because they were devised and favored by kahunas who were trained in different schools of thought. An alternative hypothesis would allow each kahuna to develop his own favorite remedies according to the guidance received from his gods and spirit guardians. Treatments, except for "the opening" and "the closing" rituals, were not as rigidly prescribed as were methods of diagnosis.

Seventh: When, in 1778 and in the years thereafter, the diseases of civilization were introduced, kāhuna lapa'au not only recognized them as being new but also searched diligently for remedies, both old and new, with which to treat them. They were much more open-minded in their search for medicines, and in their care of patients, than were foreign physicians, who clung to the approved methods they had learned from their teachers.

Eighth. Although foreign physicians would never have admitted this, native prescriptions for most ailments—except for the haoles' mercurials used in treating syphilis—must have been just as effective as were remedies used by foreigners during the eighteenth and nineteenth centuries. Indeed, the great psychological support given to native patients by their kāhuna lapa'au would have been much more effective than the meager share of it that was dispensed so casually, or not at all, by foreign physicians. They may not have been as selfish in caring only about "their personal welfare," as M. Kehukai wrote in 1866, but, for many reasons, "white doctors" certainly could not give the same kind of comforting care to native patients as native physicians did.

Ninth: Even if they were shrewd observers, excellent psychologists, and devoted attendants upon the sick, kāhuna lapa'au were woefully limited by their philosophy of medicine. Their diagnoses and prescriptions, when these are read today, seem to be aggravatingly naive. Trust in word-magic and wordplay; dependence on similarities or analogies in form or function between the afflicted parts of the body and the remedies prescribed (such as medieval Europe's herbalist-physicians respected in their "Doctrine of Signatures") or, conversely, recognition of opposites; dreams, revelations, portents, and other means of receiving messages from the spirit world, delivered either directly to the kāhuna lapa'au or through intermediaries in the material world; the omens and auguries offered by nature, encountered by chance and interpreted by intuition: all these and more were the means by which a kahuna lapaʻau divined the cause of an ailment and chose the kind of treatment he applied to a suffering patient. Prayer and ritual were the most important components in therapy because, to Hawaiians, "words bind, and words make free."

To foreign physicians (as to us today), all this sounded like a lot of nonsense, a litany of mumbo-jumbo commingled with chicanery that was both pretentious and dangerous. And yet, to be fair, it was no different, and no worse, than were the systems of folk medicine being practiced in other countries, even in those of "advanced" Europe and America, even as late as the eighteenth and nineteenth centuries. Moreover, the native Hawaiian system of medicine compared very well with those of other primitive societies: despite their isolation from all other peoples, kāhuna lapaʻau had attained a considerable degree of competence and general usefulness to their people. For this they should be commended rather than condemned. Together with all the other technological and cultural achievements of Hawaiians, their system of medicine offers further proof of their creative intellect.

Tenth: On closer analysis—and bearing in mind the fact that not all kāhuna lapaʻau were morons or frauds—the charge that their methodology was nonsensical and their terminology was nothing more than silly is lightened if many of those terms—such as "swaying-headed cuttlefish" and "newly hatched cuttlefish"—are considered as devices for remembering signs of disease, very much like the doggerel verses and mnemonic rubrics that students (and their teachers) still use in modern medical schools. For Hawaiians, a people without a written language of whom such fantastic feats of memory were required, any aids to remembering were both necessary and welcome.

Eleventh: In quality kāhuna lapaʻau ranged from the inept to the superlative. The written reports they submitted to the Hawaiian Board of Health between 1869 and 1872 show that some native physicians were pretty shallow indeed, little more than pretenders and quacks. Quite a few, however, were excellent diagnosticians. As we shall see in the next essay, the seventy case histories written in 1870–1871 by Dr. Ohule, who practiced in Kalihi Uka, Honolulu, were astute summaries, just as good as the reports from foreign physicians of the time.[89] Intelligence and medical common sense were not reserved to haoles.

Twelfth: A kahuna's claims that he had treated a patient's ailment successfully may be explained in several ways. His regimen may have achieved a cure, just as everyone hoped it would: his ministrations and remedies need not have been ineffective or dangerous. Also possible, of course, is the chance that the patient was deluded into thinking that a cure had been achieved, or the chance that a kahuna merely lied about his prowess in order to boost his reputation. In addition, as every modern physician knows, other factors could have contributed to a successful conclusion. Simple passage of time would have accounted for recovery from minor or acute ailments, but psychological support, physiotherapy, and even the good purging effected by an "opening medicine" also would have benefited many a patient.

If these factors play important parts in helping people nowadays—when, as modern physicians maintain, about 85 percent of the patients who consult them are suffering from psychogenic ailments—they certainly were just as important in helping people in the past to recover from their real or imagined illnesses. Modern physicians are only now beginning to accept the premise that very few diseases are so simple in their origin as to have only one cause. In the language of today, the concept of a "specific etiology" for a disease, which has dominated Western medicine for about a hundred years, is giving way to the concept of "multifactorial etiology." In accepting this philosophy, kāhuna lapa'au seem to have arrived at an understanding of sickness and health that was not accepted until later by the foreign physicians who disparaged and destroyed them.

Thirteenth: Most kāhuna lapa'au were sensible enough, or perhaps shrewd enough, not to attempt to treat certain kinds of afflictions, especially the advanced stages of chronic diseases for which obviously no cure was possible. This admonition, for example, was sounded often in instructions to pupils: "If it is the ma'i-'a'ai [cancer], do not treat it."

Fourteenth: For overt external ailments, like boils, burns, wounds, and broken bones, some of the kahunas' remedies were at least palliative if not curative. Washes and poultices prepared from leaves of certain plants—lau kahi (Plantago major) was a favorite choice; pōpolo (Solanum americanum) another—were much cleaner than were some of the preparations used by foreigners—chewed tobacco, for example, or mud mixed with dung. And, for all we know, they may have contained antimicrobial agents which helped to check infections, as well as fresh chlorophyll, which is believed to promote the processes of healing. Some people today, not all of whom are Hawaiians, praise the almost unbelievable speed with which kahunas' remedies can repair sprains and.broken bones.

Fifteenth: We cannot know, unfortunately, how faithfully the extant records and accounts of kāhuna lapaʻau describe the medical learning of Hawaiians before 1778. Internal evidence—references to Jehovah, "sin," bottles, and glasses, for example—shows contamination of kahunas' thoughts with haole dogma and techniques. The inclusion of a few introduced diseases in the lists of ailments—especially syphilis, gonorrhea, and leprosy—proves that the kahunas who wrote those accounts were practicing their profession long after foreigners and their diseases had come to Hawaiʻi.

Yet even if the new culture did affect the kāhuna lapaʻau's terminology and utensils, it did not seem to have had any pronounced immediate effect upon their philosophy and methodology for either diagnosis or treatment. To kahunas, the new diseases simply required new prescriptions. The foreign culture provided them only with some new words, plants, and instruments. But the loss of a person's mana was still considered to be the reason for his affliction, and an offended god, whether he bore an old name or that of the new One, was still believed to be the agent who gave health to a person or took it away. Until the end of the nineteenth century, kāhuna lapaʻau were still thinking in terms of ʻea and paʻaoʻao diseases. This in itself shows that kāhuna lapaʻau learned very little from their foreign counterparts—probably because haole doctors did not speak to kahunas, and kahunas spoke only to their gods.

Sixteenth: Because the efficacy of the many different components used as medicines by kāhuna lapaʻau lāʻau has not been established by "scientific" methods, the claims made for them by kahunas and sentimentalists remain unproved. Phytochemists and pharmacognoscists have analyzed a few of the better-known plants—but with techniques that ignore the ways in which kahunas employed them. At present, then—except for that little provided in Dr. Judd's reports to the mission in 1839 and in his lectures to medical students in 1872—there is no evidence that a practicing physician (or an inquiring antiquarian) can accept as proof that remedies used by kāhuna lapaʻau were helpful to their patients in any way other than as placebos or as palliatives.

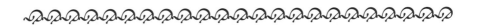

Four

Kāhuna Lapaʻau After 1778

When foreigners arrived, everything in Hawaiʻi changed. New ideas from beyond the sea challenged the power of the gods and the great chiefs who were considered to be their descendants. New diseases introduced by the visitors ravaged the populace. The Age of Faith—when the kapus of the gods and the mana of the priests were strong, the diseases were few, and cures were relatively easy to achieve (or failures even easier to explain)—came to an end. Dr. Richard Kekuni Blaisdell, a physician trained in the methodologies of modern medicine, but also a Hawaiian steeped in the lore of the people of old, summed up the inevitable fate of the native medical profession: "This highly refined, holistic and preventive health system, harmoniously integrated in their social fabric, with nature about them, and their spiritual realm beyond, was never to recover from the impact of western ways."[1]

Even before the British expedition's ships sailed away from the Sandwich Islands for the last time, kāhuna lapaʻau were seeking remedies for the venereal diseases that the visiting sailors had presented to their hospitable hosts. John Law, surgeon on HMS *Resolution* during the return visit to Kauaʻi in March 1779, wrote in his journal: "We heard today also for certain as it was confirmed afterwards by many of the Natives that when we were here the last Time [in January 1778] we gave them the venereal disease, they said they had a method of curing it but it was a long time first."[2]

But David Samwell, surgeon on HMS *Discovery* and a determined defender of the good name of Britain and her sailors, Captain Cook's above all others, insisted that Hawaiians were already thoroughly affected by "the venereal" before ever the expedition visited these islands. Moreover, he wrote, "the priests pretended to be expert at curing it, and seemed to have an established mode of treatment; which by no means implied, that it was a recent complaint among them . . . much less that it was introduced only a few months before."[3] In this opinion Samwell anticipated Captain de La Pérouse and Surgeon Rollin, who expressed the same conclusion after they visited Maui in 1786.

Despite Samwell's defense, we can conclude, with good reason, that the members of that first group of foreigners may have imparted to Hawaiians other diseases as well, although we have no specific information about them. In January 1778 both Charles Clerke, captain of HMS *Discovery* (and Cook's second in command), and William Anderson, chief surgeon aboard *Resolution,* were "far gone with the consumption." Anderson died on 3 August 1778, somewhere in the Bering Sea, after the ships had sailed northward from Kauaʻi. And in January 1779 Captain Clerke was so ill that he remained in his cabin during most of the expedition's second visit to that island. Nonetheless, in January 1778 both officers did go ashore at Waimea, Kauaʻi, and a year later Clerke went ashore at Kealakekua Bay on Hawaiʻi. Either or both of them, as well as other consumptive sailors, probably were the agents by which tuberculosis was introduced among Hawaiians.

Most members of the expedition would have been carriers of many other pathogenic microorganisms that would have been threats to Hawaiians. Even the microbes that were normal and harmless to the visiting sailors could have caused all kinds of troubles to Hawaiians who received them. William Ellis, an assistant surgeon with the expedition, observed that when the ships returned to Niʻihau and Kauaʻi in March 1779, the natives were suffering from "the venereal complaint, [and] coughs and colds, indeed, were pretty general, and one man died . . . [of] a violent griping or colic,"[4] (although this colic need not have been caused by a foreign microbe).

Assuredly a variety of strange new illnesses would have swept through the native population for months after *Resolution* and *Discovery* departed. If Cook's sailors had not introduced the microorganisms that cause colds, dysenteries, enteric fevers, meningitis, and other contagions, then certainly the foreigners who came after them would have done so. Before 1800 scores of ships had called at island ports, and every one of them was laden with many evils and few benefits. Wave after wave of sicknesses swept through the hapless islanders, and kāhuna lapaʻau were called upon to treat them.

William Shaler's comments about kāhuna lapaʻau in 1804 elevated them to a degree of competence that few other haoles, especially American missionaries, would ever allow:

Medicine is generally practiced by the priests, whose contemplative way of life has led them to the acquirement of some knowledge of botany; they understand the use and application of vomits and clysters, which are drawn from the vegetable reign, and sometimes exhibited with success. Topical bleeding is also in use, but a large share of priestcraft and mummery enters into their practice. Fortunately the good constitution and temperance of the islanders prevents their having often occasion for the skill of their physicians.[5]

This rather cavalier attitude indicates that Shaler formed his opinions before the great epidemic of 1804 wreaked its havoc.

Probably in 1804—or possibly in 1805 or 1806, for no one knows when it actually happened—a serious pestilence occurred on Oʻahu at the time when King Kamehameha I was assembling a large army in preparation for his second attempt to invade Kauaʻi. Bivouac life favored the rapid spread of the disease, which seems to have been an intestinal infection of the sort by which armies everywhere are always endangered. As has been described in an earlier essay, Hawaiians called it *ka maʻi ʻōkuʻu,* "the squatting sickness." Probably it was typhoid fever or bacillary dysentery, possibly cholera (but *not* yellow fever or bubonic plague, as some historians have claimed). Kamehameha himself was very ill with it; and so many of his supporting chiefs and warriors died that once again the invasion of Kauaʻi was prevented.

About that time, apparently in response to the people's need, the practice of the Lonopūhā kahunas was revived. Kuaʻuaʻu was a kahuna of the order of Lonopūhā, a chief of Kaʻū, Hawaiʻi, who was revered as the founder of this order. Lonopūhā kahunas, who included kāhuna hāhā, were experts in the art of healing, especially of wounds and abscesses. Kuaʻuaʻu taught this art of healing to the chiefs. "That was the beginning of the spread of this medical art, one which was famous in the time of Kamehameha I."[6]

Many years later, John Papa Iʻi recalled that anguished time, when he had been a boy serving in the household of Kamehameha I:

The method of training promising members of the court as medical kahunas is believed to have developed because of the great death rate among chiefs and commoners in the year 1806, perhaps owing to the

terrible *ʻokuʻu* disease, when the epidemic spread among all of the
chiefs and commoners of the islands. . . .

This [training] went on until all the diseases and medicines [were
mentioned] and the kinds of pigs, and the clothing suitable for offerings. All of these things composed and arranged for memorizing were
learned by all the students of the art of healing. These were the things
they recited to the medical instructors, including the name of the
ʻaumakua gods of healing from remote times. This was done in front
of the heiaus . . . , and if the recitation was perfect, it was believed
that such a person would attain skill in treating various diseases. . . .

The symptoms mentioned were chills, fever, dull headache, a pain
that shut off the breathing, and so on. If the disease was the *papaku*
(extreme constipation), or the *ʻeho* (ulcerous sore), or the *haikala* (a
severe disease accompanied by cramps), the *waiʻiki,* a mixture of green
gourd juice and *kukui* sap, was the very best medicine to use.[7]

Iʻiʻs recollections show that although frightful new diseases had
been set loose among the Hawaiian people, their physicians' philosophy of medicine and medical education remained unchanged. Nonetheless, conservative as they were, native physicians—pushed,
perhaps, by their sagacious king—seem to have been sufficiently
alarmed by the number of lives being lost to these introduced diseases
that they established a crash program for training kāhuna lapaʻau to
meet the nation's need.

Thereafter, even though for most kāhuna lapaʻau "the old ways
were best," at least some of the younger physicians must have realized that new afflictions called for new remedies. In desperation, they
turned to the strange and novel plants that foreigners were importing
almost as fast as they introduced new diseases. Don Francisco de
Paula Marin, a Spaniard who settled in Honolulu sometime in the
mid-1790s—a physician of sorts, among many other occupations,
and the first in a long series of passionate yet practical gardeners
whose activities ultimately changed the appearance of these islands—
imported many different kinds of useful plants, some of which eventually found a place in the pharmacopeia of kāhuna lapaʻau lāʻau.

The guava, for example, brought by a sea captain to Marin from
"tropical America about 1824," was generous in bearing its many-
seeded fruits. Within a few years, with the help of animals and people, guava plants were so widespread as to be almost as much of a
pest as the mosquitoes introduced at Lahaina in 1826. Tobacco and
the edible cactus also spread rapidly, as did a number of cosmopolitan weeds.

All of these plants, and more besides, in one way or another were incorporated in the growing list of remedies employed by kāhuna lapaʻau lāʻau. Preparations derived from guava fruits and leaves were used in treating "deep cuts, sprains, diarrhoea, and intestinal hemorrhage."[8] Until a generation or so ago, it was the one plant that every child who grew up in the islands knew had some medicinal value: "For constipation, eat only the seeds; for diarrhoea, eat only the rind." But nowadays few islanders are aware of the tradition, or need to test the validity of its claim. In 1934, when Handy, Pukui, and Livermore published their treatise on Hawaiian therapeutics, they concluded that kāhuna lapaʻau lāʻau had used, in some way or other, components from 317 different plants, 29 animals, and about a dozen minerals.[9]

Foreigners' ideas as well as their merchandise affected every aspect of the native society. Soon after Kamehameha I died in 1819, the kapu system by which Hawaiians had been governed for hundreds of years was overthrown at the direction of two of the dead king's imperious wives and by order of his pliable successor-son. Forty-one years of contact with foreigners who broke every kapu with impunity, who laughed at the unavenging gods, had prepared the nation for this rebellion of the mind. When the kapus were thrown aside, both gods and priests lost their power over the mana of the people. But the chiefs did not relinquish so soon their power over the bodies of their subjects.

Kāhuna lapaʻau, too, adapted their concepts of diagnosis and treatment to the new freedom. Not immediately, of course—if only because the habits of a people do not change as easily as do their numbers or their laws—but gradually, as younger generations replaced the older. Eventually native physicians learned to associate specific remedies with specific diseases. No more did they seek help in diagnosis exclusively from gods and spirit guardians; no longer did they rely for healing upon the amounts of mana present in plants, animals, or minerals. Now they began to base their judgments on observation, reasoning, and experience. In arriving at this relatively modern methodology they must have been influenced by the attitudes of newcomers in general, and especially by the examples of the few foreign physicians visiting in the islands who treated ailing haoles or chiefs, always under the scrutiny of kāhuna lapaʻau.

Nothing like a standardized system of native medicine emerged, however. Each kahuna lapaʻau still felt free to develop his own regimen of treatment, according to intuition, revelation, or experiment, while he ignored or disdained the therapies offered by other physicians, whether native or haole. But at least he treated in the same manner all cases who came to him with a specific disease, such as gonorrhea, instead of with a "personalized" medicine devised for each individual patient, according to suggestions revealed to him by his own ʻaumakua or by those of the patient. Because of this uniformity in treatment, a native physician needed to devote much less time and energy to each patient than was demanded by the older system of medicine. As a result, by the 1850s many a kahuna lapaʻau was presented with such a thriving practice that, in order to accommodate all his patients, he had to establish a modest hospital or clinic similar to the "chambers" maintained by foreign physicians in Honolulu and other port towns. During the reign of Kamehameha V (1863–1872) the Board of Health decided that it should license kāhuna lapaʻau.

Until 1820 chiefs and commoners, as well as the few foreigners who had settled in the islands—except for Don Marin, a self-taught physician and apothecary of sorts in the European tradition—were forced most of the time to rely on native kāhuna lapaʻau for treatment of their ailments. In 1816 Louis Choris, artist aboard the Russian Imperial Navy's ship *Rurik,* commanded by Lieutenant Otto von Kotzebue, saw one foreigner on Oʻahu who benefited from the ministrations of a kahuna lapaʻau:

> . . . an Englishman whom the gout had rendered entirely crippled; he could neither sit nor walk. An old native offered to cure him. . . . He made him observe from the start a most rigorous diet; after that he massaged the patient throughout the whole day, applying his hands from the waist to the feet, not ceasing even while the patient fell asleep. In six days this patient was entirely cured.[10]

To Choris, the kahuna's treatment "suggested that which hypnotism uses." To us today, the kahuna's regimen resembles a combination of diet and physiotherapy, with perhaps some assistance from "suggestion."

When a foreign vessel came to port, her doctor (if she carried one) was besieged with requests for medical care. Haole medicines of the time, except for the mercurial ointments used in treating syphilis, were scarcely better than native remedies. But no one realized this and the greater prestige of foreign therapy, added to the greater mana that foreign physicians were thought to possess, may have contributed to the recovery of local patients—when they did get well. In surgical skills, however, foreign physicians were far superior to native. Whether they dispensed medicines, performed operations, or delivered "half-white" babies, helpful ships' doctors did a great deal to promote friendly relations between visitors and natives.

During an extended visit in these islands in 1823, the Reverend William Ellis observed that chiefs and those commoners of Honolulu who "are accustomed to associate with foreigners . . . shew a decided preference to foreign medicines." Forsaking kāhuna lapaʻau, they sought help from haole physicians whenever those experts were available. But foreign doctors were never present in sufficient numbers, even when the ships that carried them were in port. Resident physicians were even rarer: in the whole kingdom, Thomas Holman of the American mission was the only doctor for little more than four months in 1820. No mission doctor replaced him until 1823, when Abraham Blatchely arrived, and he departed in 1827. The first mission physician to settle permanently in the islands was Dr. Gerrit P. Judd, who arrived in 1828.

Once in a while a ship's surgeon would stay in port long enough to be of some service to mission families, high chiefs, and resident foreigners. Under those circumstances of apportioning time to need, few commoners (except perhaps very favored retainers of important nobles) had the chance to receive any attention at all from practitioners of Western medicine. Fortunately for most commoners, as Ellis noted, they were "generally averse to our remedies, and prefer the attendance of native doctors."[11] Even so, the people died: between 1778 and 1820, when the first company of American missionaries arrived, the native population (according to estimates from those same missionaries) decreased to fewer than 135,000.

The Yankee missionaries, although they were most concerned with converting surviving Hawaiians to the somber blessings of Calvinism, were practical enough to try also to acquaint them with the advantages of civilization. Dominant among these was education according to the American philosophy. Caught between the Christian religion on the one hand, and the three Rs on the other, native medicine was doomed to eventual failure. Yet for Hawaiians their traditional form of medicine was too much a custom—and perhaps a necessity—to disappear at once. Indeed, it enjoyed a kind of renascence during the reign of Kamehameha V. Inevitably, however, the relative superiority of haole culture in general, combined with the scorn most foreigners heaped upon kahuna medicine—"superstition," they called it, if not "witchcraft," while kahunas themselves they condemned as being "ignorant" and "murderers"—eventually convinced most natives that the white man's medicine was better than their own.

The American missionaries' militant opposition to native physicians and medicines was declared almost as soon as they arrived in the islands. In April 1820, while they were detained at Kailua, Hawaiʻi, awaiting Kamehameha II's permission to settle in his kingdom, Dr. Thomas Holman, the Mission's physician—and the first American doctor who actually lived in the islands for a while—had an experience which fixed forever the missionaries' attitude toward all kāhuna lapaʻau:

> Soon after our landing, I was called upon by the King to render medical aid to one of his wives, and a number of his attendants and servants, with all of whom, by the blessing of God, I had very good success, although some of them were dangerously ill. The native Physicians were much opposed to my practice, telling my patients that I should kill them, and it is to be suspected that had I not been successful in my first setting out, the consequences might have proved unhappy for me. The native Physicians are extremely superstitious, and they know little or nothing of how to distinguish one disease from another; but generally administer the same medicine in all disorders—and if the person to whom they give medicine dies, they supposed him to have been prayed to death by some enemy. Indeed, this people do not believe in a natural death, but that they are prayed to death, killed by Ah-hoo-ah-ena [akua ʻino, evil spirits] or by some unforeseen casualty.[12]

Haole prejudice was not supported by extensive knowledge either of kāhuna lapaʻau or of their therapies. Few foreigners could even identify a kahuna lapaʻau; and most haoles were quicker to deplore kahunas' ministrations than to use them. To haoles, all native remedies were little short of being poisons, which they would rather die than try. And, for proof of their contention, they needed only to compare the rate at which Hawaiians were dying with the rate at which foreigners were thriving, amid the desolate house sites and the crowded burial pits left by the vanishing Hawaiian race.

Dr. Alonzo Chapin, a physician with the Congregational mission in Honolulu from 1834 to 1837 (whose descriptions of the town's syphilitics is presented in a later essay), held no high opinion of "the medical views and practices of the natives." These are, he wrote,

> made up of a mixture of absurdities the most ridiculous, and often dangerous. . . . Native medicines have, some of them, value, where they are skillfully employed; but, used without principle or judgment, they are . . . often the means of irremediable injury.
>
> Charms and incantations have a conspicuous place in their therapeutics, and often lead to practices the most shocking. Many [patients] have been pounded and roasted to death from a belief that their diseases were the effect of an indwelling spirit. Nor is it in all cases needful that the patient should be actually suffering with the disease; the mere apprehension of future sickness is sufficient reason for having recourse to remediate measures, and truly fortunate is he who has sufficient strength of constitution to withstand the baneful influence of their more drastic doses.[13]

By the 1830s, Yankee missionaries and the more zealous of their native converts no longer hid their antipathy toward kāhuna lapaʻau: "Most of the prayers are in vain," the Reverend J. F. Pogue huffed in 1858, "and most of the work of the *kahunas,* but it is strange that the *kahunas* still continue to this day and many people have died. Too bad!"[14]

Christianized natives, not to be outdone in this sport of vilification, turned upon native physicians, calling them "pig-eating *kahunas,*" "liars," "deifiers"—and worse.[15] Yet, because in the 1860s he was old enough to think for himself and to be disenchanted with most of the ways of most foreigners, Kamakau dared to defend kahunas: "Many times they are right, and they cure many who are sick unto death."

In the aging Kamakau, as in so many Hawaiians of his generation, the old beliefs were still strong. Through the veneer of Christian religion and haole pragmatism which they had assumed, for the same reason that they had donned haole clothing and manners (out of propriety or from a conviction thinner than a haole's silken shirt), their ʻaumakua still spoke to them, the akua still ruled from a heaven in which they had kindly allowed a bit of space for Jehovah, the newcomer:

> The ʻaumakua in this new era have become bitter enemies who punish severely the faults of their descendants, such as swearing falsely, defiling themselves by mingling with those who are unclean, eating forbid-

den food mixed with blood, eating defiled food, breaking laws, com-
mitting adultery, breaking every kind of law, the laws of God, of the
land, of parents, husband, wife, children, and relatives. It has become
a burdensome task to offer the ʻaumakua the gifts and sacrifices necessary [to atone] for the sins and errors of men. Hence a great many
more men, women, and children of this race suffer today in comparison with the past.[16]

This was one of Kamakau's several explanations—as it was of many
of his mixed-up contemporaries—for the rapid destruction of the
Hawaiian people.

ʚʚʚʚ

From about 1840 until near the end of the century, a number
of kāhuna lapaʻau, having learned how to write from missionaries
and their students, committed to notebooks, letters, and reports their
regimens for diagnosis and treatment of many of the afflictions they
tried to combat. Although these manuscripts preserve interesting
details about both native therapeutics and native physicians, they
were written too late to give a reliable account of Hawaiian medical
practices before foreigners arrived: they are suspect because they are
filled with alien words and with references to foreign utensils, medicines, and diseases—not to mention the missionaries' very punitive
Jehovah. In consequence, one who reads these manuscripts can never
be quite certain where native concepts end and foreign intrusions
begin.

Despite haole scorn and missionary preachment, kāhuna lapaʻau
continued to minister to trusting natives, especially in rural communities. In 1868, during the reign of Kamehameha V (1863–1872),
a strong-willed monarch (who shared many of his native subjects'
opinions), a second Board of Health—called "The Hawaiian Board
of Health"—was created for the purpose of licensing genuine kāhuna
lapaʻau to practice their kind of medicine. Haole residents were scandalized by this regression into "barbarism," but licensing of kāhuna
lapaʻau by the Hawaiian Board of Health continued until late in the
reign of King Kalākaua (1874–1891). Judging from the annual
reports they were required to submit, some of those licensed kāhuna
lapaʻau were excellent physicians, by medical standards of their day.
Others, unfortunately, deserved the haoles' censure. But then so did
some of the foreigners who set themselves up as physicians in the
islands.

One of the best of those native physicians, according to the evidence presented in the seventy or so case histories he submitted to the Hawaiian Board of Health on 14 March 1871, would have been the man named Ohule. He practiced at his office-hospital in Kalihi Uka, a valley community near Honolulu. His patients came to him with all kinds of ailments, from mild to severe, from curable to fatal: menstrual cramps, partial paralysis, costiveness, pain in the knee, soreness of the legs, lump in the abdomen, pulmonary discharges, dizziness, piles, burning menses, spleen trouble, ashy color of skin, constant colds, chronic stomach ache, pain in the chest, broken bones, and more—the usual kinds of miseries that prompt people to seek help from a healer they trust.

For each of these patients Dr. Ohule prepared a brief summary statement, in compliance with the Board of Health's regulations. In the statement he described the patient, the ailment (or, in many instances, the complex of several ailments), the treatment he instituted, and the effect of this regimen upon the course of the disease. Here is one of those case histories, chosen because it is relatively short:

> June 14, 1870. Puhene (male) of Kalihi-kai. . . . His sickness was kidney disease, pain in the knees, and he was unable to walk fast. In my examination and in feeling with my fingers I found that this was a customary sickness [that is, one frequently reported among Hawaiians].
>
> I gave him for medicine the leaves of the piʻialiʻi taro to cover his back for the kidney trouble. He found relief from his back to his knees. For the remainder of his trouble he was rubbed with the medicine called okiʻi. He took some internally. I took some first, then the patient took it. He regained his health and was released on the 18th day of June.[17]

Not all of Dr. Ohule's patients responded so readily. A few of them died. Ohule reported these failures too, not only because he was an honest man, but because he was confident in his many successes, and in the knowledge that, whatever happened, he was devoting all his abilities to the care of those hopeful patients. Thus, he reported about another man, after several days of treatment: "There was no relief at all. His gasping grew worse. . . . He died on the 20th day of October" [twenty-one days after treatment had begun].

Patients' average length of stay in his hospital was five days. He prescribed a variety of treatments and medications, not all of which came from the native physicians' materia medica. Dr. Ohule, well informed about haole physicians and their regimens, used their medicines where those seemed to be indicated. So, for a man afflicted with syphilis, and showing also a variety of symptoms attributed to other ailments, Dr. Ohule prescribed both Hawaiian herbs and "the white man's syphilis medicine . . . procured for one dollar a bottle." Most patients, however, received the traditional native therapies. Often these began with some kind of purgative—an "opening medicine"—either an emetic or a laxative. Sometimes the purgative was heroic in dosage and duration. For conditions needing milder remedies, poultices or unguents made from leaves, or bindings and wrappings using leaves and stems, were applied to the body.

In reading his reports, even today, we are impressed with Dr. Ohule's concern for the welfare of his patients, his acquaintance with a wide variety of medicinal plants, and his willingness to employ such newer modes of therapy as were available to him. He did not hesitate to use haole medications such as castor oil, "syphilis medicine," "Pain Killer," and other pharmaceuticals that he could buy, over the counter, at Honolulu's drugstores. (The haole doctors' pharmacies, of course, were not open to him and his fellow kāhuna lapaʻau.) But Dr. Ohule and his patients—not to mention haole physicians and their patients—did not know that Western medicines were no better than native ones. Ailing people lived or died for reasons rarely affected by the medications their doctors prescribed for them.

For all of them, physicians and patients alike, native and haole alike, the most valuable ingredient they received or disbursed would have been the psychological support the doctor offered. In this important respect, Dr. Ohule's personality, his "bedside manner," must have been paramount. He was empirical, pragmatic, undoubtedly kind, obviously concerned. He was not preoccupied with word-magic, sacred numbers, ancient rituals, and importunities to the gods, as were kāhuna lapaʻau of the older school. He was a man of the new times—even to the point of having become a convert to the religion of the new and "Most Powerful God," as he indicated in his covering letter to the Board of Health. With the confidence derived from trust in that omnipotence, he did not need to ask for help from Kāne, Kū, Lono, and Hina. No matter. He did his best to bring succor to his patients in their need.

In contrast to Dr. Ohule, Kawai Liʻiliʻi, another kahuna lapaʻau who practiced in Wailuku, Maui, in 1858, "received his knowledge through dreams." His remedy for "insanity" indicates that, at best, his therapies must have been useless, at worst, close to dangerous:

> If . . . I dream that I am told that popolo is the medicine for this disease, then I gather two handfuls of popolo, mash it fine, put it in a piece of cloth, squeeze the juice into the right ear, and into the left ear, following this treatment by roasting a white dog in the ground and permitting everyone in the house to partake of it, reserving the spleen for the patient.[18]

By the 1870s, when Mary Kawena Pukui's grandfather practiced as a kahuna lapaʻau in Kaʻū, native physicians were "giving less attention" to the signs and omens that their predecessors considered to be indications about "whether or not to proceed with a case." Furthermore, by that time surviving kahunas had decided that they were "supposed to do only what they had been trained to do." This recognition of their limitations in that troubling era of complex new diseases led many a native physician to refer certain cases to other kahuna specialists of recognized competence.[19]

Whereas in days of old all kāhuna lapaʻau believed that all sicknesses and misfortunes "came from supernatural causes," by the 1870s they were distinguishing between "god-inflicted and physically caused disabilities." In other words, they were being influenced by Westerners' attitudes toward the causes and cures of diseases. "Illness that was not caused by gods, by spirits, or by sorcery" was called *maʻi kino,* body sickness. A *maʻi kino waho,* body sickness from outside, might be caused by a sorcerer's curses, or by a wrathful god, or by an ʻaumakua. Still a third kind of illness, a *maʻi ma loko,* sickness from within, could be caused by "a persisting unpleasantness within the family, such as grudges, unresolved conflicts, and outright hostilities."[20]

Once the physician decided whether a sickness came from inside the body itself or from agencies outside it, he could accept a case or could refer it to another kahuna—even to a sorcerer (who, he hoped, would be more powerful than the baleful one who started the trouble in the first place). Thereafter, the responsible physician could choose among a number of treatments, such as the group therapy of hoʻoponopono, or medications of the kinds he favored, or prayers and rituals. All approaches were intended to placate offended gods and spirit guardians (or to implore forgiveness from Jehovah), and all tried to ease both body and spirit of the patient. A physician who prayed to the gods for help, but who used medicines as well, was called *kahuna laʻau kāhea* (because *hoʻokāhea* means to call, to pray).[21]

The new kinds of diseases that Westerners were introducing made many kāhuna lapaʻau wary of treating people so afflicted. "These ills are *maʻi malihini,* foreign sicknesses," they said. "Send the patient to the foreign doctor." Other kahunas attempted to treat people suffering with the new ailments—and got small thanks for their pains, at least from haoles. In 1860 the Reverend Dwight Baldwin, a Congregationalist minister stationed at Lahaina on Maui (who also offered whatever Western medical care he could manage to provide), complained that local kahunas were "causing unnecessary deaths" from scarlet fever.[22] (His treatment for this dreadful disease could not have been any better than were the kahunas' remedies.) Wiser kahunas refused to treat anyone suffering from a foreign disease. And, too, they declared that their skills were "no good" for ailments caused by ʻanāʻanā or hoʻopiʻopiʻo sorcerers, the ones most feared by suggestible folk.

As ever, in ability, dedication, and degrees of success kāhuna lapaʻau of the 1870s ranged from the fortunate good to the misfortuned bad. Some clever villains, seizing the chance to make a fast *kālā,* went about the countryside offering their services as physicians, even though they had received no medical training at all. These charlatans, where recognized, were called *kāhuna hoʻokohukohu,* pretenders, and of course were invited to depart, taking their wiles elsewhere. Then, too, alas, some kāhuna lapaʻau who had really been trained in their sacred profession forgot medical ethics and honorable morality: in their persuasive ways, they took advantage of patients' ignorance in order to benefit themselves. Hawaiians had a word for those crooks too: *kāhuna hoʻopunipuni,* deceivers.[23]

One confident kahuna lapaʻau did not stoop to deception, although he seems to have taken advantage in other ways of gullible patients who ventured into his consultation chambers. In 1865 he published a schedule of fees for services rendered: "For a very great sickness—$50. Small sickness—$20. Very small—$10. Attending a friend—$5. Incantation to find out disease—$3." Either he held a very high opinion of himself or was trying to scare off unwanted patients with this sliding scale of charges. In 1865 they were, to say the least, whopping.[24]

In the late 1860s, during the reign of Kamehameha V, natives' concern about receiving good medical care reached the proportions of a mild rebellion. Literate Hawaiians, having long since discovered the pleasures of writing letters to the editors of their many vernacular newspapers, expressed all sorts of opinions, ranging from complete support of the native medical profession to outright rejection of kāhuna lapaʻau in favor of foreign physicians. Thus, M. Kehukai, in 1866, rejecting kāhuna lapaʻau, advocated

> a school where Hawaiian youths can be trained for the medical profession in the way of the foreigners, because the population is greatly reduced by death. The falsehood and deceit of the idolatrous Hawaiian kahunas may be eliminated. [Meanwhile] the treating of the sick is left to white doctors who do not have the true love for this people and care only for their personal welfare.[25]

J. Nakuʻokoʻo of Pulehu in Kula on Maui wrote to the editor of *Kuokoʻa:*

> The health of the Hawaiians is a very important thing . . . that will keep us a people and make the work of being Christian progressive. Therefore I think it is not well to depend entirely on the white doctors for the health of this people but to widen the way for the Hawaiian medical kahuna to handle the diseases known to Hawaiians.
>
> There are more Hawaiian medical kahunas living on each island . . . than there are white doctors, who are perhaps mostly in Honolulu. Some of the . . . kahunas are taking care of their own families in the Hawaiian way and they are well protected. Therefore the benefits of a kahuna should be made two-fold by opening the way and not have the law bite as it does now. . . .
>
> . . . in ancient times, the population was greater, though they were ignorant and pagans, than it is in our good and proper Christian times. . . . Were there people who were never stricken by diseases? Did they have foreigners treat their diseases? Was it foreign medicines that healed them? . . . If it strikes you as being right, then prepare a petition to the Legislature at once, to widen the way.[26]

"Widen the way" became the rallying cry for people who wanted the government agencies to approve the licensing of more kāhuna lapaʻau, "and not have the law bite" them by arresting unlicensed native physicians or closing their practices.

The legislature was very much involved in defining policies and passing laws relating to all physicians, native or foreign. Among the legislators in the session of 1867 was J. K. Unauna, quintessential politician, master of verbosity and elocution, and expert at playing all sides against the safe middle. One day he rose in the House to expound his considered opinions. His speech was reported at gratifying length in *Kuokoʻa* on 2 March 1867. He supported the government's attempts to regulate the practice of medicine by licensing kāhuna lapaʻau. But, he wished to make clear, whereas delay was fatal, speed in any action would be a show of prejudice:

> This people will very quickly vanish if the medical treatment with Hawaiian plants is done away with, and all the districts of the various islands will be quickly desolated, and the dwelling of Hawaiians in their birthplace will cease, and will commence the desertion of the country districts, because we see at this time there is no foreign medicine in those districts, nor is the medicine assigned by the government sufficient, nor are the medical priests sufficient as appointed by the Board of Health. . . .
>
> Some of the representatives of the present Legislature have tried to get money to settle foreign doctors in places without medical aid, but could not, and if the treatment by Hawaiian methods is prohibited as being improper, then this race will soon become lost. It is better not to cease the practicing with Hawaiian medicine, such as are sufficiently supplied in all places where they reside.

On and on he rambled, proposing solutions requiring Yeas and Nays and Perhapses from all sides, asking that compromises be sought among all contending factions. "Let us study this problem," he urged, invoking the magical word. "Postpone decision," he advised, in the best tradition of parliamentarians, "collect information . . . prepare a textbook for preservation of prescriptions and instruction of new teachers." And finally—O prophet of the new times! O spokesman for a new age!—he recommended that a group of legislators should visit the other islands as well as Oʻahu's rural districts, to make "site inspections" (as we call them in these munificent days), "to see how things are in the country."

Most effulgent of all thoughtful citizens addressing this issue was D. W. Kalua of Honomakaʻu in Kohala, on the island of Hawaiʻi. Although he must have been a sore trial to all of the nation's harried editors, if his letter to *Kuokoʻa* presents his usual style, perhaps he helped to entertain his bored neighbors in that remotest village in the kingdom:

From the beautiful grove of my thoughts has come an idea to express my voice in the majestic field of your newspaper, that my many friends, from the sun's doorway at Haʻehaʻe to its resting place at Lehua, may see the [headline] above: "Are not some of the medical practices of the Hawaiian kahuna right?"

The body of his letter ambles on: through recapitulations of some Hawaiian herbal remedies, scoldings of white physicians for the haste with which they cut off people's wounded limbs—"the way that the Hawaiian kahuna has [with poultices and splints] is better, for no part of a person is removed from him"—and a lot of sage commentary about paʻaoʻao (one of the great unknowns in kahunas' lore), and "diseases caused by unfulfilled oaths, by family gods, and the like." His peroration and conclusion, incontrovertible in any language, are pulled from the same windy verbiage as his beginning:

There are many kinds of diseases that are healed by Hawaiian kahunas and some which are impossible, are not. So it is with white doctors, some diseases are curable, some are not, and diseases that are fatal end in death. . . .

With friendly aloha to the editor and to the boys who set the type, D. W. Kalua.[27]

Happily, *Kuokoʻa* received letters from more reasoning men. W. H. Uaua of Wailuku, Maui, on 2 March 1867, sent in his answer to the important question:

I can state positively, there are among Hawaiian relatives here . . . a body of skilled priests who by feeling or massaging can ascertain the ailment within a person, and they will foretell his sickness and the suitable medicines also. . . . This skilled practice was the medical treatment of Hawaii, not joining with sorcery and idolatry.[28]

In an attempt to counteract this medical if not spiritual backsliding (and prompted to do so by Dr. Gerrit P. Judd, once a physician-member of their Mission), the American missionaries in the islands at their annual meeting in 1867 proposed that the government should establish a school for training young Hawaiians in the art of haole medicine. The legislature of 1868, seeing merit in the proposal, appropriated the sum of $4,000 "for the medical education of Hawaiian youth." For two years nothing was done by anyone to start the medical school. In 1870, after the legislature renewed the appropriation of $4,000, and impatient with the bureaucratic inefficiency and clandestine opposition to the whole idea among entrenched for-eigners, Dr. Judd himself established the medical school. To the dis-pleasure of the Board of Education, themselves hostile to the plan, but to the satisfaction of some Hawaiians, Judd actually succeeded in starting it on 9 November 1870.

For almost two years Dr. Judd alone was the school's faculty and administration. In his private hospital and dispensary on Punchbowl Street (just inland from the present city hall, Honolulu Hale), and in the wards of The Queen's Hospital nearby, he taught "ten carefully chosen Hawaiian youths" how to be physicians in the haole style. Probably his school was just as good as were most one-man institu-tions of its kind and time in America or Europe, and quite possibly it was better than many, because of his extensive medical experience and his abilities as a teacher.

In 1872, soon after the school's first class of students was gradu-ated and licensed to practice—by the Hawaiian Board of Health, of course, opposition from haole physicians being too strong for him to overcome—Dr. Judd suffered a stroke. The Board of Education was disinclined to find anyone to take his place, or even to ask the legisla-ture to renew its appropriation. Thus Hawaiʻi's first medical school was allowed to die even before Dr. Judd did. The ten young Hawai-ian physicians were assigned to remote districts on the outer islands —far enough removed to offer no threat of competition to haole phy-sicians in the towns. Nothing is known about their subsequent careers. They may have been useful to the sparse native population still surviving in those rural areas; probably, because they were denied status, support, or subsidy, they did not practice haole medi-cine for long.[29]

⌘⌘⌘⌘

Kāhuna lapaʻau of the time must have drawn a wry satisfac-tion from the death of the haole medical school long before their own profession expired. Nonetheless, by 1900 haole medicine had com-pleted its triumph over native. Neither Dr. Judd nor his medical stu-dents were responsible for the demise of the native medical profes-sion. Haole certitude in every thought and action achieved that: the uncombative kahunas were crushed under the weight of foreigners' ridicule and antipathy. Haoles and all things haole enjoyed the insu-perable advantage of being on the winning side: everywhere about them, in every aspect of life, natives could see how they and their culture were doomed and dying, succumbing to the diseases, the ideas, the artifacts of supercilious foreigners. Presented with such overwhelming evidence of weakness, natives and their kahunas became increasingly defensive and embittered.

Haoles never ceased to condemn the native medical profession. Predictably, an American missionary, stationed at Lahainaluna High School at the time, expressed his opinion of kāhuna lapaʻau in his version of Hawaiʻi's history, *Ka Moolelo Hawaii*, published in Hawaiian in 1858:

> Most of the invocations were evil, and the performance of the priests was worst. But the strange thing is that these evil practices of the priests are continuing in our present time, and many people have died. What pity! When will these evil practices in ignorance cease in these islands?[30]

And yet the strange discovery to emerge from his condemnation is the fact that, in themselves, those invocations and practices are not at all evil to us who read them in this more liberal age. To Christian preachers like the Reverend Mr. Pogue they were evil simply because they called upon "false gods" for help, not upon the one true Jehovah.

An article in *The Friend* for July 1892, entitled "The Lanai Horror," referring to the death of several people on Lānaʻi who were said to have died because of the ministrations of kāhuna lapaʻau, revealed both the haoles' attitude toward native physicians and the relentlessness of their campaign to exterminate "kahunaism" by any means they could invent:

> There is reason to believe that such murders constitute no small percentage of the causes of death that are swelling the immense mortality among Hawaiians. . . . The kahuna domination paralyzes the efforts of our skilled physicians to heal the people. The government employs physicians at great expense, but most of the people are prevented from obeying their prescriptions by the orders of the exorcisers to whose violent and destructive treatment they timidly submit. . . . The kahuna is the deadly enemy of Christianity and civilization. . . . They cannot think reasonably nor entertain sound opinions.

The snide sniper who wrote that article in *The Friend* did not consider the plain fact that most Hawaiians who depended upon kāhuna lapaʻau for medical care had no other physicians to turn to. In all rural areas, and certainly on Lānaʻi in 1892, haole physicians were not to be found. Foreign doctors, always scarce at any time before the 1920s, lived and practiced in the towns. Patients of any ethnic group, not only Hawaiians, had to travel to the towns for medical attention—if they could afford to make the trip and pay the doctors' fees. Until the era of the sugarcane plantation hospitals began in the 1890s, most country people lived and died without ever seeing a haole doctor.

ᐁᐧᐁᐧᐁᐧᐁᐧ

Fifty more years of haole domination had to pass before a haole physician in Hawaiʻi could see that sort of vicious propaganda in perspective: "The knowledge of Old Hawaiian medical lore," wrote Nils P. Larsen, M.D., at last, in 1944, "has been buried under a pile of Anglo-Saxon prejudice and pompousness, the usual trimmings of the superiority complex."[31] But Larsen, much too romantical about matters Hawaiian, went to the other extreme, and praised kāhuna lapaʻau and their remedies more than they deserved.

More than anything else, the establishing of the germ theory of disease in Europe during the 1880s, with its attendant changes in methods of diagnosis and therapy, dealt kāhuna lapaʻau the death blow. Even a dweller in the backcountry could be impressed by the miracles of rescue achieved by the new kind of foreign physician who came to live in the islands after 1890. Faced with such unbeatable competition, lacking patients and students, kāhuna lapaʻau knew that they were needed no more. As they died, much of their lore and most of their strengths perished with them.

Today, sometimes, some of the medicaments remembered from the olden days are still used, not only in rural districts in Hawaiʻi. Nevertheless, in this age of miracle drugs, gleaming hospitals, physician-specialists of the new dispensation, and health insurance plans, the true kahuna lapaʻau has vanished, as have most of his people. Ironically, now that surviving Hawaiians have all but forgotten the medical lore of their ancestors, haole scientists have become intensely interested in it—not to revive it, but to retrieve from its pharmacopeia any ingredients which might be of value in modern medicine. Only very recently—when finding some of the kahunas' rarer medicinal herbs on these bulldozed islands is almost impossible—phytochemists and pharmacognosists have got around to analyzing the collectible ones for components which might be added to the materia medica of tomorrow's physicians. In "the land of Niolopua," where dwell the shades of kāhuna lapaʻau and those resistant Hawaiians who do not share heaven with converts of Christian missionaries, sighs of grieving must be lightened with ghostly mirth and snorts of exasperation.

ಌಌಌಌ

Although the materia medica used by kāhuna lapaʻau lāʻau have been much praised by some people (whose partiality toward things Hawaiian often outweighs good sense or knowledge), those medicines—except for ʻawa—have never been studied properly and their worth has yet to be established. In all probability they will never be evaluated "scientifically"—that is to say, in controlled tests on sufficient numbers of animal and human subjects, employing the medicines in the combinations and methods of application prescribed by kāhuna lapaʻau—if only because they are no longer needed in this age of chemotherapeutic marvels.

By comparing the Hawaiian pharmacopeia with those of other primitive peoples, scholars of today can easily find reason to decide that most medications were useless, or at best placebos, but that perhaps some regimens were effective in easing the conditions for which they were applied. Native physicians in any primitive society were not entirely stupid. More often than not they were shrewd observers as well as dedicated healers; and, in the quiet, unhurried centuries before Western civilization intruded upon them, they had lots of time for experimentation and many generations of patients on whom to test their empirical formulations.

As Europeans and Americans have realized only lately, much to their surprise, China's herbalists long ago discovered ma huang, which contains the salutary principle now called ephedrine; India's physicians have prescribed for hundreds of years the tranquilizing hypotensive agents in snakeroot, *Rauwolfia serpentina,* one of which we call reserpine; before the Spanish conquistadores arrived, the medicine men of Peru found quinine, still used as a specific drug for treating malaria, in the bark of cinchona trees; and healers in the Orinoco basin were adepts in the uses of curare as well as the complex techniques by which it is extracted and prepared. And "primitive herbalists" the world around have long been acquainted with the whole array of narcotic and hallucinogenic drugs, from marijuana and hashish, derived from Indian hemp, to opium and its relatives, obtained from the Oriental poppy, and mescaline, psilocybin, and other compounds present in certain species of mushrooms and cacti. As far as we know, Hawaiʻi's indigenous plants did not yield any hallucinogens. The nearest thing to a disorienting substance of that sort was the narcotizing agent in ʻawa, extracted (or perfused) from *Piper methysticum*. Colonizing Hawaiians brought starts of that plant from islands in central Polynesia.

The only medications used by Hawaiian kahunas about which we possess some knowledge of their physiological effects are ʻawa and the cathartics from raw kukui nuts *(Aleurites moluccana)*, from the bitter gourd *(Lagenaria siceraria* var.), and from moa *(Psilotum nudum)*. Innumerable claims, opinions, and denunciations, many of them more imagined than informed, have been directed upon ʻawa. Those physiological effects of ʻawa which have been substantiated by scientists were summarized by R. Hänsel, of the Institute of Pharmacognosy at the Freie Universität in Berlin, in "modern scientific language":

> Apparently, *ʻawa* for the Polynesians was a stimulant, an anesthetic, and an effective medicine. . . . (1) It removes tension and anxiety. (2) It is an analgesic. (3) Small doses relax the muscles of the extremities, while larger doses paralyze through relaxation, without, however, causing a decrease in consciousness or will power. (4) The reversible relaxation or paralysis of the muscles of the extremities is not as pronounced as it is with curare; it also probably acts on the central nervous system. (5) The drug is active against various skin diseases. (6) Consumption of *kawa* may lead to photophobia.[32]

In addition, we can safely assume that most of the kahunas' medicines contained some vitamins of modest therapeutic value and that poultices prepared from fresh green leaves may have helped to heal wounds, and to check infections, because of their content of chlorophyll and perhaps other antimicrobial agents as well. A few toxic plants are known, but kahunas did not seem to use them, not even the maleficent sorcerers. Their horrendous terrifying curses were potent enough.

All the rest remain mysteries. Is the tea prepared from the stems and roots of the *ʻuhaloa (Waltheria indica)* really analgesic, as some people today insist? Did kāhuna lapaʻau use remedies that were the equivalents of today's hypotensives, tranquilizers, energizers, febrifuges, and vermifuges? Did they really know agents that acted as contraceptives and abortifacients? Had they discovered anything that acts as a hallucinogen? We do not know the answers to these questions, because the last kahuna lapaʻau was dead before anyone thought to ask about those aspects of his profession.

Among the many foreign physicians who practiced medicine in Hawaiʻi during the nineteenth century, Dr. Gerrit P. Judd seems to have been the only one who did not instantly oppose native physicians or disdain their remedies. He was overworked enough—and yet enlightened enough—to be interested in the kahunas' pharmacopeia if not in their prayers; indeed, he actually tested some native remedies on himself and used them in treating native patients.

Dr. Judd arrived in Honolulu in 1828 as a physician-member of the Third Company of Congregationalist missionaries assigned to the Sandwich Islands by the American Board of Commissioners for Foreign Missions, in Boston. For several years he was the only resident physician in the entire kingdom. Overburdened with patients foreign and native, commoner as well as royal; and always in need of medicines, assistance, and time, he realized very quickly that neither kāhuna lapaʻau nor their remedies could be dismissed with the scorn that foreigners usually heaped upon them.

With characteristic forthrightness, Judd stated his opinion in a report to the Sandwich Islands Mission written in the fall of 1839:

> It has been an object with me not to oppose the practice of the native physicians in mass, but to endeavor by the best means in my power to correct and modify their practice so that it shall save, not kill, the people. It is my intention, if possible, the coming year to make Hookano [a young man who had attended Lahainaluna High School for six years, whom Dr. Judd took as a medical assistant early in 1839] acquainted with the native practice as it now exists and make him the agent for collecting facts upon the subject. It is out of the question for us to think of putting down the native practice unless we will attend to all the sick ourselves, since it is not human nature to be sick and die without seeking some means of alleviation. The idea of improving the native doctors has therefore suggested itself to me as an exceedingly important one demanding immediate attention.[33]

Before the end of that year, in another report to the Mission, he wrote:

> I commenced the investigation of the native practice and by the aid of these two assistants [Hookano and a youth named Kalili] obtained from several natives the various doctrines and practices of the art

which have come down through the legalized channels *mai ka wa kahiko mai* [from the old times].

The results of these investigations have been embodied in their proper order and committed to writing in a Book kept for the purpose.

These investigations occupied several weeks of the year and have been continued as opportunity afforded. We also instituted a series of experiments on native medicines which resulted pretty much as all experiments of the kind usually do. We found we could prepare from the native Gourd alone [*Lagenaria siceraria*], or combined with *koali* [*Ipomoea* spp.] or *pipa* [*Mucuna gigantea*], an extract which could physic most delightfully and like Brandreth's Pills to any amount which might be desirable. But there being no regular source whence the materials can be derived and preparation of them being attended with some trouble, we have neglected to use them, it being easier to take from the shelves what was already at hand and good enough without seeking for anything better.

If, however, it is thought desirable to supply the stations with the article it can be done at a rate somewhat cheaper than similar foreign articles.

About 3 quarts of Pills have been made during the year, of which half proved to have been damaged in boiling the gourds. The rest have been disposed of to advantage.

I have been unable to prepare an account of the Native Practice in the English language.[34]

The "Book" in which someone committed those observations to writing is not present as such in any of the several archives in Hawaiʻi. If it still exists, and if it can be found, those notes would be the best possible aid to understanding the native medical profession and the value of their materia medica at a time when kāhuna lapaʻau were at the height of their power.

Until that book is found, Dr. Judd's comments on a few native medicines, expressed when he was the sole teacher in Hawaiʻi's first haole medical school, provide the only direct information about their efficacy. A notebook written in Hawaiian by one of his native students shows that, to the end of his life, Kauka Judd retained his interest in therapeutics used by kāhuna lapaʻau. Thus, on 9 February 1871 they discussed

Kahoukapu's diagnosis and treatment of Kamiki, a woman from Waimanalo, suffering from a condition the kahuna called *paʻaoʻao*. An infusion prepared from *moa* [*Psilotum nudum*] pounded and boiled in a pot [was mixed] with cooked sweet potatoes. This was the food she ate until her bowels were purged. Kauka said: I know what the *moa* weed is . . . I've boiled it in water and sweetened it with sugar and given it to people to drink. I have drunk it myself also. It does act on the bowels, but not very well, and it gives such a griping stomach-ache.

On 10 February Kauka said: "Gargling with mountain-apple juice [a decoction of mountain-apple leaves and bark, pounded and placed in water] is good for sore mouth. It is like alum."[35]

Possibly, however, "the missing book" has been made available in other forms. In 1858–1859 "a series of articles" appeared in *Ka Hae Hawaiʻi,* a vernacular newspaper, that was based upon a book "copied for G. P. Judd and recorded by Kahookano [Hookano?]." The articles (and presumably the book) presented the philosophy and practices of kāhuna lapaʻau "as told by a native informant named Kekaha in 1837."[36] These newspaper articles are "the earliest native Hawaiian account of medical concepts and practices." Thus stated Blaisdell in his foreword to Chun's book,[37] which presents an English translation of the articles printed in Hawaiian. As Chun demonstrated, they were a primary source of information about the native medical profession for both Kamakau and Iʻi when they wrote their accounts in the late 1860s.

The articles provide further evidence for the part that kahunas' prayers for spiritual guidance played in their efforts to diagnose and treat assorted ailments among their patients. Moreover, because they are derived from thoughts current in the mid-1830s, they show how foreign ideas as well as introduced infectious diseases were strongly influencing kāhuna lapaʻau's responses to medical problems. Already the Westerners' idea of specificity in treatment was being accepted by native physicians. And, in consequence, they were relying upon available plant and animal resources for the specific remedies they prescribed in the treatment of certain identifiable diseases.

ぐ-ぐ-ぐ-ぐ

More recent investigators of native materia medica have been neither as daring nor as well informed as Dr. Judd. With laudable zeal for discovering something useful in modern therapy—but with regrettable indifference to kāhuna lapaʻau's prescriptions—bacteriologists, chemists, and pharmacognosists have squeezed, ground, pressed, extracted, eluted, and fractionated in assorted ways all kinds of ingredients ripped from the tissues of plants and marine animals found in Hawaiʻi. While these brutal techniques may be dictated by the methodologies of their several disciplines—and of course are necessary in order to provide researchers with more or less "purified" preparations for testing in laboratory experiments—they also do violence both to the composition of kāhuna lapaʻau's remedies and to the manner in which they employed them. In their determination to study only one variable at a time, scientists have never used combinations of several ingredients, as kahunas did so often. And, moreover, no scientist has ever invoked the help of the gods of healing with reverent prayers, hallowed rituals, "opening medicines," "closing medicines," and all those other religious and psychological preparations which played such important parts in the methodology of a kahuna lapaʻau and the responses of his patients.

Useful as such research projects may prove to be, in terms of modern science and better medications, by their very nature they are incapable of evaluating the remedies employed by kāhuna lapaʻau. The day has long since passed when that evaluation could be made. Today's physicians and pharmacognosists, doubly bound by the rules of analytical science and by the scruples of medical ethics, are prevented from testing on human subjects any compounds having unknown properties. And, although in Hawaiʻi, even in Honolulu, a few people who have preserved some knowledge of the old ways are using remedies of the kind developed by kāhuna lapaʻau, they are not talking—for obvious reasons.

The "last genuine" kahuna lapaʻau is believed to have been a kahuna hāhā named Kamaliʻikane. In 1901 he was living on the island of Hawaiʻi, in the district of Kaʻū—near the site of the heiau hoʻōla of Hono-a-Kāne—practicing his profession for the benefit of the few natives and even fewer foreigners who lived in that remote region. Mary Kawena Pukui, the Bishop Museum's incomparable informant on matters concerning Hawaiʻi's natives and their culture, was born and raised in Kaʻū, and in the 1960s she remembered Kamaliʻikane very well, because he treated her and members of her family. In 1901, she recalled, "he cured my father's insomnia with a bath of warm water and dodder."[38] Her father, we should know, was Henry Nathaniel Wiggin, born and raised in Salem, Massachusetts.

In the late 1960s, a Hawaiian man "skilled in the use of native

medicines," as was his father before him, was licensed by the State
Board of Health to dispense those remedies to clients in Honolulu. In
order to avoid complications with the laws of the state (and with resident physicians graduated from approved American, European, or
Asian medical schools), he was called a "naturopath," not a kahuna
lapaʻau. The Yellow Pages of Hawaiian Telephone Company's 1989
directory list thirteen "Physicians—Naturopathic."

ぐぐぐぐ

   Much altered, undoubtedly debased, remnants of the ancient
lore persist in unlicensed people, especially among Hawaiians who
live in rural areas. These remnants are supplemented—and confused
—by borrowings from the folk medicines of other ethnic groups now
living in the islands, European and American as well as Chinese, Japanese, Korean, Filipino, and, most recently, Vietnamese, Laotian,
Samoan, and Tongan. Apart from these amateur—and rather free-
lance—transmitters of folklore, those who live in Hawaiʻi can also
turn for help to genuine professionals from Asian countries who have
been trained there in their specialties. Foremost among these are herbalists from Japan, China, and Southeast Asia and experts in acu-
puncture, who often supplement that kind of treatment with mox-
ibustion and prescriptions using herbs.

Most young islanders know little (and care not at all) about the
virtues of herbs or other natural substances as therapeutic agents.
Repudiating the old ways, they put their trust in Western medicine,
its physicians, and its medications, conveniently if expensively dispensed at urban pharmacies. In general, those islanders who do
resort to folk remedies, Hawaiian or otherwise, are old or middle-
aged people or recent immigrants from other Pacific islands or Southeast Asia. They collect and prepare the ingredients for these medicines according to prescriptions they learned as children from
grandparents, parents, or neighbors. Usually they treat only themselves or members of the immediate family, and do not extend their
care to friends or neighbors.

In some communities, however, a knowledgeable elder—often a
grandmotherly sort of woman—acts as an adviser or counselor in
matters of sickness or distress for neighbors as well as for relatives
who believe in the power of her mana and have faith in the efficacy of
her remedies. "She will tell you what to do," as people say who know
about her. By this they mean that she will suggest the remedies to be

taken and the way they are to be used. Ordinarily, she herself will not prepare those remedies. She is circumspect not because she fears the law—about which she is apt to be unaware—but rather because she believes that an important part of the cure lies in her client's involvement in the process of preparing his medicine. Perhaps, too, she is a bit sensitive to the contempt for her knowledge that haoles in the past have expressed. She will help her petitioners with advice about wrongs which must be righted, about offenses against spirit guardians or against people which must be corrected: hoʻoponopono, "setting things aright," the psychological easing of a sufferer, is still an important step in the quest for health of body and peace of mind. And who can say that in this she is wrong?

She is, as probably one of her near ancestors will have been, a valuable combination of healer and priestess. Nowadays she is called a *"kupuna lapaʻau,"* an "elder healer."[39] And she is wise enough to know her limitations. She will suggest treatments only for simple ailments which can be helped with simple means. People with serious illnesses beyond her ability to help (if she recognizes such conditions) are referred to physicians trained in modern medical schools. In most instances, she does little harm and probably does a great deal of good. In matters of the spirit she can be a powerful force—just as, in the old days, a kahuna lapaʻau could be. She, more than anyone else, is the nearest thing to being a legitimate successor to the kāhuna lapaʻau of old. She has her counterparts among the older people of other ethnic groups. For most immigrants, as well as for some native Hawaiians, such ties with the past are still strong.

All the "legitimate" kāhuna lapaʻau died long ago, of course, and, if personal observation can be trusted, so have most of the partly trained and thoroughly confused disciples they acquired along the way. Their students, in turn, even unto the fourth and fifth generations, have so modified the teachings of genuine kahunas that almost nothing survives any more to continue the philosophy and practices of ancient times. Following the examples of physicians trained in Western medicine, and influenced during the 1960s by uninformed "hippies" and other newcomers wanting to return to the use of "natural" and "organic" herb medicines in the manner of simpler times, this newer breed of "kahunas" shows an alarming tendency to prescribe simpleminded concoctions based on entirely spurious notions about what the people of old believed and taught.

Having heard somehow about Western medicine's principles of

specificity as they relate to the assorted causes of diseases and to the selection of medications for the treatment of certain diseases, now these younger "kahunas" mouth the catchphrases of Western-style physicians. "For every sickness," they intone piously, "there is a remedy." And so, determined to be "scientific," they actually do prescribe a specific remedy for a specific disease. Thus, according to some modern kāhuna lapaʻau, a tea brewed from *māmaki* leaves is the sole remedy for diabetes. Other healers will recommend some other kind of herbal therapy for the same ailment. Gullible patients swallow them, as instructed. And no one among these hopeful folk, whether kahuna or patient, has learned yet that Western physicians no longer place such great emphasis on the principle of specificity. That is a concept from the first half of the twentieth century. Nowadays, the accepted doctrine speaks about "multifactorial agencies"—and multifactorial treatments. (Allopaths, alas, are always one step or two ahead of naturopaths.)

Nonetheless, people being as needful (or as trusting) as they are, perhaps some patients are benefited by the kind attentions of their concerned kāhuna lapaʻau. The placebo effect; the psychological rewards to hoʻoponopono and hoʻomalu, even, possibly, some chemical component that is present in the herbal remedy, may explain why some of these patients do feel better after they have taken the recommended medicines.

Whether or not this new approach to sickness and to cure is effective is not the point at issue here. The point is that the fundamental belief of the modern naturopath is different from that professed by kāhuna lapaʻau in days of old. Although today Jehovah may be invoked in prayers beseeching his help, the many gods of old have been forgotten. And forgotten too have been the quotas of the mana that are incorporated in their *kino lau,* their physical manifestations, which are the plants and animals and minerals they have put in this world for our benefit, in more ways than one.

Even though at least some of the materia medica of the kāhuna lapaʻau are being used today, we still do not know how effective they are. Even more to be regretted is the lack of interest in those medicines—and in the lore of the older people who know how to use them —that is shown by younger members of a community or of a family fortunate enough to have one of these kūpuna lapaʻau in its midst. Inasmuch as no scientist can ever learn from her what she can tell, only a younger member of her family can receive those confidences

which are of such interest to sociologists, psychologists, pharmacognosists, and historians, if not to physicians.

Although we know very little about the pharmacological
value of their materia medica, the kāhuna lapaʻau of old knew even
less about their efficacy. Only the fact that certain remedies were prescribed for a particular ailment, while other medicines were used for
different diseases, suggests that native physicians may have had some
knowledge about the relative effects of their potions or poultices on
the conditions being treated. Not every kahuna lapaʻau would have
been grossly stupid; the generations of priest-physicians could not
have been consistently unobservant. During the course of many centuries of empirical experience, they would have acquired considerable information about both the effects of their prescriptions and the
responses of patients. No doubt, with them as with medicine men in
other primitive societies, some of their treatments were actually helpful, some were harmful, and most were ineffective. For ailing Hawaiians, as for ailing people everywhere, an important ingredient in the
physician's ministrations was the very fact that he was treating them.

Moreover, for most patients, then as now, recovery came sooner
or later, by natural processes of healing or, in cases of psychogenic
illness, from the comfort of being reassured. When health was
restored, both patient and physician could rejoice—and, if they were
wise, would give more thanks to the clemency of their gods than to
the skill of the priest-physician. When a cure was not achieved, both
patient and physician knew that the sick person was beyond the care
of mere mortals. Whereupon, with the acquiescence of fatalists, they
submitted to the will of the gods.

Even though kāhuna lapaʻau were not experts in chemistry or
pathology, they were beyond all doubt masters in applied psychology. They were able to convince patients and the general populace
that, either as prescribers of treatment or as intercessors between
gods and mortals, they could bring care to the afflicted and cure to
the fortunate. They were able to convince other people because they
themselves were persuaded that they had received their powers from
the gods. All things were possible to humble people who had faith in
the gods. Quacks may have betrayed this faith for gain, and sorcerers
may have used their powers to wreak evil rather than to do good, but
kāhuna lapaʻau in general seem to have been honest and honorable

men, as reputable and as devoted to their profession as are the majority of physicians in any society. Even after foreign physicians had introduced to Hawaiʻi the principles and the simples of Western medicine, and by their disapproval had heaped opprobrium on "native witch-doctors," kāhuna lapaʻau continued faithfully to serve their people. Some persisted doggedly in the old ways; others tried to adapt to the new by developing new medicines or by imitating the regimens of their haole rivals. As the infectious diseases of haoles were introduced, one after the deadly other, kāhuna lapaʻau were quick to incorporate awareness of them in their system of medicine while striving to find native remedies—and the right gods—with which to combat these alien entities. The open-mindedness, the adaptability, of the kahunas is unquestioned—and is much more commendable than was the small-minded antipathy with which foreigners regarded the native medical profession.

But whatever course the kahunas chose to follow proved inadequate to meet the needs of their people. They were cut down, not by their ignorance (as foreigners asserted), but by ruthless adversaries which neither native nor foreign physicians could vanquish: the disease-producing microorganisms introduced among Hawaiians by foreigners, aggravated by the extreme susceptibility of the Hawaiian people to those invisible invaders. Before foreigners arrived, with their poxes and pyrexias, native physicians with their methods of diagnosis and regimes of therapy apparently were providing adequate care for the ailments of indigenous Hawaiians. The kāhuna lapaʻau's concepts of sickness and treatment may have been naive, in contrast with those of Western physicians, but the native physicians themselves were not failures: they met the needs of aboriginal Hawaiians, and therefore must be considered as having been successful for their time and place.

FIVE

1778: An End, and a Beginning

Once again the faithful Makaliʻi, those six little eyes in the heavens, rose above the eastern horizon as the sun sank in the west, to tell star-watching priests that a new year would soon begin. On all the islands "flags were displayed from the temples, to announce the coming of the Makahiki festival; the services at the royal heiaus were suspended, and the chiefs and people . . . betook themselves to sports, games, and the pursuit of pleasure."[1]

The Makahiki was a time of peace, when chiefs put aside for a while the plottings and the fighting by which they hoped to gain lands and power. For four months the great temples were closed, war was forbidden, and the weight of the most stringent kapus was lifted from the people. With this relief from worry, when even ruling chiefs must pretend to be kind, Hawaiians remembered the benevolence of Lono-i-ka-Makahiki, a chief of Kaʻū and Puna. In his youth he was quick-tempered and haughty, but when age quieted him he "tended to the affairs of his kingdom" and "earned the gratitude of his subjects."[2]

In the two centuries and more since the death of the good chief Lono, "his name was made famous through the Makahiki god, Lono-i-ka-ʻou-aliʻi, and [he] was thus thought of as a god of the Makahiki celebration."[3]

ಉಉಉಉ

So did the years pass, each as like to the others as are the leaves on a kukui tree, with nothing to distinguish one from another as they fell out of memory into nothingness. Until one day, near the end of a certain Makahiki season, the time came which was unlike all others that had gone before.

132

Across the sea from beyond the southern horizon moved things such as the people of Kauaʻi had never seen: two floating islands, whose tall and branching trees had caught the clouds of Lono from out of the sky:

> Chiefs and commoners saw the wonderful sight and marveled at it. Some were terrified and shrieked with fear. . . . One asked another, "What are those branching things?", and the other answered, "They are trees moving about on the sea. . . ." A certain *kahuna* named Kuʻohu declared, "That can be nothing else than the *heiau* of Lono, the tower of Ke-o-lewa, and the place of sacrifice at the altar."[4]

When at last they understood that these were not forested islands drifting upon the sea, but great ships fitted with "sails shaped like a gigantic sting-ray . . . the valley of Waimea rang with the shouts of the excited people. . . ."[5] "Lono! It is Lono!" they cried, seeing "the resemblance the sails of his ship bore to the *kapa* of the god."[6]

ʻoʻoʻoʻoʻo

"The god enters, man cannot enter in. . . ." So sang the poets, seated before the great temples, as they intoned the verses of the *Kumulipo*. But on that misfortuned day, when at last the ocean-moat had been crossed, when the barriers of space and time had been leveled, not only the god entered in. Man, too, entered in—lustful, carnal, heedless, and diseased man rushed in, thrusting aside all the guardian deities of Heaven and Earth. "The source of the darkness that made darkness" had come.

ʻoʻoʻoʻoʻo

Their sails bright against the blue of sea and sky, the two ships moved grandly toward Waimea. They were HMS *Resolution* and HMS *Discovery,* and Captain James Cook, England's great explorer, was their commander. The expedition was sailing from Borabora for Alaska, to search for a northern passage across the top of America, when, at daybreak of Sunday, 18 January 1778, *Resolution*'s lookout saw two islands rising high from the sea: Oʻahu far to the right, and Kauaʻi to the left.

Twenty-four hours later Captain Cook's flagship *Resolution* was close enough to shore to receive visitors from Kauaʻi. The explorers in their turn, astonished by the presence of these high islands in the broadest part of the Great Ocean, marveled even more at the numbers of friendly "Indians" who lived on them. Captain Cook wrote in his journal: "We were agreeably surprised to find them of the same Nation as the people of Otaheite and the other islands we had lately visited. . . . How shall we account for this Nation spreading it self so far over this Vast ocean?"[7]

Early in the morning of Tuesday, 20 January, *Resolution* stood in for the bay of Waimea, on Kaua'i's southern shore. "Several Canoes filled with people" met the ship,

> and some of them took courage and ventured on board. I never saw Indians so much astonished at the entering a ship before, their eyes were continually flying from object to object, the wildness of thier [sic] looks and actions fully express'd their surprise . . . and evinced that they never had been aboard a ship before.[8]

No one other than Captain Cook recognized the elements of tragedy gathering at Waimea on that fateful Tuesday morning, amid the joyful greetings from hundreds of natives drawn to Waimea's shore from miles around, amid the ribald anticipations of *Resolution*'s sailors as they neared the alluring shore. All others present at that meeting indulged in more pleasing thoughts. The sailors were eager to enjoy all the delights of "refreshment and recruitment," as the eighteenth century's more genteel folk called eating and fornicating. And the friendly "Indians" were offering honor to Lono-i-ka-Makahiki, returning to them at last, as long ago he had promised to do. The companion-gods who stood with him on that immense vessel also attracted the Indians' admiration. As did the ship itself, so laden with iron, so full of wonders beyond imagining.

When sailors from those great ships stepped upon Waimea's sands and, mingling with fascinated Hawaiians, clasped their hands in greeting, rubbed noses in the native manner, spoke with them face to face, they unloosed upon the friendly Indians hordes of new germs that in time would prove to be more deadly than were all the cannon and muskets the expedition's marines could have trained upon them.

Even before *Resolution* dropped anchor, and during the whole course of the explorers' visit, Captain Cook worried about protecting the innocent Indians from the greatest evil his sailors could inflict upon their unsuspecting hosts:

> As there were some venereal complaints on board both the Ships, in order to prevent its being communicated to these people, I gave orders that no Women, on any account whatever were to be admitted on

board the Ships, I also forbid all manner of connection with them and ordered that none [of the sailors] who had the venereal upon them should go out of the ships.[9]

Knowing the interests of his sailors, and the cordiality of Polynesia's women, the humane captain hoped for success in his endeavor even as he doubted the efficacy of his measures:

But whether these regulations had the desired effect or no time can only discover. It is no more than what I did when I first visited the Friendly Islands yet I afterwards found it did not succeed, and I am much afraid this will always be the case where it is necessary to have a number of [ship's] people on shore; the oppertunities [*sic*] and inducements to an intercourse between the sex[es], are there too many to be guarded against.[10]

All commanders of lecherous men in those years should have entertained these same fears and reached the same conclusions. Yet few commanders allowed themselves to be so concerned. Captain Cook, however, was no ordinary officer: above all else, he was an observer, a thinker, a *scientist* in the true sense of the word. From his knowledge of sailors he could fear that his regulations would fail to control them; and because of his interest in the diseases of men he was able to explain exactly why, despite all good intentions, his regulations were too liable to fail. No other captain in Britain's Royal Navy at that time, and very few of its physicians, would have been capable of this feat of reasoning:

It is also a doubt with me, that the most skilful of the [medical] Faculty can tell whether every man who has had the venereal is so far cured as not to communicate it further, I think I could mention some instances to the contrary. It is likewise well known that amongst a number of men, there will be found some who will endeavour to conceal this desorder, and there are some again who care not [whether they] communicate it.[11]

At that time in medical history neither the victims of venereal diseases nor the physicians who treated them understood that syphilis and gonorrhea are two different infections. Symptoms which today are accepted as characterizing each infection were considered then to be varied manifestations of one disease. Educated people called it "the venereal distemper," "the venereal disorder," or simply "the venereal." In England the vulgar called it by a number of names, of which "the clap" (for gonorrhea) and "the great pox" (for syphilis) were the most distinctive.

In 1770 Great Britain's famous (and eccentric) physician-philosopher, Dr. John Hunter, confused everyone—and delayed differential diagnosis for about sixty years—when he contracted both syphilis and gonorrhea after inoculating himself with pus taken from a case he thought was one of gonorrhea alone. Hunter's error, presumably, arose from the fact that the donor of the pus was a prostitute infected with both diseases. Such double infections must have been frequent, and not only in Hunter's time and country. Probably a few of Captain Cook's promiscuous sailors had contracted both diseases before they reached the Pacific Ocean, although most of those who had what the ships' surgeons usually called "the venereal disorder" may have shown the symptoms of only one infection—or no symptoms at all—when they were examined before being allowed to go ashore at Kaua'i.

Many physicians among Dr. John Hunter's contemporaries questioned his pronouncement that syphilis and gonorrhea were different manifestations of a single disease. Naturally, controversy raged in medical circles, and at least three schools of thought kept it going until, in 1838, Dr. Philippe Ricord of Paris finally showed that syphilis and gonorrhea are two different diseases, each characterized by a distinctive set of symptoms. In 1879 Albert Neisser, one of Europe's first bacteriologists, demonstrated the presence of gonococci, the bacteria that cause gonorrhea, in stained preparations of gonorrheal pus. And in 1885 Bumm proved that these bacteria (now known as *Neisseria gonorrhoeae*) caused clinical disease in human volunteers. The spirochete that causes syphilis, *Treponema pallidum,* was discovered in matter from syphilitic lesions by Schaudinn and Hoffmann in 1905.

Because Cook's expedition would have stayed for only a short time at any one anchorage, those of its members who wrote about the appearance of "the venereal distemper" in Hawaiians would have seen evidences of gonorrhea rather than syphilis. The incubation period of gonorrhea is short—from three to five days in most cases—while that of syphilis ranges from four to six weeks in most individuals and can extend to thirteen or fourteen weeks in a few hardy people.

ぐ・ぐ・ぐ・ぐ

In spite of expressions of aloha from Kaua'i's women, who "us'd all their Arts to entice them into their houses," those ready sailors were prevented for a while from "meddling with them on the shore,"[12] less by Captain Cook's regulations than by "the utmost vigilance" of his officers. Even so, the inviting women were spared the venereal disorder for only a day or two longer. As they always contrive to do, lecherous sailors and wanton women found ways to meet, under the cover of darkness in the warm tropic nights, if not in heat of day, aboard the anchored ships, if not under bushes or in thatched huts on shore. "The great eagerness of the Women, concurring with the Desires of the Men, it became impossible to keep them from each other."[13] Some women, as unclad as mermaids, swam out to the ships, while others arrived in canoes paddled by fathers, or brothers, or husbands. Eagerness to receive the mana—and the gifts —of Lono made prostitutes or panders of all. Mana was passed in a touch. Greed was appeased with a nail, a small mirror, a cheap kerchief, a button.

Not entirely unaware of these happenings, Cook and those officers who shared his concern tried—by exhortations, daily physical examinations, and threats of punishment—to keep sailors who showed symptoms of "the venereal" from "having connexion" with Kaua'i's women. These efforts too were made in vain. Thomas Roberts, *Resolution*'s quartermaster, added one more name to history's long list of infamous little men when he noted in his journal that, on 25 January 1778, "Will Bradlyey" received two dozen lashes at Captain Cook's direction "for disobeying orders . . . and having connections with women knowing himself to be injured with the Veneral disorder."[14]

Bradley was not the only culprit: according to William Charlton, a midshipman on *Resolution,* "Jno. Grant and Benjm. Syon [were] punished with 12 lashes each for absenting themselves from the boat when on Shore, and Wm. Nash with one Dozn for Disobeying orders."[15] More than likely all the sailors assigned to the shore party took turns at work and at forbidden play, but only those four were so unalert as to be caught.

One Will Bradley would have been enough. Unfortunately he was not the only sailor who transmitted the venereal distemper to Waimea's women—or to agreeable men, whether *aikāne* or *māhū*. Most of the expedition's 170 members, including midshipmen and lesser officers, evaded Captain Cook's regulations just as fecklessly as did irresponsible Will. Not everyone in the ships was diseased, of course; but, as Cook feared, enough among them were carriers of gonococci, or of syphilis spirochetes, or of both, to share with Bradley the blame for passing on "the clap" and "the pox" to Kaua'i's hospitable people.

The "great eagerness of the women" was an irresistible counter-force to Cook's orders. If those women (and men) had been less forward, or simply more chaste, Cook's regulations might possibly have tempered the lusts of his men and spared Waimea's people the troubles they invited. But chastity was unknown among Polynesians, who believed that the pleasures of sex should be enjoyed, not repressed, and who put this belief most openly into practice, in any form, at any time, and in any place. Almost every journal-keeper in the British ships remarked this promiscuity, just as almost everyone happily took advantage of it. Captain Clerke wrote of it with disapproval:

> They are profligate to a most shameful degree in the indulgence of their lusts and passions, the Women are much more common than at any place we ever saw before . . . every Aree according to his rank keeps so many women and so many young men (I'car'nies [*aikāne*] as they call them), for the amusement of their leisure hours; they talk of this infernal practice with all the indifference in the world, nor do I suppose they imagine any degree of infamy in it.[16]

Surgeon Ellis was equally clear with his opinion:

> There are no people in the world who indulge themselves more in their sexual appetites than these. . . . The ladies are very lavish of their favours, but are far from being so mercenary as those of the Friendly and Society Isles, and some of their attachments seemed purely the effect of affection. They are initiated in this way of life at a very early period; we saw some, who could not be more than ten years old.[17]

Those frolicking sailors, those women so free with their favors, did not know how appalling would be the consequences of their venery. The gadabout folk of Waimea quickly conveyed the news about the return of Lono, along with their venereal infections, to friends on O'ahu, who in turn relayed news and germs to people of all other windward islands in the archipelago.

The price of hospitality was horrendous. By 1800 it was recognized in Europe. A missionary who, in writing a *Historical Sketch of the Otaheitian Islands* included in his book a short digression about the Sandwich Islands, arraigned Britain's sailors for what they had done to the Hawaiian people:

> Notwithstanding all the precautions which Captain COOK had taken to prevent it, these friendly islanders were contaminated with the venereal disease, of which great numbers had already died [before February 1779]. Cruel memorial of the British name! The first boon of *civilization* to the *Barbarians* of the South Seas![18]

Those first tourists to wander into a Hawaiian landscape wanted the same things that most visitors to any foreign country seek: food and water first; a bit of sex, preferably illicit; and then, the physiological self having been quieted, a quick sortie for souvenirs and a glance or two at the scenery.

Although his sailors earnestly hoped to rearrange the priorities in these interests, Captain Cook, always the provident commander—and the only certified celibate in the expedition, as Surgeon Samwell asserted—put them to work under his own inhibiting eye. He ordered *Resolution* and *Discovery* moved to positions closer to land. When they were safely anchored he went "ashore with three boats, to look at the water and try the desposition of the natives, several hundreds of whom were assembled on a sandy beach before the village."[19]

Awed by the arrival of Lono himself, those hundreds of natives "all fell flat on their faces" the instant he stepped ashore, "and remained in that humble posture till [he] made signs to them to rise."[20] Honoring Lono, they brought him "a great many small pigs . . . presented . . . with plantain trees, in a ceremonious way as is usual on such like occasions." Although the greeters asked nothing in return, the tactful captain "ratified these marks of friendship by presenting them with such things as I had with me." After he ascertained that Waimea stream's water was "very good and convenient to come at," he returned to *Resolution* "and gave orders for everything to be in readiness for Watering in the morning."[21]

The sailors, to the last man, were delighted with that green oasis in the ocean-desert: fresh from the Amorous Isles of Tahiti and Borabora, these wanderers knew that in the agreeable women of

Kaua'i, so friendly and so generous, they had discovered not a tribe of Indians, certainly not a band of angels, but yet another set of houris to welcome heroes come in from warring with the sea.

The lure of all that half-covered flesh proved to be more than mere men could resist. Even so, for most of them connection of a venereal sort did not occur the moment they landed on Waimea's golden sands. The commander's regulations, if not his own watchful eye, seem to have restrained them yet a while. Until on Friday, 23 January, when the ships were "standing off and on" because of freshening winds and a choppy sea, three smallboats were dispatched to shore for water and victuals. Neither captains nor lieutenants went along to ensure that traffic with the natives would be strictly economic rather than commercial in the broad sense. That was the day when Will Bradley and several other sailors added the germs of gonorrhea and syphilis to the many others that they and their shipmates had bestowed in earlier meetings with the islanders. Two days later, on the summary Sabbath, Will Bradley was whipped at *Resolution*'s mast for disobeying Captain Cook's orders. As usual, punishment was meted out too late: the damage was done—not only as Captain Cook feared but even more than he expected. Never again would Hawaiians—or their visitors, wherever they came from—be able to enjoy the disportings of venery without fear of catching one or more of the venereal diseases. Civilization at its worst had come to stay. And with it, as a French wit has said about so many other despoiled places, came "the diseases of syphilization."

Too late to save the people of Kaua'i, the northeast winds increased in strength, driving the ships from their anchorage. For several days they fought to remain in the bight of Waimea until, on Tuesday, 27 January, *Resolution* raised the signal flag telling *Discovery* to withdraw. Both ships retreated to the lee of Ni'ihau, Kaua'i's little neighbor. To a smaller and duller audience the visitors repeated the performances they had given at Waimea. William Bligh, *Resolution*'s master, took a boatload of sailors ashore on 29 January and, martinet that he was, brought them off safely (and continent) with a supply of water and yams. On the following day Lieutenant John Gore's party was marooned on the island by strong winds and crashing waves. During that ill-famed night gentle John Gore lost control over his men, and some of them presented the venereal distemper to their dusky comforters.

Captain Cook, foiled in his hope of protecting the people of

Ni'ihau, no longer hid his disappointment. "Thus the very thing happened," he wrote, "that I had above all others wished to prevent."[22] On 2 February, unable to take aboard any more provisions from Ni'ihau or Kaua'i, the mariners stood away northward, resuming their course for Alaska. Settling into the routine of a long journey, sailors took up their duties as they warmed themselves with memories, and officers and midshipmen took out their logs and journals inditing impressions of the islands they did not expect to see again.

Among all the members of the expedition only Captain Cook wrote down at that time his thoughts about the effects their visit might have had on the naive islanders. Yet even he could not foresee what havoc he and his companions had wrought. He guessed, all too correctly, that his men had brought new diseases to assail the bodies of a people most susceptible. But how could he foretell that by their every act, by their very presence, as godlike creatures who commanded marvels and broke every kapu without fear, he and his companions had caused Hawaiians to doubt the power of their ancient gods and to question the rule of the chiefs and priests who held them in thrall? How could he know that, in the instant he and his men appeared off Waimea, they began to thrust upon a people not yet ready to cope with them so many of the benefits and almost all the evils of the whole modern world that the visitors took so much for granted?

As the fragile ships bore off to the north, "again launched into that extensive ocean that separates America and Asia," wrote John Ledyard, still another American colonial,[23] Captain Cook, looking back, named these newest of his geographical discoveries the Sandwich Islands, in honor of his powerful patron, Sir John Montague, fourth Earl of Sandwich and First Lord of the Commissioners for executing the Office of Lord High Admiral of Great Britain and Ireland.

ぐぐぐぐぐ

In November 1778 the two battered ships, their weary crews, and their care-worn commander came back across the roughened sea. Balked by barriers of ice in their search for the Northern Passage, driven from the Arctic Ocean by threatening winter, they fled to the warm south, to the Sandwich Islands they had every reason to remember with longing, if not with ardor. This time they came upon the islands from the northeast, and were given the rest of the archipelago to enter on their charts. Maui was their first landfall, at day-break on Thursday, 26 November, and that afternoon they saw smaller Moloka'i to the west.

Once again they arrived during the Makahiki season. As before, the islands' inhabitants crowded to the shores to see Lono's floating islands passing by. Aboard the ships sailors and officers gazed across the water to the land, hoping to enjoy its bounty soon.

In the afternoon, as they cruised along Maui's northern coast look-ing for a harbor or a safe anchorage, several canoes approached. The Indians "came into the Ships without the least hesitation. They were of the same nation as those of the leeward islands . . . and they knew of our being there. Indeed," Captain Cook continued, "it appeared rather too evident, as these people had got amongst [them] the Veneral distemper, and I as yet knew of no other way they could come by it."[24]

Lieutenant King was more forthright about this evidence than his captain, or than any other journal-keeper in the expedition: "They had a Clap, their Penis was much swelled & inflamed."[25] (The signs of acute gonorrhea are unmistakable, and practically diagnostic to anyone who has seen them before: a copious discharge of thick yel-low-green pus flowing from an inflamed and swollen penis or from a vagina similarly affected.)

Aboard *Discovery* Captain Clerke learned how the venereal disor-der had reached the people of Maui so quickly: "The first Man that came aboard told me he knew the Ship very well & had been aboard her at [Kaua'i] . . . & related some Anecdotes, which convinced me of his Veracity."[26] Such an explanation could not quiet Captain Cook's distress, nor did it persuade him to rescind his order forbid-ding women to board the ships. Sadly he wrote in his journal: "The evil I meant to prevent by this I found had already got amongst them."[27]

ぐぐぐぐ

On 30 November the ships rounded Maui's northeastern-most point, to discover the vast body of yet another island looming above the sea—Hawai'i. While they skirted past Maui's rugged east-ern coast, so near and yet so unreachable, more natives came out in canoes, bringing food and water to trade for iron. Some of those men too showed signs of having "the clap."

Leaving Maui, the ships headed across the channel for Hawai'i, the southernmost and largest island in the archipelago. For seven more weeks the leaking ships, with their hungry tantalized passengers, beat their way along Hawai'i's coasts, past its eastern cape, around its southern point, up the barren western shore, seeking the harbor they so desperately needed. "We begin to be in want," Cook noted on 30 December 1778, when they were off the eastern cape.[28] Tempers were as frayed as the stays in the ships' rigging. The sailors, impatient for more meaty pleasures, refused to drink "the very palatable beer" brewed from Maui's sugarcane that Captain Cook, in his unremitting efforts to keep his men "free from that dreadful distemper the Scurvy," ordered the quartermasters to serve instead of grog.

Under the accumulating stresses of three and a half years of exploring in unknown seas, aggravated by those weeks of frustration off Maui and Hawai'i, everything was falling apart: the ships, their equipment, the discipline and spirit of the crews, and—most tragic of all—the tight control that Cook had imposed on himself above all others in the expedition. Even his standing order to prohibit women from boarding the ships was no longer enforced, "as it was out of our power to leave [the Indians] in a worse state than we found them," wrote William Ellis, surgeon's second mate on *Discovery*.[29] To the austere captain this was one more galling proof of the power of animal instincts to betray the best intentions of rational men.

At long last, on Saturday, 16 January 1779, they came abreast of a bay cut deep into the island's flank, sheltered on the south by a point of black lava, on the north by a grim precipice looking as if it were stained with dried blood. Kealakekua the place was called, "the Way of the God," because from there, many generations before, Lono-i-ka-Makahiki had sailed away to a destination beyond knowing, from which he promised to return some day. Mr. Bligh, sent in a smallboat to examine the bay, pronounced it "a good anchorage [with] water tolerable easy to come at."[30]

On Sunday morning the two ships, under reduced sail, moved slowly into the bay of Kealakekua. Excited Indians crowded into almost a thousand canoes, and uncountable others, swimming along the canoes or lying upon surfboards, escorted them in. "I have no where in this Sea seen such a number of people assembled at one place," wrote Captain Cook in the last entry his journal would receive from his own hand. "Besides those in the Canoes all the Shore of the bay was covered with people and hundreds were swimming about the ships like shoals of fish."[31]

The people, in all their thousands, "were full of joy. . . . Their happiness knew no bounds; they leaped for joy [shouting]: 'Now shall our bones live; our god has come back. These are his *kapu* days and he has returned!' "[32]

ʊʊʊʊ

The final act of this drama swept relentlessly to its climax. Opening in splendor and ritual ceremony honoring Lono returned, it progressed through disillusion, distrust, and disgust, until Death entered in to end it. On the fourth Sunday, after much triumphal pageantry on his arrival, the same warriors who had worshiped him in Lono's Heiau of Hikiau, at the innermost curve of Kealakekua Bay, turned in fury upon Captain Cook. With spear points and daggers made from English iron they killed him and four Royal Marines on the rocky beach at Kaʻawaloa, beneath the blood-red precipice. No one knows how many Hawaiians died in the retaliatory affrays that followed.

The visitors had proved to be too human. They had stayed too long, eaten too much, wenched too freely—and, in exchange for hospitality, had given their hosts several new diseases, cheap trinkets that lost their glamor too soon, and many many troubling thoughts. Familiarity had bred contempt among the people on the land and aboard the ships. The Hawaiians, scorning men who showed all too clearly that they were not gods, demonstrated again and again that they were "prodigious expert at thieving." Their theft of *Discovery*'s cutter before dawn on that Sunday morning of 14 February 1779 was only the latest in a series of annoyances, and provoked the confrontation that brought the drama to its bloody finish. In trying to take King Kalaniʻōpuʻu as hostage against the return of the stolen cutter, Captain Cook's very human action drew upon his mortal self the rage of disillusioned men.

With his death yet another hero was destroyed, a modern Prometheus who strove to combat ignorance with knowledge, and who therefore was struck down—by jealous Jehovah, as some of his countrymen would say, for his presumption and his pride. But even before he fell another longer and more relentless tragedy had begun: the destruction of the Hawaiian people.

They were to be destroyed in many ways, by many different agencies, some derived from themselves, most brought to them by successive waves of foreigners who came to their islands after the world learned that they existed. Among the agents introduced by foreigners, by far the most destructive were the microorganisms that cause infectious diseases. And of those pathogens that came early, by far the most deadly were the germs that cause syphilis, gonorrhea, tuberculosis, and the intestinal infections.

ଔଔଔଔ

   Much has been written—and said—about the part that Captain Cook's sailors played in transmitting the venereal diseases to the people of Hawai'i. The literature concerned with this problem started with Cook himself. And it continues to increase, although the rate of growth is slower now than it was during the nineteenth century, when clucking moralizers found it so useful a subject for their preachments.

According to the opinions they expressed, those writers can be classified in three groups. The first, with the largest representation, agrees that the venereal diseases were introduced by Cook's sailors. The disappointed captain himself accepted this as a fact and so did most of his associates. Captain Clerke, for example, a worldly man not given to hypocrisy or excuses, wrote in March 1779, when the expedition returned to Waimea, Kaua'i, fourteen months after its first visit:

> Here are many of these good Folks both Men and Women about the Ship miserably afflicted with the Venereal disease, which they accuse us of introducing among them during our last visit, they say it does not go away, that they have no Antidote for it, but that they grow worse and worse, explaining the different symptoms in the progress of the disorder till it totally destroys them. Captain Cook did take such preventive methods as I hop'd and flatter'd myself would prove effectual, but our Seamen are in these matters so infernal and dissolute a Crew that for the gratification of the present passion that affects them they would entail universal destruction upon the whole of the Human species. . . . It is certainly a most unfortunate and ever to be lamented incident, here's a most miserable curse entailed upon these poor Creatures which can never end but with the general dissolution of Nature.[33]

With the important exception of *Discovery*'s surgeon David Samwell, most of Clerke's fellow officers shared his belief. Lieutenant King's comment, entered in his log on 1 March 1779, about the man from Kaua'i who, without being asked, "told us that we had left a disorder amongst their women," from which he himself was suffering, has already been quoted in full. The poor man's "feeling terms" convinced King that "we were the authors of the disease in this place." The authors of this "sad havoc" brought troubles to some of their shipmates as well: in an unwanted form of reciprocity, the infected women, as generous with their newly acquired germs as with their favors, gave over both of the venereal diseases to many of the expedition's sailors who were free of them when the ships first reached Kaua'i in 1778.[34]

Captain Clerke's remarks about the virulence with which the venereal distemper attacked Hawaiians give further support to the belief that it was new to them. He explained the phenomenon according to the medical philosophy of his century:

> That it should rage more violently, and its dreadful Symptoms operate more expeditiously here than at the Friendly or Society Isles [Tonga and Tahiti] I suppose may be attributed in a great measure to the quantity of Salt these people make use of in their customary diet.[35]

Today we can recognize in such fulminating symptoms the responses of a population not to salt but to microbes they had not encountered before. Syphilis had produced similar "expeditious" effects on Europeans in the sixteenth century, either because the disease was only recently introduced among them (by Columbus' sailors coming home from America, according to one hoary theory) or (according to more modern thoughts) because increasingly virulent strains of the syphilis spirochete were being evolved during that period of intense social upheaval. In 1778 the venereal diseases were newly introduced among inhabitants of Tonga and Tahiti also, but the effects of syphilis spirochetes there may have been reduced to some extent by the fact that many people in the islands of the South Pacific were also infected with the spirochetes that cause yaws. Because the two species of spirochetes are closely related and cause very similar lesions, modern epidemiologists believe that infection with yaws helps to immunize an individual against syphilis.[36]

After reading many statements of early explorers, such as those of Clerke and King, after learning that exactly the same series of sickening events occurred at all the Pacific islands visited by European ships, both before and after Cook's three voyages, one can hardly doubt that Cook's sailors, because they were the first foreigners to come to Hawai'i of whom we have a record, must have transmitted the venereal diseases to the people of these islands. And yet, although we must regret the effects these diseases were to cause among Hawaiians, we cannot honestly accuse those common sailors from Europe and America of being *willing* agents of destruction when they themselves knew nothing about the harmful germs they carried and were even less aware of the terrible effects those microbes would have upon the peoples of the Pacific—or, indeed, upon themselves, eventually.

Only recently have writers upon this subject been sufficiently informed to realize that the introduction of all kinds of new infections was an inevitable consequence of contact between seafarers from countries in which those diseases were endemic and healthy islanders whose isolation had spared them any acquaintance with those contagions. These recent writers, instructed in the principles of microbiology, epidemiology, psychology, and sociology, concede that no regulations could possibly have saved Hawai'i's people from contracting the many different communicable diseases for which Cook's sailors were infectious carriers. In the course of the expedition's two visits, some Hawaiians contracted not only the venereal diseases but also infections caused by tubercle bacilli, streptococci, enteric pathogens, at least the commoner viruses, and probably other microbes as well. This conclusion is supported by the fact that these pathogens are "normally" present in the bodies of at least a few individuals in any "normal population" as large as was the complement of sailors aboard *Resolution* and *Discovery.*

We need not wonder how those mariners could have achieved such microbiological mayhem during so short a stay. Think of them, turned loose on Waimea's sandy beach or on Kealakekua's rocky strand, as they coughed, hawked, and spat when the impulse arose, just as they and their contemporaries did at home in Europe and America. Picture them urinating and defecating almost wherever and certainly whenever they pleased, without bothering (as Hawaiians did) to dig catholes in which to bury their bodies' dangerous wastes. Then as now—as all too often the people-pigs among us forget— those unhygienic practices were exceedingly hazardous to the health of everyone exposed to them.

Today, as we lament the deadly effects of Hawaiians' contact with foreigners, we must also accept their inevitability—and not only for Hawai'i's natives. The people of all other isolated societies suffered exactly the same consequences. Even late in the twentieth century, despite all that has been learned about epidemiology, isolated tribes in South America, Africa, and Papua New Guinea are still being attacked by microorganisms taken among them unwittingly by visitors coming from places outside their borders. Nowadays, as in the eighteenth century, the only way to protect primitive peoples from the afflictions of "civilization" is to prevent them from having any contact at all with its representatives.

Throughout the nineteenth century, however, before the role of microorganisms as causative agents of infectious diseases was established and the varied manners of their transmission were understood, most writers about Hawai'i who discussed the delicate subject of venereal diseases were caught up in prejudices and polemics. According to their sympathies (and usually with complete disregard for all the sources of information available to them), either they accused Captain Cook of criminal carelessness in *permitting* his sailors to transmit the venereal diseases to innocent Hawaiians, or they defended him, with mindless devotion, as a great man much traduced, who did everything in his power to prevent the introduction of those foul contagions, only to be defeated in that endeavor by his "dissolute" sailors and all those "awful immoral" women. Not one of these writers, strange to say, seems to have understood the human animal for what it is—or to have accepted the basic fact (which surely cannot have escaped the notice of all but the most academic of writers) that in most people the sexual urge is an irresistible force beyond control by commandments and good intentions.

Some propagandists, resorting to a logic based on emotions rather than documents, went so far as to accuse Captain Cook personally of being as immoral and wicked as the worst of his sailors. Kamakau's colossal snarl, published in *Ka Nupepa Kuoko'a* for 16 February 1867, set the tone for these attacks:

> [Captain Cook] had been but a short time in Hawaii when God punished him for his sin. It was not the fault of the Hawaiian people that they held him sacred and paid him honor as a god worshiped by the Hawaiian people. But because he killed the people he was killed by them without mercy, and his entrails were used to rope off the arena, and the palms of his hands used for fly swatters at a cock fight. Such is the end of a transgressor. The seeds that he planted here have sprouted, grown, and become the parents of others that have caused the decrease of the native population. . . . Such are gonorrhea, and other social disease; prostitution; the illusion of his being a god [which led to] worship of him; fleas and mosquitoes; epidemics. All of these

things have led to changes in the air which we breathe; the coming of things which weaken the body; changes in plant life; changes in religion; changes in the art of healing; and changes in the laws by which the land is governed.[37]

Bigots of this breed are busy still in Hawai'i: determinedly uninformed, certitudinous beyond instruction, they prefer to blame the blameless captain for the faults of commoner men and common women.

Indeed, even in the 1990s some Hawaiian activists are so bitter that they accuse *all* haoles, without exception, of deliberately destroying *kānaka maoli,* the "true," or "genuine," or "native" Hawaiian people (the present fashion for distinguishing them from all alien intruders—who, by implication, are somewhat less than perfect). One of these revisionists has summed up the entire course of Hawaiian history since 1778 in a single sentence: "Dose focking [sic] haoles: dey come heah, dey keel us all off, dey steal all ouah lan'." She may be right about the end result of Hawaiians' contacts with haoles and their taking ways. But she is most unfair in her unwillingness to interpret the events of the past in terms of the knowledge of the people in the past, who, all unwittingly, achieved the effects she decries.

ᘓᘓᘓᘓ

The second group of writers insisted that the venereal diseases were already present among Hawaiians before 1778, and that therefore Captain Cook and his sailors were not responsible for introducing those infections. David Samwell, surgeon's mate aboard HMS *Resolution* until Dr. Anderson died of tuberculosis on 3 August 1778, when Captain Cook promoted him to be surgeon of *Discovery,* was the first to propose this face-saving argument in print, but he was not the only member of the expedition to believe it. The thesis was a persuasive one, for his time. He maintained that the sailors who were allowed to go ashore, after physical inspection by the ships' surgeons, showed no symptoms of disease and that the testimony of Hawaiians (especially of that pain-racked man who spoke with Lieutenant King at Waimea) was unreliable—not because they lied but because they answered inquiries put to them with replies intended to please their questioners and because Hawaiian physicians "seemed to have an established mode of treatment; which by no means implied, that it was a recent complaint among them, much less that it was introduced only a few months before."[38]

For these reasons (and perhaps for others he did not mention), Samwell thought himself "warranted in saying, that there are by no means sufficient proofs of our having first introduced it; but that, on the contrary . . . they were afflicted with it before we discovered these islands."[39] Samwell's argument was readily accepted by Englishmen who admired Captain Cook, and by all those who wished to absolve Britain's clean-cut sailor lads of all censure for "entailing upon Hawaiians so dreadful a curse." But that kind of absolution is a matter of faith that in this case is not sustained by facts. Moreover, it is weakened by Samwell's prejudices.

Samwell can hardly be criticized for not knowing what we know today about the etiology and epidemiology of venereal diseases. To be specific, he did not realize (or possibly he chose to ignore, as Cook did not) the fact that some people who appear to be healthy can be carriers of viable microbes that may infect other persons. Yet Captain Cook, who was not a physician, did deduce this fact from his observations upon the varieties of human specimens who traveled with him on those voyages of exploration—and, most pertinently, upon their experiences in successive ports of call. But Surgeon Samwell, like most physicians of his era, did not possess Cook's powers of reasoning. Proof of the existence of the "carrier state" in humans and animals would not be achieved until more than a hundred years after 1778. In short, mere visual examination of sailors' genitals, which Samwell and his fellow surgeons relied on in 1778, did not determine whether or not they were still infectious. That determination can be reached definitively only by modern laboratory tests.

And, of course, Samwell did not know that centuries of isolation had spared Hawaiians from not only the venereal ailments but also from all of the major infectious diseases that afflicted Europeans during the eighteenth century. He can be censured, however, for not admitting that feckless men like Will Bradley who, "knowing himself to be injured with the Veneral disorder," willfully disobeyed Captain Cook's regulations. Furthermore, Samwell's motives in writing his little tract are questionable. His regard for Captain Cook amounted to veneration, as the loyal Welshman himself disclosed in a letter to a friend on 26 February 1781: "His great Qualities I admired beyond any thing I can express—I gloried in him—and my heart bleeds to this Day whenever I think of his Fate."[40]

Samwell was very much aware, too, of the foolish controversy that excited Europe's chauvinist intellectuals after the survivors of Captain Cook's expedition finally got home to England in 1780. Who were responsible, those closet philosophers demanded, for introducing the venereal distemper into Tahiti? Were they Britain's men, sailing on *Dolphin* with Captain Samuel Wallis, when they discovered that lovely island on 18 June 1767? Were they sailors from France aboard *Boudeuse,* commanded by Captain Louis de Bougainville, who discovered Tahiti for themselves on 2 April 1768—and who called it "La Nouvelle Cythère" because of the boundless delights they enjoyed in that island inhabited by tawny sons and daughters of Venus? Or were they the latecomers from Spain who, aboard Don Domingo Boenechea's frigate *Aguila,* reached Tahiti on 8 November 1773, intending to found a colony there?

Today we can be sure that, if Britain's sailors were in fact the first foreigners to reach Tahiti, then they must be charged with having introduced the venereal diseases among Tahiti's people when they introduced Tahiti to the world. And we can be equally sure that the sailors of France and of Spain—as well as those of every other nation who touched at New Cythera—contributed their shares of germs and genes to the people who dwelled in "the Amorous Isles."

Naturally, in the 1770s and 1780s no honor-defending nationalist could endure the thought that his countrymen sowed disease and "sin" wherever they went. Few Europeans were as honest, or as outspoken, as Denis Diderot. But then he was no chauvinist. He knew very well how sailors from any country behaved, at home as well as abroad. His warning to Tahitians, that they ought better to weep over the coming of France's explorers in 1768 than grieve over their departure, was advice that Polynesians never heard—and would not have heeded.

Neither did Europe's disputatious academics. Once again almost everyone blamed everyone else, just as they had done in the sixteenth century, when the first pandemic of syphilis raged through Europe: Frenchmen then called it "the Spanish evil," Italians named it "the Gallic sickness," Germans dubbed it "the Italian ill," and Englishmen, with their genius for bland generalizations, settled upon "the Great Pox" for an epithet. Knowing all this, Dr. Samwell tried to spare his hero the opprobrium that was being directed upon Wallis, de Bougainville, and Boenechea. Samwell may be esteemed for his loyalty, but his arguments must be rejected because they were both erroneous and partisan.

Not so easily dismissed, however, are the statements made by

France's Captain de La Pérouse and his chief surgeon, M. Rollin. During the few hours they spent on the leeward shore of Maui in 1786, they were convinced that the miserable Hawaiians living there were seriously afflicted with syphilis in its late stages, as well as with a condition the Frenchmen thought was leprosy. As has been discussed in an earlier essay, their comments are puzzling because they were not confirmed by observations from any other Westerners who followed them. Nonetheless, they cannot be ignored entirely. The French explorers may have come upon a forlorn colony of syphilitics and lepers who must have been infected before Cook's sailors reached Hawai'i. Or, possibly, as is suggested in that earlier essay, those few Hawaiians may have been afflicted with an assortment of other diseases that together mimicked the symptoms of syphilis and of leprosy.

The third group of writers, mercifully a small one, was little more than a clutch of caponized ostriches, with heads thrust deep into the sands of prudery. Ignoring the raw facts of life, in which lusts play a very large part, these innocents insisted that anyone who claimed that the venereal diseases were introduced by Cook's sailors or were already present among Hawaiians was sadly mistaken. These sheltered apologists, Defenders of Virtue, products of gelded Christianity in the Victorian Age, simply would not believe that some of Hawai'i's women behaved like wantons and that most of Cook's sailors did not comport themselves like bishops. Knowing nothing about the pathology of infections, and pathetically ignorant of mariners' morality, they conjured up yaws, or yellow fever, or bubonic plague, or almost anything else in the way of a nonvenereal ailment in their determination to preserve untarnished the shining name of COOK and the purity of Hawai'i's women. Still other defenders maintained that the venereal diseases "arose *de novo*" among libertine Polynesians. One of the most recent of these naive strainings of the imagination was proposed by an Anglican prelate in Honolulu in 1928, during the sesquicentennial celebrations commemorating the British expedition's visit to the Hawaiian Islands.[41]

The effects of the British voyagers' visit upon Hawaiians were profound. The very structure of their society was shattered, even as, all too often, their bodies sickened and died from the ravages of infections new to them.

When the British explorers sailed away for the last time they left behind them diseases and doubts. The diseases, not all of which were venereal, spread at alarming rates through the sociable people, affecting not only adults but their offspring as well. "The abundant stock of children"[42] that Captain Clerke had seen was soon reduced: never again would indigenous Hawaiians' birth rates exceed their death rates. Hoping to stop the spread of these foreign sicknesses, native physicians tried to find new medicines with which to treat them, if not new methods of diagnosis or new prayers for placating offended deities.

Small changes in the native way of life foretold greater changes to come. The most obvious innovations replaced implements of wood and stone with iron or steel axes, hatchets, knives, daggers, spear heads, and fishhooks. More subtle, and much more insidious, were the new thoughts stirring in the minds of the people, whether of high station or low. They began to question the kapus which bound them to each other, to the priests and chiefs, and to the many gods who until then had ruled the narrow realm of the eight islands beneath the Eye of Kāne. After the people at Waimea and Kealakekua learned to know the British, they said: "These are not gods; these are men, white men from the land of Kahiki."[43] When they saw how white men and Hawaiians together broke so many kapus without divine punishment, they no longer went in fear of the gods. Thereafter they feared only priests and chiefs, who were only men; and thereupon the authority of priests and chiefs began to crumble slowly away. As respect for them weakened, belief in the gods was doomed. The gods did not die: slowly they withdrew from the people, who no longer honored them. But when, at last, they departed, nothing was left to guide the people, to give them rules to live by and purpose in living, to hold them together in the Four Kingdoms of Hawai'i nei.

Yet not all of the effects caused by the foreigners were blighting. Among the good things they left behind were tools of iron and steel, mirrors of glass, pieces of cloth: these objects, these treasures to Hawaiians at first, told them that beyond the far horizons lay wondrous countries inhabited by other kinds of people, who made much greater marvels, such as those they had seen and touched and coveted aboard the visitors' ships.

The explorers from Britain also left other mementos of their stay, although they did not see these, and probably never wasted a thought on them: the few half-haole children who were born to some women from Waimea and the communities around Kealakekua Bay—and who survived beyond infancy. Samuel Kamakau, writing in 1867, disdainfully called these children " *'opala haole,* foreign rubbish."[44] Possibly some of those infants, as unwanted as rubbish, were killed at birth. Others would have died soon after birth, just as children of unmixed blood succumbed to the new sicknesses, or to neglect. But a few managed to survive beyond that dangerous period. Accepted and loved by their mothers' families, in the manner of generous Hawaiians, and with their assortment of attributes and features, some of which might have recalled the far-wandering fathers, they grew up to be the first representatives of the "Part-Hawaiians" who are preserving now some of the ancestral genes.

ᘓᘓᘓᘓ

Aboard *Resolution* and *Discovery* officers and sailors rejoiced at having escaped the fate of Captain Cook and the four marines, whose bodies lay in the cold depths of Kealakekua Bay. The living were glad to be alive, moving once more toward home, after making a last attempt to find the Northern Passage.

Captain Clerke, having become the expedition's commander, noted how his sailors had changed:

> That idea of turning Indian ["going native"] which was once so prevalent among them as to give us a great deal of trouble is now quite subsided, and you could not inflict a greater punishment upon those who were the warmest advocates of this curious innovation in life than to oblige them to take that step which 16 or 18 months ago seemed to be the ultimate wish of their Hearts, & which some of them went so far as to attempt at the risk of death itself.[45]

Poor Captain Clerke. He, too, would "come home to port no more." On 22 August 1779—the day after the expedition, driven once again from the Arctic Sea by winter's advance, sighted the coast of Kamchatka—tuberculosis, the enemy he could not escape, killed him.

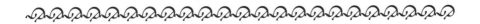

Six

Exploration and Exploitation: 1786–1825

"If Otaheite is call'd the Queen of the S<u>o</u> sea Isles," Lieutenant James King wrote when HMS *Resolution* and HMS *Discovery* departed for the last time from Kaua'i in March 1779, "& the Society Isles the most amiable group, Owhyhee may be term'd the King of the S<u>o</u> sea, & these Islands the most capable of being made useful."[1]

Lieutenant King's appraisal of Owhyhee's value to Europeans did not appear in the official narrative of Captain Cook's third and last voyage to the Pacific Ocean. When they read the text in the three large quarto volumes that presented the approved distillation of all those ships' logs and impounded private journals, most Englishmen searched for descriptions of the exciting adventures in distant parts of the world and accounts of the titillating encounters with "noble savages" and tempting women that remained in Canon John Douglas's discreet redactions. Righteous Christian folk, sternly rejecting the perverse wickednesses of freethinkers as much as the profligacy of sailors, deplored the decline and fall of Captain Cook and prayed for the sinning heathen who dwelled in those benighted albeit beautiful isles.

But London's merchants, thoroughly practical men, studied very carefully the navigators' charts in the folio *Atlas of Illustrations* that supplemented the three volumes of narration. And they too felt the thrill of discovery when they found, in the last paragraph on the last page of Volume II, in stately measured phrases purporting to be Captain Cook's, although actually written by Canon Douglas, the Admiralty's tribute not to the glamor of the Sandwich Islands but to their convenient position in the earth's broadest sea:

Perhaps there were few on board who now lamented our having failed in our endeavours to find a Northern Passage homeward, last summer.

To this disappointment we owed our having it in our power to revisit the Sandwich Islands, and to enrich our voyage with a discovery which, though the last, seemed in many respects, to be the most important that had hitherto been made by Europeans, throughout the extent of the Pacific Ocean.[2]

In itself such praise for the high island of Hawai'i would not have aroused the interest of those far-seeing men of business. That was stirred only in the concluding pages of Volume III, where Lieutenant King's narrative (transmuted by Canon Douglas) told them how eagerly Chinese merchants in Macao bought furs and pelts the explorers had picked up, almost incidentally, as mementos of Nootka and Prince William's Sound in northwestern America.

Within the year several of London's traders had sent two ships into the wide empty hemisphere that Captain Cook had opened up and charted for their exploitation. They chose Nathaniel Portlock and George Dixon, both of whom had sailed with Cook on his last voyage, to command *King George,* a vessel of 320 tons burden, and *Queen Charlotte,* a snow of 200 tons. Between 1785 and 1788 these ships, favored by trade winds, shuttled forth and back across the Pacific, by way of the well-placed Sandwich Islands, carrying furs from the shores of northwestern America to the teeming coastal cities of China. Pelts from Alaska, from western Canada, and from the lands now called Washington and Oregon were exchanged for teas, silks, and porcelains of the Celestial Empire. And from there, richly laden with such treasures of the Orient, other ships sailed home to England and to profits most rewarding.

Attracted by such success, European and American competitors hurried to take their shares of it. The great era of the China Trade began. Although in the general preoccupation with the rewards of commerce no one foresaw this consequence, when those merchant ships moved into the Pacific they carried with them the seeds of death and destruction for the hapless people of Polynesia. Miss Charlotte Beverley's screams for revenge were about to be answered. And more than just the few Hawaiian warriors who killed Captain Cook were going to suffer for that bloody deed. "Descend Nemesis!" implored the maiden fury, anguished in London-town:

> Descend Nemesis! and in wrath divine,
> Punish the horrid wretches for their crime.
> Roll! Thunders roll! and skies upon them pour,

The greatest plagues that vengeance has in store.
Britons arise! and animated save
The fame of COOK from drear oblivion's grave . . .[3]

The French government also, not willing to be outdone by the British foe and determined not to be shut out, sent their official expedition to explore the Pacific, in the name of Science and for the glory of France and of Louis XVI, her most Christian King. Under the command of Captain the Count Jean-François de Galaup de La Pérouse, the frigates *Astrolabe* and *Boussole* sailed from Brest on 1 August 1785.

Toward the end of May 1786, having made the long track north-by-west from Easter Island, the French explorers raised the island of Hawai'i. La Pérouse's description of their approach to the neighboring island of Maui captured as has no other voyager's account the joy and the yearning of weary mariners when, at last, after weeks of hardship on the pitiless sea, they arrive before the very portals of Paradise:

> We beheld water falling in cascades from the mountains, and running in streams to the sea, after having watered the habitations of the natives, which are so numerous that a space of three or four leagues may be taken for a single village. . . . The trees which crowned the mountains, and the verdure of the banana plants that surrounded the habitations, produced inexpressible charms to our senses, but the sea beat upon the coast with the utmost violence, and kept us in the situation of Tantalus, to desire and devour with our eyes what it was impossible for us to attain.[4]

After Captain Cook's survivors departed in 1779, La Pérouse and his associates were the second group of Europeans to call at the Sandwich Islands and leave a record of their visit. They stayed for only a few hours, at a cove on Maui's southwestern coast now called La Pérouse Bay. Hot, dry, almost waterless, "made hideous by an ancient lava flow," as La Pérouse described it, and inhabited by a meager group of people and animals all so foully diseased that the Frenchmen could not get away from them fast enough, this ghastly place was a great disappointment after the verdant prospect that had so enchanted them only the day before.

Nevertheless, the visitors dutifully observed the repulsive people, the measly hogs and mangy dogs, before fleeing back to their ships. M. Rollin, *Boussole*'s surgeon-major, was convinced that "the leprosy and venereal disease . . . the most humiliating and most destructive [scourges] with which the human race are afflicted," were both prevalent and virulent among Maui's people. "The advanced state of the disorder" led him to believe that syphilis "existed in these islands before the discovery of them" by Captain Cook.[5]

Appalled by what they found on Maui, they did not care to set foot on any of its neighboring islands: within two days they sailed past them, escaped into the open sea, and set a course for Alaska. Unlike Cook and his company, they did not return to the Sandwich Islands when they completed their survey of North America's western coasts.

ởởởở

On 24 May 1786, four days before La Pérouse's expedition appeared off Maui's southwestern shores, Captain Portlock aboard *King George* and Captain Dixon aboard *Queen Charlotte* made a much more pleasant landing on the southeastern coast of O'ahu. The British ships were lying in the lee of Koko Head when *Boussole* and *Astrolabe* sailed past O'ahu, too far out to be seen. As the first foreigners to land on that southern part of O'ahu, the British traders were received with much interest by the friendly natives. The Hawaiians had heard about Captain Cook and his great ships; and some of them may have known that, in 1779, Captain Clerke, Lieutenant Gore, and Lieutenant King, together with a number of sailors from *Resolution* and *Discovery,* had spent a few hours at Waimea Bay, at the farther end of O'ahu. Although southern O'ahu's people were willing to supply the English traders with food and water, the ships, hove-to about a mile offshore, lay too far out for ready provisioning. Portlock decided to sail for Ni'ihau, where, he remembered, yams and water could be obtained with relative ease. He went regretfully, having seen enough of "Woahoo," as he wrote later, to declare that it was "the finest island in the group, and the most capable of being turned to advantage, were it settled by Europeans, than any of the rest; there being scarcely a spot which does not appear fertile."[6]

Although Portlock, Dixon, and La Pérouse were the only captains who wrote accounts of their visits to the Sandwich Islands in the years immediately following Cook's discovery of this archipelago, quite possibly they were not the first foreigners after 1779 to take advantage of the group's location. Kamakau, borrowing from

Pogue's *History* published in 1858, mentioned a number of ships, giving details about them that he had no reason to invent:

> Not five years [after Cook's visit] there arrived at Kauai a boat called *Olomakani* or *Olo* because it was the first boat to bring strings of beads (called *olo*) as ornaments for the neck. Next there landed at Hawaii the ship called *Kanikani,* which brought the first knives called *kanikani* and *hanaoi.* . . . Then came the *Kane,* the boat that took Kai-ana Ahu-ula to foreign lands. . . . Most of these boats were ships of war or ships looking for new lands. Some among them were friendly, others were bent on destroying men and governments.[7]

Kamakau's names for these (and other) vessels were fanciful appellations given them by Hawaiians, not those by which they were known to their crews. His *Kane,* for example, actually was *Nootka,* a trading ship of British registry, commanded by Captain John Meares, who did take her to Kaua'i in 1787. She can be identified because Meares, too, wrote a book about his experiences, in which Ka'iana 'Ahu'ula, a young chief from Kaua'i—and the first Hawaiian tourist to travel abroad in first-class accommodations—played a prominent part.

Between 1786 and 1799 inclusive, according to Bernice Judd's annotated list of *Voyages to Hawaii Before 1860,* forty-five different foreign vessels visited the Hawaiian Islands whose arrivals or departures are recorded in accounts written either by their masters or by other mariners who were present in Hawaiian waters at about the same time. Every one of those forty-five vessels, and every man aboard her, meant some kind of trouble for the Hawaiian people:

> Aboard these ships [wrote the Reverend John Pogue in 1858] were all manner of men with all manner of faces. If these men were to separate according to their consciences, there would be only two groups; those who kept the commandments of God, and those who did not. . . .
> . . . Some were good, some were of an evil disposition. The greatest benefit derived therefrom is the word of God; other justifiable benefits were: clothing, iron, whale oil and its products, things which make for a better life among the people. The deadly and evil impediments were: rum, gin, barley [brandy?], tobacco, and the many incumbrances and sensuous amusements.[8]

ararar

Following in the wake of explorers and fur traders came ships of other kinds, bearing men who expressed identical needs although they may have pursued different goals: merchants looking for sandal-wood; whalermen hunting for oil; captains of warships imposing law and order upon primitive islanders to the advantage of foreigners; even, on occasion, pirates with stolen ships and little booty, or eager scientists collecting everything they could lay their hands on and carry away. The Sandwich Islands became one great caravanserai for flitting ships; and, without being asked, Hawaiians were thrust into many new roles—as hosts, chandlers, panders, and whores, fore-most among them, to mariners from countries half a world away in space and 5,000 years ahead in time.

Once again Hawai'i's islands and their people were subjected to a new invasion and another kind of conquest. But this time, under this new sort of attack, Hawaiians had no refuge to which they might run. Whether or not they intended to be so, all visitors, since the beginning, have been agents of change for Hawai'i. These changes have not yet ended, nor will they cease until the last restless traveler has reached those shores, or the islands themselves have sunk back into the sea from which they emerged. In consequence of this last and continued invasion, Hawai'i's people, its plants and animals, the very appearance of its islands, have been altered forever.

To native Hawaiians, the nineteenth century was a time of trou-bles, a time of dying. As the people of old perished, and their shades went to join those of their ancestors, "there to sleep the long sleep of Niolopua," the islands they left behind gave room to new breeds of men coming to fill their places. Almost everything those Hawaiians had known, every living creature, from insects in the soil to birds in the air, would be affected. And many other things around them, from the foods they ate to the colors they saw in men's eyes and skins, would be different. Even the hills and the mountains would change, not at first in their shapes but in the green garb they assumed, fashioned of new species of trees, shrubs, vines, and grasses.

ぐぐぐぐぐ

Hawaiians learned many lessons from foreigners. Not all captains were as considerate as James Cook, or as diabolical as Simon Metcalfe, who perpetrated the Massacre of Olowalu, in 1790. And, assuredly, not all Hawaiians were as generous as Kalani'ōpu'u, "the King of Owhyhee," or as proud as Kame'eiamoku, that vengeful chief of Kona, who killed Simon Metcalfe's son and all but one of his shipmates. Common sailors, differing not a whit from crew to crew, served mutual interests with natives in the indulging of their common appetites; and the usual run of ships' mates and lesser officers were not above meeting both natives and sailors at that human level. As John Boit, fifth mate on the American trader *Columbia,* observed in 1792, when welcome hordes of women boarded her while she lay off the island of Hawai'i, "not many of the . . . crew proved to be *Josephs.*" Boit, seventeen years old at the time, responded like a true sailor to "these beautiful isles, the inhabitants of which appeared to me to be the happiest people in the world. Indeed, there was something in them so frank and chearful that you could not help feeling prepossessed in their favor."[9]

Captains, on the other hand, weighted with responsibilities, looked upon all Hawaiians as creatures to be used. Inasmuch as their chiefs had been using them for centuries, commoners never thought to complain. Captains and chiefs alike exploited them, as provisioners, laborers, servants, prostitutes, and, after a time, as deck-hands shanghaied or recruited to replace crewmen who had deserted or died.[10] In exchange for these varied services, foreigners usually paid in goods or in coins, with incidental supplements in germs and genes.

Islanders, in their turn, having lost their awe of haoles—as, in the beginning, they called all strangers—looked upon them as providers of things they wanted. Commoners were happy to receive tools or bits of iron (that could be shaped into fishhooks, chisels, or nails), pieces of cloth, and pretty trinkets. Chiefs accepted all these things and more—especially guns, powder, and ball, which helped them to wage their interminable wars, while they coveted (but did not get) ships which could transport soldiers from one island to another.

By 1802 John Turnbull, in charge of cargo and trade for the British ship *Margaret,* found Honolulu's natives much shrewder bargainers than he had expected, charging higher prices than he liked. He blamed Americans for this, of course, yet gave them grudging (and prophetic) respect, acknowledging that they "will do more than any other nation in raising [Hawaiians] to an eminent degree of civilization."[11] Gone forever were the good old days of Captain Cook's time, when a single nail could buy a hog six feet long.

American traders were not the only reasons for the high cost of haole living. Early in 1789, several months before the first American ship reached the Sandwich Islands, Captain William Douglas of the

British vessel *Iphigenia* encountered a most unlikely price-setter at Waimea, Kaua'i. "A couple of hatchets, or 18 inches of bar iron, was expected even for a hog but of a middle size," complained Douglas. "This exorbitant disposition arose principally from the suggestion of a boy, whose name was Samuel Hitchcock, who had run away from Captain Colnett [of the *Prince of Wales*] and was become a great favorite with Taheo himself [Ka'eo, the ruling chief of Kaua'i]."[12]

By 1804, Russian Captain Urey Lisiansky noted, cloth and items of clothing had replaced iron as favored trade goods.[13] And Archibald Campbell remembered, from his stay in Honolulu in 1809–1810:

> These islanders have acquired many of the useful arts and are making rapid progress toward civilization. Much must be ascribed, no doubt, to their natural ingenuity and universal industry, but great part of the merit must also be ascribed to the unceasing exertions of Tamaahmaah, whose enlarged mind has enabled him to appreciate the advantages resulting from an intercourse with Europeans.[14]

Fortunately for everyone, relationships between foreigners and natives usually were friendly. On only a few occasions did greed or spite lead to violence and murder.

Premeditated attacks on foreigners were surprisingly rare, considering the relative helplessness of visitors and the incentives for assault and robbery they offered. Despite the wealth of treasures that foreigners carried on their persons and in their ships, despite frequent provocations by common sailors if not by captains, Hawaiians proved to be remarkably restrained, even long suffering, in their meetings with haoles. They could have been saved from endless troubles if, like bellicose Fijians or fierce Samoans, they had massacred every haole who ever attempted to set foot upon any Hawaiian shore. Instead, they rushed to the beaches, welcoming foreigners as though they were bearers of gladsome tidings rather than unwitting carriers of diseases and disasters. After 1796—when Hawaiians made the last *planned* assault upon visitors—foreigners, and Hawaiians, would be murdered often enough, but always they died in consequence of acts of unpremeditated violence. Crimes of passion, drunken brawls, sudden rages, burglings and robberies, smoldering antipathies took their victims, as they still do even today.

Although Captain Cook found a people living in a "stone age culture," as later anthropologists would call it, by 1820 many members of that primitive society were adjusting intelligently to the impact of the new civilization being introduced among them.

Western culture affected Hawaiians both physically and psychologically, forcing them to make a very wide range of responses, and to a degree almost inconceivable today. In general, Hawaiians adjusted to the new culture with remarkable success in every way but one. This one exception—their susceptibility to introduced infectious diseases and their inability to survive the invisible enemies that caused them—lay beyond the power of mind or body to control. And therefore, because it was beyond control, so mysterious, so implacable, so powerful, eventually it affected all others of their responses, turning them in upon themselves at immeasurable cost to the spirit.

❦❦❦❦

With no other instruction than the example and the needs of foreigners to guide them, yet with an enterprise their visitors both deplored and commended, shrewd chiefs and clever commoners learned to set up markets where their produce could be bartered for trade goods; to sell their women as whores, their men as laborers; to put an adjustable price upon each article of commerce, according to the basic principle of supply and demand; to anticipate the requirements of an increasing number of visitors by growing greater quantities of foodstuffs; and to develop new businesses that would attract more vessels to the several island ports. At first these new ventures were related primarily to provisioning ships and entertaining their crews. But, as the years passed, and more foreigners discovered the islands' safest offshore anchorages and their one available sheltered harbor, Hawaiians flocked in great numbers to those favored places and, by their presence, enlarged fishing camps into ugly little towns. By 1800 most foreign vessels called at one port on the leeward coast of each major island: Kealakekua Bay on Hawai'i, Lahaina on Maui, Waimea on Kaua'i, and, busiest of all, Honolulu on O'ahu.

❦❦❦❦

Honolulu exists because foreigners created it, on the muddy shore beside the tiny harbor of Kou. Before foreigners arrived at Kou, in their great white-winged ships, most commoners avoided that little pocket of nothing, that pouch on O'ahu's bottom, which even coral shunned because of the mud and the fresh water issuing from Nuʻuanu's stream. Some sun-baked fisherfolk lived there, in thatched huts shaded by the few scraggly trees which like such hot, dry places, and in the little community of Kapuʻukolo, close by the mouth of Nuʻuanu stream.

But the chiefs could not always shun the land of Kou. There stood the famed heiau of Pākākā, the temple served by the most powerful priests of Oʻahu, its high walls "adorned all around with the heads of men offered in sacrifice." Also in Kou was "the great ʻulu maika place for the gathering of the chiefs." At certain times of the year these lordly ones, attended by retainers and servants, would meet at Kou to settle problems of governance, to learn from the priests the wishes of the gods. When that consulting was done, they would drink ʻawa, play kōnane, bowl on the ʻulu maika field, or ride their boards in the surf of Māmala, just as, many generations before, the chiefess Māmala had enjoyed doing with her first husband, the shark-man Ouha.

Commoners agreed that Kou might be a nice place to visit, very briefly, provided you attended a chief who would protect you. But they also felt that no one with any sense could want to live there permanently. It was too hot, too dry, and, beyond all doubt, too dangerous. "Man-eating sharks," as people called the priests of Pākākā and their prowling minions, hunted prey in the land of Kou, to offer up in sacrifice within the ramparts of the heiau. The waters of Māmala, although they might be home to sharks of the sea, were safer than was the solid earth of Kou.

Southern Oʻahu's chiefs and commoners much preferred to live at Waikīkī, with its groves of tall coconut palms, and its swamp lands in which taro could be grown and captive fish. Waikīkī was made comfortable by "the cool sea-breezes of ʻAinahau" and the clean ocean beyond. There, without fear of sharks, whether animal or priestly, a man could fish, or swim, or, while lying on a long, narrow, heavy board, ride the waves from their cresting on the reef to their breaking on the wide sandy beach.

Other people chose to dwell in the green valleys of Nuʻuanu, Pauoa, and Mānoa, where the water of Kāne flowed in plenty. At the time when Kakuhihewa was king, amid the taro lands of Nuʻuanu about a mile inland from Kou (near the place where today School Street crosses Liliha Street) lived a high chief named Honolulu. Perhaps because he was a good chief, "a sheltering presence" to his people, or perhaps because his household stood within protecting groves of koa and kukui trees, this portion of Oʻahu's district of Kona was known as Honolulu, which is to say, "an abundance of peace."

Low against Oʻahu's soaring mountains, hidden behind spray tossed up by the surf crashing upon its reef, the harbor of Kou was not easily seen from foreigners' vessels out at sea. Sailors from Captain Portlock's ship almost discovered it in June 1786. Hoping to find a safe anchorage, Portlock sent third mate Samuel Hayward in a sail-rigged longboat to explore Oʻahu's southern coast. Hayward's search took him around Diamond Head as far west as Waikīkī, less than two miles short of Kou. Because Hayward found no harbor, and Waikīkī's bight was no better than were the roads off King George's Bay, in the lee of Koko Head, Portlock decided to sail for Niʻihau.

During the next eight years many foreign ships sailed past Kou without finding it. Then, at last, a very whimsical fate gave the prize to Captain William Brown, an English trader. On 12 November 1794 he brought his *Jackall* in, through the high surf of Mamala, through the harbor's narrow throat, into the calm waters of Kou, stilled between reef and shore. Later that same day *Prince Lee Boo,* commanded by Brown's partner and friend, Captain Gordon, dropped anchor beside *Jackall,* only a short cable's length from the huts of Kou. On 3 December an American trader, Captain John Kendrick, master of *Lady Washington,* joined the two in their haven.

To them, and to all seafarers who followed, this little inlet in Oʻahu's southern shore was a discovery second in importance only to that of the Sandwich Islands themselves. For Kou provided the only safe harbor in all Hawaiʻi—and, therefore, in all the wide expanse of the northern Pacific Ocean. Another and much larger anchorage, about five miles to the west, awaited its discovery by foreigners; but a barrier reef denied all ships entry to Wai Momi, as Hawaiians called the place, and Pearl Harbor would lie beyond the reach of large vessels for 106 years more.

Captain Brown was pleased with the convenience of his harbor and enchanted with the countryside around it. As he looked beyond *Jackall's* rail he must have seen Oʻahu as, half a century later, Samuel Kamakau remembered it from the days of his youth: "a pleasant land looking toward the west—a fat land with flowing streams and springs of water, abundant water for taro patches, mists resting inland breathed softly on the flowers of the *hala*."[15] Claiming the right of a discoverer, Brown named the harbor "Fair Haven"—a poetical Englishman's way, it so happened, of saying "Honolulu."

He and his fellow captains did not enjoy this refuge for long. When Kalanikūpule, Oʻahu's embattled king, asked for assistance in his war with Kaʻeo, king of Kauaʻi, Captain Brown sent guns, powder and ball, and nine volunteer sailors to help Oʻahu's army repel the invaders. In the decisive battle, waged near ʻAiea on 12 December 1794, Kaʻeo was killed and his army was routed.

The next day, when news of the victory reached Captain Brown at Fair Haven, he ordered *Jackall*'s guns fired in celebration. One of the cannon was loaded with grapeshot, rather than with powder alone. The grapeshot passed through the side of Captain Kendrick's ship, killing him as he sat at dinner in his cabin, and several sailors of his crew.

Captain Brown's grim Nemesis had one more exaction to make of him. Ungrateful Kalanikūpule, thinking to increase his strength for the contest he plotted against Kamehameha, king of Hawaiʻi, decided to seize the ships of his foreign allies. On New Year's day of 1795, his warriors attacked *Jackall* and *Prince Lee Boo,* murdered both captains, and captured the two ships with their crews. So died the first three foreign captains who, so trustingly, brought their ships into the haven of Honolulu.

This was the last of Kalanikūpule's victories. When Kamehameha, at Kealakekua Bay, learned that Kalanikūpule intended to use the stolen ships in making war, he saw that his time for triumph had arrived. Within three months he had conquered Maui and Molokaʻi, winning with them Lānaʻi and Kahoʻolawe. In the fourth month, at the decisive battle of Nuʻuanu Valley, he defeated Kalanikūpule and added Oʻahu to his kingdom.

The three sacrificed captains were avenged. But Captain Brown's Fair Haven would know peace no more. Because of its harbor, the village of Kou would grow into the town of Honolulu. Because of Honolulu, the name of the island beyond it would gain a new meaning. No longer would Hawaiians think of it by its ancient name, Oʻahu, "the garment." Henceforth, they would regard it as ʻO-ahu, "the gathering place." (However, the older name, Oʻahu, is still the official one.)[16]

To Oʻahu most of all, more than to the other islands, the haoles came. Honolulu would be the port through which most foreigners entered this island realm. They did not arrive in great numbers at first. But as the years passed their numbers swelled, and by 1900 more than a million foreigners had come through this entry. And still they pour in. In 1989 more than 6 million tourists swarmed in, during that single year, almost all of them coming through Honolulu's International Airport.

Although many sailors said they were eager to enjoy the assorted liberties of "going native," few of them succeeded in jumping ship, and even fewer were strong enough to cut permanently the ties that bound them to home—or to the wanderlust that made them leave home for the first time. "Culture shock," as we call it today, "homesickness" as they thought of it, was as hurtful then as it is now. And boredom, too, the surest arouser of wanderlust, drove many a sailor back to the sea. Nonetheless, after 1790 the numbers of "deserters, vagabonds, and renegadoes" who did make the break grew steadily. In 1810 Archibald Campbell knew about sixty foreigners living on Oʻahu alone.[17] By that time each of the larger islands must have had its share of expatriates, who preferred to endure the occasional whims of chiefs rather than cope with the unrelenting hardships of life at sea. "Many inducements were held out to sailors to remain" in the islands, Campbell remembered, when he got home to Britain.

They supported themselves by working for King Kamehameha or for his vassal chiefs as carpenters, joiners, masons, blacksmiths, gunners, boatwrights, "physicians," and interpreters. Hospitable Hawaiians made room for all, provided each with at least one "wife," a thatched hut to live in, aloha for their varicolored children, and a growing market for the articles they produced or the skills they shared.

In those early years any foreigner was a haole to Hawaiians. The word itself was merely descriptive then, conveying none of the racist prejudices that are associated with it today. Later, as the number and diversity of foreign types increased, the epithet was applied exclusively to white people, especially to Americans and Englishmen. Other malihini, or newcomers, acquired labels more specifically their own. Chinese, for example, were called "Pākē," probably because the first settlers from China addressed each other, in jest or in respect, as "pai kei," a Cantonese colloquialism for father.[18]

By 1820 many ships called each year at island ports, stopping for profitable trade and for "rest and recruitment." Hawaiians, slow to learn about the dangers they risked, proved to be agreeable hosts—

and remarkably adept pupils of their guests. By 1819, Captain Louis de Freycinet observed, natives had learned about money as a measure of value and were as ready to abandon the primitive system of bartering as they had discarded the stone tools of their parents. They accepted good hard coins derived from any country, but favored "Spanish dollars" and American gold or silver pieces above all others.

❦❦❦❦

     Somewhat to Kamehameha's annoyance, Honolulu became the most important place in his kingdom. He preferred to live at Kailua on the island of Hawai'i, or at Lahaina on Maui, or, if ever he had to visit conquered O'ahu, at palm-shaded Waikīkī. Not for the first time, Hawaiians wondered at the strange predilections of haoles and yielded to their will.

Perforce, in 1803 Kamehameha moved to Honolulu, the better to keep a ruler's eye on both foreigners and subjects—and, incidentally, to prepare for his second attempt to invade Kaua'i. Where Kamehameha lived, there was the center of his kingdom; when he moved, the government moved with him. His many wives and several younger children, as well as the high chiefs and powerful priests who were his lieutenants and administrators, together with their families, retainers, and servants, "thousands of mouths" in all, took about two years to follow him from Kailua on Hawai'i to his new capital in Honolulu.[19]

The villages of Kou and Kapu'ukolo were lost in the tides of people. Along the harbor's shore, from the mouth of Nu'uanu stream eastward to the near edge of Kaka'ako and inland for more than a furlong, grass huts rose up, outnumbering the trees; temples of stone were built to honor Kāne, Lono, and Kū; new fields were laid out for games of 'ulu maika, *kilu,* and spear-throwing, and for warriors clad in loincloths learning to drill with muskets. Scattered throughout the growing town were storehouses, some made of thatch and wood, for keeping the things of old used in each day's living, some made of stone or adobe, for keeping the new things fashioned of cloth, glass, china, foreign woods and tarnishing metals, objects of exotic shapes and alien names, which everyone wanted to possess but no one really knew what to do with, all disgorged from the holds of trading ships gathering in Honolulu's harbor.

Kamehameha and the royal family lived in a compound of many thatched houses, wrote Kamakau, "surrounded by a palisade, distinguished by the British colors and a battery of 16 carriage guns belonging to his ship . . . which lay unrigged in the harbor." This "palace," as foreigners insisted on calling it, stood near the curve of the shore (about where Pier 11 is today), giving the king a clear view of all vessels moored there and all the haoles going to and from them. Within 500 yards of the palace, east and west, on call whenever he wanted to confer with them, lived the important chiefs of his government and two of the three haoles who were his trusted advisers, Isaac Davis and Don Francisco de Paula Marin.

Adjoining the king's palace to the west (in the area now bounded by Fort and Nu'uanu Streets) lay the muddy shore called Nihoa, where "natives build ships under the direction of haoles." Kamehameha knew the worth of ships, both in war and in commerce, and in those days so many were being made for him at any one time that they were "lined up on shore like canoes."

To haoles Nihoa was known as "the Beach." Upon this muddy trampled stinking shore thousands of foreigners, and the many things they brought from the world beyond, including their germs, would make their entry into Hawai'i.

ぴぴぴぴ

While most seafarers thought of the Sandwich Islands as being nothing more than a resting place in midocean, a few far-sighted British navigators tried to persuade their government in London to claim these islands for the Crown. Lieutenant King's estimate, Canon Douglas's sonorous accolade, Captain Portlock's praise, Captain Meares's certainty that "Providence intended them to belong to Great Britain," aroused no interest at all either in King George III or in his ministers. Only London's merchants saw how the Sandwich Islands could serve commerce, and through it the people of the British nation.

Even so, a number of other Britons continued the attempts to persuade their government that the Sandwich Islands were worth the taking. Captain George Vancouver, who led the first of Britain's exploring surveys into the American northwest after Cook's death, brought his three ships to spend the winter months in Hawaiian waters in 1792, 1793, and 1794. Convinced that Britain should acquire the archipelago, in 1794 he actually arranged a treaty with Kamehameha, whereby that pragmatic chief ceded his island of Hawai'i to George III in return for expected benefits both tangible and political. Vancouver considered this arrangement "the most solemn cession possible of the Island of Owhyhee to His Britannic Majesty . . . and [Kamehameha] with the attending chiefs unanimously acknowledged themselves subject to the British crown."[20] But King George's ministers would not accept the cession: they simply did not want to claim a sea-girt mountain of useless volcanic rock lying about as far from London as any place on earth could be, and they neither ratified hopeful Vancouver's treaty nor kept the promises he had given to Kamehameha in King George's name.

Thomas Manby, master of Vancouver's flagship *Discovery,* agreeing with his captain, explained how the islands, developed into a colony, could supply provisions, rum, and sugar to British settlements in northwest America as well as to "the Chinese market. The whole process might be executed at a very easy and cheap rate, as the islanders are particularly fond of being employed in your service, and show a great readiness in learning everything you will undertake to teach them."[21]

Alexander M'Konochie, a former commander in the Royal Navy, was as seigneurial as Manby had been in his disposition of Hawaiian lives and labor: "A very important supply of natives could be procured for our service," he wrote in 1816. The commercial advantages to be obtained from such a colony would derive from agriculture, whaling, trading, the fur trade with China, banking, the refurbishing of ships, and the recruiting of their crews.[22]

These earnest recommendations, and others as well, aroused no interest in London. Once again, Great Britain declined to accept a prize that was hers for the taking.

ৼৼৼৼৼ

Two other European powers also missed the chance to acquire the Sandwich Islands. In 1789 Ensign E. J. Martinez, having heard about them from fur traders he met on the northwestern coast of America, wrote a report to the viceroy of New Spain, suggesting that the Spanish government should "make a settlement on the islands, for the purpose of conquering the Hawaiians and preventing other nations from using the islands to the disadvantage of Spain."[23] The viceroy sent Lieutenant Manuel Quimper on the *Princesa Real* to look over the islands in April 1791 but, unconvinced by either Martinez or Quimper, made no effort to take them for Spain.

In 1816–1817, Georg Anton Scheffer (né Schaeffer), a bumptious Bavarian "Doctor of Medicine and of Natural Sciences" employed by the Russian-American Trading Company, did his considerable best to take the islands for Russia. Although he was instructed to establish trading posts only, Scheffer proceeded to build fortresses at Honolulu and at Waimea and Hanalei on Kaua'i. Russia's flag was flying over these militant trading posts before annoyed merchants from other nations realized what was happening. They soon informed King Kamehameha, rusticating at Kailua on Hawai'i, of Scheffer's machinations. Kamehameha ordered his vassal chiefs to expel Scheffer, troops, and trade goods. Confronted with threats of force, Scheffer and his henchmen departed, leaving their forts behind them. Ultimately, Russia's higher officials, from Alexander Baranov, governor of the Russian-American Trading Company's headquarters at New Archangel in Alaska, to Czar Alexander I in St. Petersburg, repudiated Scheffer's intentions and actions. Once again Hawaiians and their islands sank back into an uncertain peace.

The era of island-grabbing in Oceania had to await more imperialist, if not more enlightened, ministries in Paris as well as in London. By that time the Sandwich Islands were beyond the grasp of Europe's powers: the American eagle, hovering above the vast Pacific, was watching them with a jealous eye.

めめめめめ

Meanwhile, planning ahead, some captains were introducing useful plants and animals "at those places where they might add to the comfort of inhabitants or promise to supply . . . future navigators . . . with the necessary refreshments."[24]

Such interest in improvements were not common: in general, navigators wasted little effort upon the welfare of anyone but themselves and their crews. Few captains cared to clutter deck space with stinking unsteady animals and the fodder to maintain them for the sake of brown-skinned "savages" or white-skinned competitors. And often enough those who did take the trouble lost most of their plant and animal cargoes during the many weeks spent at sea. Captain Meares, for example, lost all the goats aboard *Felice* when they were killed "in one day by a sudden roll of the ship."[25] On other vessels many of the livestock they carried were slaughtered in order to provide food for hungry sailors kept too long at sea by unfavorable weather. The few captains who did succeed in enriching Hawai'i with useful animals or plants deserve the gratitude of everyone, native or foreign, who benefited from their forethought and persistence.

Vancouver brought in the animals that caused the greatest disturbances in Hawai'i's ecosystems. He is the prime example of the well-meaning foreigner who thrust troubles upon these islands even as he tried to help their people. Wary, if not actually afraid, because while serving as a very young midshipman aboard HMS *Discovery* he had been beaten by angry warriors at Kealakekua Bay on the morning of Captain Cook's murder in 1779, an anxious demanding martinet, "universally obnoxious" to his crews when in 1792–1794 he returned to the Sandwich Islands as commander of his own expedition,[26] Vancouver could not forget for a moment how dangerous his hosts might be. Despite his continual state of alarm, he was still human enough to feel an affection for Hawaiians comparable to that which a tolerant schoolmaster might conceive for a mob of athletic youths about to become men. And he was patriot enough to want to claim them, along with their islands, for his country.

Vancouver moved among Hawaiians like a plump little missionary amid cannibals, warding off political and social entanglements with paternal counsel and magisterial deportment, giving potted plants and packets of seeds to chiefs interested only in acquiring guns. "It is not right to sell things or to kill people," he admonished. "Stop making war; live in peace; be friends with each other," he urged, like a latter-day Lono-i-ka-Makahiki. In the presence of such earnestness, such inflexible decency, even ferocious chiefs minded their manners. Of them all, Kamehameha, the warlord of Kona and Kohala, was most impressed. Not then but later—when after years of intestine warfare and a conquerors' despotism he had made himself acknowledged king of all Hawai'i and could afford to be a statesman rather than only a grasping chieftain—Kamehameha would heed Vancouver's admonitions and imitate his virtues. Succeeding generations of Hawaiians, grateful for Vancouver's tempering influence upon their first monarch as well as for his many gifts to their islands, would honor him as "a Christian and a true Englishman," calling him "the father of the Hawaiian people."[27]

In 1793, as a gift for Kamehameha, Vancouver put ashore at Kealakekua Bay five cows, two ewes, and a ram. About eleven months later, on his last visit, he added to Kamehameha's wealth "a bull and two cows, with two bull calves, three rams and three ewes from California, which with all that were landed last year we have no doubt but that the islands will . . . be well stocked with these useful animals."[28]

These herbivorous animals proved to be both the best and the worst of all imports from abroad. Following Vancouver's advice, Kamehameha placed them under a kapu for ten years, "not to be touched or slaughtered," as Stephen Reynolds remembered, "except the males should become too numerous. Then the King might kill for his own, and the Queens' and Chiefs' eating. The women . . . were to have a separate animal."[29] Kamehameha sent this little herd to the plain of Waimea, above Kawaihae, "a great tract of luxuriant, natural pasturage, . . . there to roam unrestrained, to 'increase and multiply' far from the sight of strangers."[30]

In that "very rich and productive" setting, without winters or predators to reduce their number, the animals multiplied prodigiously. Even when the protecting kapu was lifted, "few cattle were killed until after 1830," according to Reynolds.[31] By 1850 they had proliferated to an alarming number: R. C. Wyllie estimated that "at least 25,000 wild cattle and 10,000 tame ones [were distributed among] the various islands of the group." By 1852 "the whole number . . . was estimated at more than 40,000, including at least 12,000 wild ones, and the opinion was expressed that cattle (and horses) were increasing at a ruinous rate."[32]

In giving Hawai'i's residents the means for developing a cattle industry, Vancouver certainly benefited both the people and the economy of the struggling little kingdom. Natives and visitors enjoyed welcome additions to their diets in beef, veal, lamb, mutton, and goat meat; homesick Americans could appease their longing for milk (although not for several generations did Hawaiians acquire a taste for the stuff); and exports of meat, hides, and tallow drew modest returns in goods or in money.

Nevertheless, Vancouver's generosity introduced the agents which most upset the ecological balance among Hawai'i's endemic plants, animals, and people. Unrestricted grazing in forests and plains, rather than in enclosed pastures, allowed the cattle to eat every plant they could reach. In doing so they destroyed the ground cover, consisting of native grasses, ferns, shrubs, and smaller trees, to such an extent that many indigenous plants, devoured down to the last specimen, became extinct.

In those days, nobody knew about ecology and ecosystems, the delicate interdependence that Nature has imposed upon all living creatures, including human beings themselves, and their environment. Because our sapient race was younger then, and uninstructed, people thought that Earth was maternal and gracious, that it would remain forever as they were discovering it, commodious, unreproving, unpolluted, unspoiled. To Europeans and Americans, but not to Hawaiians, Earth was a thing to be used, a treasury to be plundered, an immense expanse of sea and land given to them for their enriching and their pleasure, which they could rearrange to suit their convenience and exploit to increase their profit. Because they knew as little about it as about themselves, they believed that Earth was infinitely adaptable, inexhaustible. They did not yet know how wrong they were. Nor did they dream how soon the planet they set out to ravage would sicken because of the grievous wounds they and their descendants would inflict upon it. That realization would be attained only in a more ruinous age.

No places on earth have suffered the consequences of exploitation faster or more extensively than have the islands of Hawai‘i. And still the despoliation continues. Vancouver and his gifts are not the sole causes of these changes, of course. Many other well-intentioned men and women since his time have helped to "upset the balance of nature," as ecologists say.

With the loss of certain flowering plants, indigenous birds and insects were deprived of the specific sources of foods upon which they depended for existence. As a result, many species of birds and insects became extinct or have been so severely reduced in number and habitat that they have almost vanished. In 1948 entomologist E. C. Zimmerman thought that "to say a third or more of the [native insect fauna] are now extinct would be no exaggeration."[33] Although the destruction of plant and insect foods is not the only reason for the disappearance of native birds, zoologist Andrew Berger maintained that "a higher percentage of species of birds have become extinct in Hawaii than in any other region of the world. Approximately 40 percent of the endemic Hawaiian birds are believed to be extinct, and 25 of the 60 birds in the 1968 list of *Rare and Endangered Birds of the United States* are Hawaiian."[34]

The slide toward extinction does not end. For animals and plants, too, as well as for native Hawaiian people, the sliding way of death is inescapable. In 1970, of the sixty-nine species of indigenous birds, twenty-five were extinct, twenty-five others were endangered, and only nineteen seemed to be surviving.[35] By 1989, thirty-one species were "listed as endangered."[36]

The disappearance or jeopardy of Hawai'i's indigenous birds are direct consequences of the introduction of foreign people and foreign animals. These have caused the destruction of many habitats or led to competition for places in habitats not yet lost. Foreign birds, introduced intentionally or released accidentally, serve not only as competitors but also as carriers of microorganisms that cause avian malaria and avian pox. Moreover, rats, mongooses, and feral cats make continual attacks on adult birds, their nesting young, and their eggs.[37]

ᘒᘒᘒᘒ

With the loss of ground cover and protecting shrubs, the land itself suffered: water and winds eroded the bared earth, and new streams joined the old in staining the sea with precious soil.

Cattle caused other and more immediate troubles. They ate crops in gardens and fields, sown in hope but not always harvested. As cattle strayed and munched, they provoked innumerable disputes between careless owners and exasperated victims. A few of these "cow cases," carried for judgment first to local chiefs and later to the kingdom's courts by contentious haoles, such as Britain's consul Richard Charlton, threw Honolulu's residents and justice into perpetual turmoil. In some districts, such as Waialua and Kahuku on O'ahu, depredations by cattle and horses more than once brought the country folk close to famine.[38] Not until the middle of the nineteenth century did the Legislative Assembly finally enact laws requiring construction of fences, paddocks, and other devices for controlling livestock either domesticated or wild. And many more years passed before all these barriers were completed.

Today the wild beef cattle have been rounded up or annihilated, but sheep still roam the higher slopes of Mauna Kea on Hawai'i, and wild goats and pigs, not to mention feral dogs and cats, have found habitats in mountain ranges on all the islands.

ᘒᘒᘒᘒ

Of the large domestic animals, horses were the last to arrive. On 24 June 1803 William Shaler, master of *Lelia Byrd,* landed a mare and a foal for John Young at Kawaihae—"the first horses that ever trod the soil of Owhyhee," as Shaler said. Two days later, at Lahaina, Maui, he presented King Kamehameha with a stallion and a mare. "Their beauty and mettle excited the wonder and admiration of the natives."[39] These valued creatures, also protected by royal kapu, multiplied manyfold in a few years. Later ships brought cargoes of new stock to supplement the progeny of the first imports. Stephen Reynolds, cherishing a Lamarckian belief that pleased haole residents and annoys geneticists, declared that "horses born and reared on the islands are superior in all respects to those imported from California—better limbs, better spirits, and tougher animals. But slight attention has been given to procure good studs."[40]

By the 1830s horses were of paramount importance in the Hawaiian way of life. Natives, from dignified elders to screeching urchins, became as expert at horsemanship as at swimming. Almost every family, native or foreign, owned at least one patient nag, if not half a dozen spirited steeds. People no longer walked when they could ride. Often enough they rode without saddle or stirrups, using only a rope noose for a bridle. At times everybody seemed to be out riding at once, in happy noisy cavalcades, amid clouds of dust, going nowhere in particular, but thoroughly enjoying the fun of being on the move. "Furious riding" became the first traffic offense in the towns, and runaway horses the first hazards.

The roads, muddy or dusty according to the daily rainfall, were little more than paths among dwellings and fields. They followed the whims of people rather than any planned pattern. Around these casual byways the little towns just sort of grew.

No wheeled vehicle rolled along the roads of Honolulu "until about 1825 or 1826," according to Stephen Reynolds. Probably he referred to "the coaches recently brought from America" that the Reverend C. S. Stewart mentioned in his *Journal*. They belonged to two enterprising young men, Mr. Elwell and James Hunnewell, who, "having trained their horses to the harness," provided the first means of public transportation to townsfolk. On Saturday, 12 June 1825, they called at the mission compound to take the Stewart family for "an evening airing. . . . The plain affords a beautiful drive, but we little thought, on our first arrival, to see it enlivened and ornamented by so neat and genteel an equipage."[41]

Levi Chamberlain, business agent for the American missionaries, waited almost three years for the cart he asked the ABCFM to order for the mission. Shipped from Boston in 1825, it finally reached Honolulu in April 1827. "A strong well made & excellent carriage, just what we want to bear the beating of Honolulu, it is constructed for a horse or for oxen by having fills and a tongue to ship & unship at pleasure."[42] This entry confirms Reynolds' statement that the missionaries were the first to use oxen as beasts of burden. "Jersey wagons came in about a year later."[43]

No chronicler, resident or transient, recorded the arrival of the first cat or the first foreign dog. Probably every sailing vessel, beginning with Captain Cook's, carried at least one cat as a control for the rats infesting her. And many a crew must have kept a dog or two as pets. Captain Vancouver's ship *Discovery,* for example, carried a Newfoundland dog, which so excited the admiration of Hawaiians that they offered three hogs for it. Vancouver's surgeon-naturalist, Archibald Menzies, believed that their interest "shows that these people are much more anxious to improve or augment their present stock of animals and vegetables than the indolent natives of Tahiti, who seem to consider the produce of their own island as fully sufficient for every purpose of ease and luxury."[44]

Like all other creatures that survived the long sea voyages and made the last great leap from ship to shore, cats and dogs too found another home in Hawai'i. After the usual nine days' excitement, Hawaiians made room for them in houses and bellies. Before long the native "poi dog," somewhat like Alice's Cheshire cat, began to fade from the scene. F. D. Bennett, a British zoologist who visited Hawai'i in 1834–1835, observed that "the aboriginal, or poe dog, characterized by its small size, brown color, foxy head, long back, crooked or bandy fore-legs, and sluggish disposition, is now a rare, and will probably be soon an extinct species . . . lost amid a mongrel race of dogs, partaking of every foreign variety."[45] No one noticed, or cared, when the last native dog died, because Hawaiians did not need the breed any more as a source of meat. With its passing one more creature indigenous to Polynesia vanished.

Nor did anyone remark the arrival of the lesser domestic animals, or new breeds of the bigger species. From one quarter or another, by intention or by accident, they came, ferried by ships that were virtual arks. Rats, mice, cats, and dogs slinking ashore; cows, horses, pigs, goats, hares, and rabbits; geese, turkeys, chickens, ducks, doves, and pigeons—all bestowed with haole generosity, all brought their vermin with them. New kinds of worms and flukes which can infest human as well as animal hosts—such as beef tapeworm, dog tape-worm, and probably the roundworms of swine that cause trichinosis and ascariasis—arrived during this period. And only heaven knows how many kinds of pathogenic bacteria and viruses accompanied those animal importations. More than likely a number of *Salmonella* species and serotypes, bacteria which are often present in rodents, fowl, cattle, swine, cats, and dogs, were introduced, to afflict not only their usual animal hosts but also humans as well.

In the late 1980s, cases of *Salmonella* infections, or of "food poisonings" caused by toxins released by *Salmonella* organisms, occurred much too frequently among both residents and visitors: Hawai'i enjoys the distinction of showing the highest incidence of salmonelloses in the nation. Epidemiologists explain that this pre-eminence arises not from the slovenliness of people who provide and prepare our foods for hotels, restaurants, and carnivals, but is proof, rather, of the diligence with which our medical and public health ser-vices report such cases and identify the causative bacteria.

Even so, in the old days the islands' remoteness and the slowness of sailing vessels spared Hawai'i's people many diseases to which their brethren in foreign lands were subject. Foremost among these were bubonic plague, smallpox, measles, tularemia, schistosomiasis, the rickettsial diseases, and rabies. Moreover, because mosquitoes did not arrive until 1826, Hawaiians did not have to contend with filariasis, yellow fever, dengue fever, the several virus encephalitides, and malaria. Native birds, too, escaped for a while the viral and malarial infections which are presumed to have destroyed so many of them after mosquitoes and introduced foreign birds, as carriers of those infectious microbes, were established in the islands.

According to J. F. Illingworth, an entomologist, houseflies, head lice, and body lice were brought to Hawai'i before 1778. Although early foreigners mentioned them, most such visitors were more impressed by the beautiful feathered hand kahilis, which they called "fly-flaps," than by the flies themselves. Presumably, said Illing-worth, cockroaches and fleas were here too, although no one thought to write about them until Kotzebue did so in 1816. No one can know when scabies mites arrived, but "the itch" they caused was noticed soon after 1778. Other kinds of pests came later, centipedes and scorpions "about 1835." These, and others no doubt, like mos-quitoes, came from ports in Mexico.[46]

Many other kinds of pests arrived aboard foreigners' ships, in an unplanned invasion that still continues. Almost every airplane and steamship that lands in these islands brings uninvited stowaways of this sort. The majority of these represent species that are already established here. But several times in each year new kinds of pests do arrive, and manage to find places for themselves in a hospitable area. Snails minuscule or giant, slugs, spiders, cockroaches, moths, butterflies, grasshoppers, leafhoppers, beetles, weevils, aphids, mealy bugs, thrips, nematodes, ants, termites, midges, gnats, lizards, geckos, skinks, frogs, and toads: creeping, crawling, flying, biting, burrowing, free-living or parasitic, creatures of every phylum and almost every family found a wide-open home in these indulgent isles. Even the bottoms of ships, fouled with seaweeds, barnacles, and the spores, eggs, cysts, and larvae of a variety of marine creatures from other seas, brought many exotic species to dwell in warm Hawaiian waters.

Yet, by the mercy of Providence, no one has released—so far!—harmful snakes or other reptiles in these islands. One attempt to introduce snakes, probably harmless ones, came very close to succeeding in the early 1840s. A physician (or perhaps a reverend), identified only as "Dr. B," went to call on Mrs. Gerrit P. Judd and her children soon after he had arrived in Honolulu. Long afterward Elizabeth Judd Wight remembered the occasion:

> "Mrs. Judd," he said, "I have brought you something beautiful," and, carefully unrolling a package, produced a glass jar full of live snakes. . . . "I am going to put them in the taro-patches up Manoa Valley."
>
> "No, you are not; those snakes shall never leave this house alive. If the Lord had intended us to have snakes He would have put them there Himself." And, taking the jar, my mother went into the kitchen, closely followed by Dr. B., where, without a word, she emptied them into a kettle of boiling water. "I think that you have made a great mistake," angrily remarked the doctor; "They would have been such an addition to these islands."[47]

Dr. B's indifference to the Lord's intention is shared all too often by too many people. Either willfully or carelessly, they have brought in creatures, among both plants and animals, that Hawai'i could very well do without. The giant African snail, Cuban thrips, termites, fruit flies, and many a rampageous weed (like "Koster's curse") are only a few of the obvious examples of such interlopers.

One small inoffensive little blind snake did arrive by accident in the early 1930s. It looks so much like an earthworm that most people do not recognize it as a snake. It came in soil around the roots of plants imported from the Philippine Islands that were intended for use in landscaping the new campus of the Kamehameha Schools on Kapālama Heights. Enthusiastic gardeners, busily sharing plants, have succeeded in distributing this harmless creature throughout all the islands.

Although occasionally a big snake has arrived at a Hawaiian port by accident, coiled up in a packing crate or slithering out from under a cargo skip—and once in a rare while a venomous yellow sea serpent from Southeast Asia has actually been found swimming in the ocean off Oʻahu—so far these larger reptiles, whether venomous or safe, have not been established in the islands. Hawaiʻi's reprieve, however, is not likely to last. The state is in greatest danger from the brown tree snake, a native of Papua New Guinea and Melanesia. Already this omnivorous reptile has been introduced by accident into several Pacific islands east of Melanesia. It is a very serious pest on Guam—which is only one stop away from Hawaiʻi, whether by ship or by airplane.[48]

ʒʒʒʒʒ

New kinds of plants arrived oftener than did novel kinds of animals. The earliest planned importations brought seeds or rooted stocks yielding edible vegetables and fruits. The obvious need for providing dependable supplies of fresh (and familiar) foods in this midocean oasis led some captains to be generous with such gifts and interested Hawaiians to take care of them. Not until food supplies were assured in plenty did anyone give much thought to improving the Hawaiian landscape with ornamental flowers, shrubs, and trees.

For most of these early introductions neither the dates of arrival nor the names of their bringers are known. Like so many of the men who came to Hawaiʻi, the plants appeared by chance at one port or another. Some sank roots into the new land and made themselves at home. Others, like the fruit trees from temperate zones, unable to adapt to the perpetual summer of the islands' coastal plains and valleys, languished and died, until, much later, people thought to grow them at higher elevations.

Along with the plants of economic value came the weeds. Hardy as always, meeting little competition from the native flora and fauna, they spread even more rapidly than did the food plants. Whether or not they were wanted, they filled the empty spaces provided by nature, grazing animals, or the activities of people. Whether or not they were valued, they were useful: they brightened raw lands with touches of color; helped to hold soil in place against the bite of winds and water; gave kāhuna lapaʻau lāʻau new medications to try in hope; and, when their brief life was ended, added their bodies to the earth, enriching with humus the ground from which they had drawn their sustenance.

Among these uninvited settlers would have been the cosmopolitan species that dominated the islands' weed patches until recently: the "Jamaican vervain," the spiny amaranth, the several kinds of "Spanish needles" belonging to the genus *Bidens,* and numerous species of grasses. Moreover, some of the desirable plants escaped from cultivation to become as widespread as weeds. The earliest of those would have been tobacco, the edible cactus, guava, and wild tomatoes. Now those too are being overcome by newer arrivals.

Then, sometime between 1791 and 1795, Don Francisco de Paula Marin came to stay, changing uncertain hope for imported plants to surety of success. Until his death in 1837, Don Francisco was practically a one-man agricultural bureau, the self-appointed expert who assumed almost entirely the responsibility and the pleasures of establishing new kinds of plants in Honolulu.

Don Marin's vineyard was a verdant garden in the desert of Honolulu. None of the town's other resident foreigners ever bothered to plant a tree for the sake of shade or fruit—although some did try to grow vegetables for their families—and throughout all Hawaiʻi no haole followed Marin's fine example for the sake of profit. A few haoles, like John Young and Isaac Davis, put retainers to growing fruits and kitchen vegetables for use in their own households. Once in a while, apparently, a derelict off a ship pulled himself together long enough to show an interested Hawaiian how to cultivate and harvest a new kind of crop.

ぐぐぐぐ

Honolulu in 1820 was an ugly, barren, hot, and feculent town, a straggle of grass huts and a very few stone or adobe houses. Its residents sweltered amid clouds of dust or skidded along in mud, often ankle-deep, according to the amount of rain Lono-of-the-Long-Clouds bestowed upon them. Foreigners might sweat and complain, but they did nothing to improve the place. They were too busy making a living—or too impatient for an early escape from this dismal port—to care about beauty, or comfort, or civic pride. Natives, knowing nothing about towns in other parts of the world, thought that this was how all seaports must be, and therefore how Honolulu would always be.

Honolulu grew only because it offered a convenience for ships and sailors, not because it provided solace and comforts to its inhabitants. The people who were condemned to live here matched the town. Without a source of fresh water other than muddy Nuʻuanu stream, a few distant springs and brackish wells, or rain caught as it flowed off a roof, they thirsted and they stank. Hawaiian commoners, if they still were concerned about grooming their persons, bathed perforce in the dirty river or in the turbid harbor, amid the refuse dumped overboard from ships moored there. Chiefs, and perhaps the more favored among their retainers (as John Iʻi remembered), enjoyed the few spring-fed ponds, such as the bathing pool at Honokaʻupu.[49] (That pool was situated near the present intersection of Queen and Alakea streets.) Haoles, not much given to bathing in those days, in any part of their large world, must have been as odorous as were Honolulu's lanes and byways.

Those "streets," not yet rutted by wheels or swept by brooms, served as the town's open market, transportation network, and sewage and garbage disposal systems. Scavenging pigs, dogs, goats, cats, rats, and chickens devoured whatever was edible, leaving the residue to be trampled into the dirt, or just to lie there until it disintegrated. (But at least those things were "biodegradable," as we say in the jargon of today, unlike the perdurable litter—aluminum cans, plastic containers, pieces of glass, and rusting parts of dead machines—that we strew so generously about our landscapes in this our modern age.)

From the beginning Honolulu's residents seemed determined to earn for their town the name by which eventually it was known to sailors throughout the seven seas: The Cesspit of the Pacific. For the assorted discomforts and affronts to all the senses, the foreigners had only themselves to thank. Unlike Hawaiians, they did not know about kapus of hygiene and sanitation for individuals, households, and communities—or, if they did know better, they did not bother with them any more. They were accustomed to dirt, disorder, and ugliness, to the smells of unwashed bodies, the stench of rotting garbage and decomposing ordure, the stinks of civilization such as they lived in at home. Wherever they went they flaunted their disdain for even the most elementary precepts of hygiene and sanitation, not to mention those of morality and decency. And, because most of them believed that soon they would be going back to whatever place they called home, they gave neither thought nor effort to improving the port towns to which chance and the ceaseless quest for money (or adventure) might take them.

Wherever they congregated, pollution followed. They contaminated everything, as did the flock of harpies Jason's Argonauts saw, not only with their wastes but also with their behavior. The worst of their despoilings affected the minds and attitudes of natives. Left to themselves, Hawaiians would not have dared to show such disrespect for their many deities by befouling earth, air, and water in the ways that haoles did. But when they saw how the foreigners behaved, Hawaiians marveled. And then they imitated the men who disdained so fearlessly the gods and their kapus.

Pollution took many forms: haole excrement, and with that haole germs, was not the only abomination heaped upon Honolulu's earth and tossed into its water. The signs of foreigners' presence piled up around their stores and habitations: rubbish, junk, the debris of wrappings, crates, barrels, papers, jute bags, and rags that once had protected their precious trade goods; empty bottles, jugs, jars, crocks, shards of glass; the scabrous shops, warehouses, and sheds; the raucous rancid grogshops and whorehouses; the two "inns"; the dismantled hulks of dead ships rotting in the harbor; the one pitiable cemetery near Kaka'ako in which the husks of dead haoles were dumped and soon forgotten: all these advertisements for the superior Western civilization made of Honolulu too a noisome midden, alive with maggots, flies, vermin, and with the least admirable specimens of mankind, foul-mouthed, diseased, and indomitable, lurching through the town in search of rum and women. Every port town in the world, and many a nation's larger cities, exhibited the same horrific scenery, animated by the same kinds of swaggering unwashed heroes.

Less obvious signs of pollution derived from haoles' demands for food, firewood, water, women, and workers. Hawaiians supplied these easily enough, at first under orders from chiefs, later under the stimulus of gain for themselves. In order to serve ever increasing numbers of haoles, people from villages far and near, even from other islands, left their quiet homes for the fleshpots of Honolulu.

Most of them did not go home again. If death did not claim them soon, the town's lures of pleasures and profits kept them there for yet a while. Those few who managed to go home usually went back to die of diseases they contracted in this sink of iniquity. And, inevitably, before they died all of them passed their germs along to relatives and friends.

John Cook, a haole who lived on Kaua'i in the late 1840s, noticed this dismal cycle that had begun long before his arrival: "Many's the time one could see a fine healthy, strapping young girl, with fresh clear complexion, leave Kauai and return in six months or so with her face all blotched and sodden, an utter physical wreck, who would help to further spread the disease like wildfire through the countryside."[50] In this way the lasting miseries of the venereal diseases, tuberculosis, and the intestinal infections were disseminated among country folk who never saw Honolulu.

As the number of ships calling at Honolulu increased with each year, so too did the resident population needed for servicing them and their crews. By 1820 it was a miniature market town, operating more to suit the purposes of foreigners aboard their ships than for the sake of the people who lived there, whether haole or Hawaiian. And, inevitably, especially after 1819, when the American whaling ships began to make their long cruises through the Pacific, Honolulu was destined to become a depot town, an entrepôt where items of commerce could be stored until they were transported to other destinations. All this, and more, as Adelbert Chamisso, aboard the Russian brig *Rurik,* predicted in 1816, was "fitted to the pattern of history."

The need for firewood, used in ships' galleys and for kitchen fires in the town, called for more woodcutters and charcoal makers. Eventually they denuded the plains and nearby hills of trees and shrubs, down to the last twig. Grazing horses and cattle, erosion by wind and water, completed the destruction of the ground cover. Soon the plains east of Honolulu, once green, yielded nothing but dust, and the lower slopes of Kalihi, Nu'uanu, Pauoa, Makiki, and Mānoa became as barren as Punchbowl and Diamond Head had always been. They would remain bare and sere until long after the development of modern systems for delivering gas and electricity into Honolulu's homes eliminated the need for kitchen fires. Not until the 1930s would the slopes of Pauoa and Makiki Round Top become green again, with a cover of new kinds of weeds and trees. The process of natural reforestation, almost unaided by human intervention, continues slowly even now, and has only begun on Punchbowl and Diamond Head.

Least obvious of the haoles' effects, but ultimately the most devastating, were the encroachments upon the spirit which corrupted and demoralized Hawaiians, both as individuals and as members of their society. Even though most of the foreigners who came to Hawai'i were not the best specimens of their societies, they were nonetheless representatives of a civilization that possessed material things and controlled mechanical power to a degree far superior to anything the Hawaiian culture had been able to achieve. The contrast between an ax made of steel and an adze shaped from stone, or between a wooden spear and a musket, or between a dugout canoe and a swift schooner, was so impressive that Hawaiians did not need to be told how primitive they and their artifacts were.

Lieutenant King, in 1778, during the very first encounter between Hawaiians and haoles, noticed how "their behavior in general shewed a sense of their inferiority, & the advantages we had over them."[51] Unfortunately for Hawaiians, that sense, understandable in 1778, did not diminish with further exposure to haole technology— or to haole self-assurance. Every time a ship arrived, laden with so much wealth and bearing foreigners so arrogant in their authority, so confident in their knowledge, the lesson was driven home. As it always must, the world around, the weaker society gave way to the forces of the superior. In this Hawaiians were like the people of what fortunate Westerners today are pleased to call "Undeveloped Countries" or "the Third World." Hawaiians were being subjected to the same scarifying experiences, displacements, corruptions that beset "primitive"—and therefore "disadvantaged"—societies everywhere on earth, and at all times, even today.

Hawaiians paid a high price for this development, by any standard. The Reverend Sheldon Dibble in 1843 appraised the cost from a missionary's exacting level: "Cheating, trade in arms and rum, physical violence, murder, arrogance, and general exploitation are also the white man's contribution to Hawaiian civilization . . . new modes of crime and new modes of accelerated destruction were introduced from Christian countries."[52] He did not include the diseases and vices consequent upon "licentiousness" in this arraignment because he had already devoted several pages in his *History* to that distressing subject.

As they admired, and coveted, and emulated, and imitated, taking as their models the men and the things coming from those advanced societies beyond the seas, Hawaiians abandoned the ways of old by which their lives had been regulated for so many centuries. They were corrupted not so much by evil men as by their own desire to possess the good things the foreigners brought. They were demoralized not because they accepted the moral code of foreigners who were immoral, but rather because the foreigners, in their freedoms of behavior, presented them with so many exemplars to choose among that Hawaiians became thoroughly confused and therefore found no single moral code to accept in place of the one they were discarding. They needed teachers who would show them what to do and tell them how to think in the manner of foreigners. But, except for dogged, didactic Vancouver and theorizing Golovnin, no foreigner took such a role because no one else recognized that such teaching was needed immediately. And, among the ruling ali'i, no one except King Kamehameha and Kalanimoku saw what was happening to their people and understood what the people must do to save themselves from disaster.

Not all foreigners, of course, were evil men. Some were as moral and as decent as mothers and pastors at home wanted them to be. They read the Bible, said their prayers, "kept themselves pure," minded their manners when, during shore leaves, they went a-wandering among cheerful natives and picturesque landscapes. But, the world of men being the way it is, such examples of virtue, few to begin with at the start of a voyage, almost disappeared from a ship's company during the long run to the Sandwich Islands. And the few decent sailors who managed to endure the voyage were lost in the ebb and flow of the wanton many.

The flagrant boast of American whalermen—"We hang our consciences on the Horn, and we pick 'em up again on our way home"— had not yet been proclaimed. But the attitudes that their bragging advertised were common early in the nineteenth century, influencing the minds and manners of sailors from any nation who entrusted themselves to ships that ventured out upon the sea.

While he lived, King Kamehameha held the nation together. This was the true measure of his greatness: not his prowess as a warrior, nor his power as the conqueror, but his wisdom made him a noble king. Gained in part from Captain Vancouver's schoolmasterly righteousness, but most of all from his own shrewd appraisal of good men and bad, both Hawaiian and haole, Kamehameha's wisdom resembled that of Israel's David in the years of his age. War was put aside. Tyranny was tempered with justice. An autocrat's despotism yielded to a leader's concern for the welfare of all his people. And the approach of death gave him the vision of a prophet: "Keep the kapus," he enjoined them. "Respect the gods," he warned. He knew how much people need to respect and to fear and to obey powers greater than themselves, if they are to survive.

While he lived most of his people obeyed him, more out of habit by then, or in fear of him, than from belief in the gods or in the potency of their kapus. Yet long before he died the gods were being put aside, their kapus were being evaded. More than once, as he saw how his people were being suborned and corrupted, Kamehameha must have grieved over the fate that would befall them when he was gone.

In this willingness to adopt the best of the ideas that foreigners brought from their greater world, and in his insistence upon keeping the best ideas and the guarding kapus that his precursors had evolved for their smaller world, Kamehameha established his greatness. Later in the nineteenth century certain admirers of his military conquests thought to honor him with the grandiloquent (and inappropriate) title "Napoleon of the Pacific." He deserves higher praise, for other and better achievements in peacetime, for his great mana. And as the only genius whom, so far, the people living in these islands have produced.

♂♂♂♂

The first important kapu to be broken by commoners, if not by ruling chiefs and their retainers, was the one that forbade women to eat with men. Haoles laughed at a rule they considered stupid; how could the women they took to the sleeping-mats not join them at the eating-mats? And when those women (as well as their men) found that breaking one kapu brought down no punishment upon them, from either gods or priests, how could they resist the cajolings of haoles to break other kapus?

When women served as harlots to haoles, and men labored for foreigners on their ships and on the beach at Nihoa, families were disrupted, children were neglected, the very fields and gardens in which the people should have been growing the foodstuffs to sustain their communities were no longer cultivated. Hunger, always a lingering threat even in normal times, entered many a household, along with the nails, pieces of iron, tarnished mirrors, lengths of sleazy cloth, and the diseases that were the haoles' payments for services rendered. Neglected children died, or ran wild in the towns; infants were not born, or did not survive the first few weeks of life.

ຂາ∕ຂາ∕ຂາ∕ຂາ∕

Sexual experience was not in itself an evil thing to Hawaiians. Like all sensible Polynesians, they were rather relaxed about premarital and extramarital sexual activities. Commoners, at least, put no price upon virginity, thought chastity a most unnatural state, and seldom evolved a jealous lover. Among maka'āinana the mad maniacal possessiveness of passion or frustration was neither a theme for poets nor a cause for complaint to partners at love. Despite this great degree of sexual freedom in youth—and probably because of it —most couples who decided to join in a permanent union achieved reasonably happy lives; and, with maturity, many attained the consolations of mutual respect and affection which distinguish successful marriages in any society.

Before 1778 their license to experiment and to enjoy the pleasures of sex brought no complications of any kind. Prostitutes were not needed; an illegitimate child did not exist. "A child born too soon" simply joined his mother's family, as welcome a member of the group as were her siblings, or he was "given" to another family, to be raised either as an adopted child or as a foster child. Among commoners nobody worried about bastardy or the purity of bloodlines. That special form of arrogance was reserved to high chiefs—and to proud aristocrats in Europe and America.

The presence of foreigners did not change the attitudes of Hawaiians toward sex. But foreigners did introduce complications with which Hawaiians had not contended before 1778. The first of these was the demand for women as full-time companions to sailors while they remained in port. This demand—and the payments the women received for their favors—created the genuine prostitute, a class and an occupation new to Hawai'i. A girl who once or twice lay with a transient mariner would not have been scorned; but a wife or mother who forsook home, husband, and children in order to consort with sailors was a harlot to Hawaiians as well as to the haoles who used her. The effects of absence—even if it was only temporary, even if her family considered the woman to be "gainfully employed" and she went home with a small fortune in trinkets and trade goods—hurt more people than herself alone.

In November 1816, the Russian Imperial Navy brig *Rurik,* commanded by Lieutenant Otto von Kotzebue, arrived in Hawai'i. Serving aboard her were Louis Choris (the artist whose portraits give us likenesses of Kamehameha I, his favorite wife Ka'ahumanu, and several other Hawaiians), and Adelbert von Chamisso, a naturalist during this early stage in his extraordinary career. Although sympathetic toward the Hawaiians he saw, Chamisso deplored the evidence that they were becoming "commercial and mercantile," especially in matters of sex. When, inevitably, he wrote his book about *Rurik's* voyage, Chamisso delivered himself of a philosopher's balanced epigram: "Shame appears to be born in man, but chastity is only a virtue, according to our law." But, he continued, to Hawaiians "chastity as a virtue was foreign; we have inoculated it with covetousness and greed and stripped it of modesty."[53] He foresaw too the time when "sooner or later, fitted to the pattern of history, the large islands of the Pacific Ocean will be joined to the world of our civilization."[54]

Three years later Jacques Arago, a witty and observant artist with Captain Louis de Freycinet's exploring expedition, reached Honolulu. His saucy comments about pompous chiefs and certain resident foreigners gave way to sentiments closer to compassion when he looked at the town's commoners:

> The condition of women here is truly wretched . . . they are treated like beings perfectly useless, except to propagate the species. . . .
>
> Strangers . . . have little difficulty in meeting with female companions. They enter a hut, and for a handkerchief, a necklace of glass beads, one or two shining buttons, or similar trifles, they are at liberty to make their choice.[55]

The second set of complications introduced by foreigners were unmitigated disasters for everyone. These were the microorganisms that cause the several venereal diseases and the other chronic infections, such as tuberculosis, as well as the germs that cause the swifter, short-term acute infections, such as the many virus diseases and the "enteric fevers." As is usual with unprepared populations, Hawaiians who contracted foreigners' ailments all too often suffered intense and rapid bouts of sickness, most of which quickly terminated in death. If a diseased woman lived long enough to bear a child, often it was stillborn, or afflicted with congenital syphilis or gonorrheal ophthalmia or physical defects, or all three conditions together. To say that infants blighted in this way did not have much of a chance to live is an obvious understatement. Furthermore, because of the destructive effects of syphilis spirochetes and gonococci upon reproductive organs in both males and females, the few adults who appeared to have recovered from these venereal infections were barren in many instances. Wrote the Reverend Sheldon Dibble in 1843:

> Sin and death were the first commodities imported to the Sandwich Islands. As though their former ruin were not sufficient, Christian nations superadded a deadlier evil [the venereal diseases]. That evil is sweeping the population to the grave with amazing rapidity. And it is yet to be seen whether the influences of Christianity on the rising race shall stay that desolation.[56]

All these contagions, complicated by physical, physiological, and psychological damages, led to a rapid decline in the birth rate and to an appalling mortality among natives of all ages. Moreover, the rates of sickness and of death would have been increased by the almost total disturbance of social and biological ecosystems in the port towns. When Hawaiians went to live in the towns, they abandoned the practices of personal hygiene and community sanitation that for so long had protected them from indigenous germs. In the relatively crowded confines of Honolulu, for example, they could not very well trot a mile or more (or even a furlong or two) in order to find a secluded spot in which to relieve themselves whenever they felt the need to do so. Once again coarse haole example showed them how to meet these problems of urgency—and, naturally, added to them even greater problems of filth and pollution.

The esthetics of pollution troubled no one, native or foreign, in those mephitic times. But the microbial content of human excrement affected everyone, even haoles. The virulent bacteria and viruses that cause enteric fevers, diarrheas, and dysenteries, the ova of parasitic worms, the cysts of pathogenic amoebas, would have been widely distributed in water and soil, and therefore in foodstuffs. If Hawaiians before 1778 did not suffer from "bowel fevers" and "bloody fluxes," or from infestations with hookworms, pinworms, threadworms, and roundworms, they most certainly did experience these afflictions after Honolulu began to grow.

"Pure water, Man's greatest need," as Honolulu's Board of Water Supply proclaims, which we today take for granted and waste so thoughtlessly, was not available then to most residents. Only the few families fortunate enough to have access to a protected well or spring had safe water to drink. No public water supply was provided, or even imagined. Households sent someone each day to fetch water from the nearest stream, irrigation ditch, or taro patch. The precious fluid was carried home in calabashes, stoppered gourds, and—the latest convenience offered by civilization—in glass bottles or clay jugs retrieved from the rubbish heaps of grogshops. No family ever had enough water for all its needs. And rarely was that water safe to drink.

Inasmuch as human and animal feces were not disposed of safely, disease-causing germs got into the water at its very sources, as well as into those varied containers at every stage of transportation and storage. Honolulu, in effect, became a permanent bivouac, in which the same opportunities for distributing intestinal pathogens that brought on the maʻi ʻōkuʻu epidemic in 1804 were repeated and perpetuated. The town's populace demonstrated once again that, as sanitary engineers and microbiologists would be saying a hundred years later, a community's source of drinking water can be a direct connection between a sick man's guts and a hale man's mouth. Gastrointestinal infections—diarrheas, hepatitis, dysenteries, enteric fevers—would have been epidemic and almost unending. Honolulu's residents endured frequent outbreaks of typhoid and paratyphoid fevers until the 1890s, when finally governmental agencies provided parts of the inner city with drinking water from protected sources. Before that time, as annual reports from the Board of Health indicate, enteric fevers were the main causes of death for Honolulu's inhabitants. The same dangers occurred in Hilo, Lahaina, and Waimea on Kauaʻi, as well as in smaller towns and villages on all the islands. Indeed, Lahaina, supplied with water from an unprotected surface reservoir, was a notorious locus of typhoid fever until after World War II.[57]

In 1989, epidemiologists with the State Department of Health warned that human carriers of typhoid bacilli are found "in some ethnic communities [and] therefore the potential for prolonged carrier states and epidemics still exists."[58] The term "ethnic communities" is the safe way for bureaucrats to refer to recent immigrants from countries in Southeast Asia and from other Pacific islands. Meanwhile, we should not forget, related enteric pathogens derived from animal sources, such as swine, poultry, and rodents either raised locally or imported from mainland areas, are always about, ready to harry Hawai'i's human residents regardless of ethnicity.

During the period under consideration, Honolulu's haoles, whether permanent residents or transient, would have been naturally immunized by previous exposures to infections in foreign places before they reached Hawai'i and, therefore, were relatively protected against microbial pathogens they encountered here. So also were the few Hawaiians who had traveled abroad or who managed to live through the first hazardous weeks they spent in the town. But death rates for natives newly arrived from rural districts must have been very high.

Haoles, whether "good" or "bad," by their behavior and in their attitudes, with their possessions and demands, began to erode every aspect of the Hawaiians' culture, gradually stripping them of trust in every one of their ancient customs, habits, beliefs, and illusions. Yet, to be fair to those haoles, they did not know how much harm they were causing. They knew no other way to live, especially when they were out in the world, far from home. Nor did they have any idea that many of the sicknesses from which they suffered could be passed on so easily to friendly islanders. In those years few people anywhere even suspected that infectious diseases are caused by "contagions," living agents, the minute creatures that today we call "germs."

Ninety-nine percent of the sailors who came to Hawai'i in those times were rough, ignorant, filthy, and mean, if not actually vicious. They had to be little more than brutes, in order to endure the hardships of service aboard vessels at sea and the tumults of the ports in which they gained for a while refuge from the sea if not escape from their brutish companions. The few good and decent men among them (Herman Melville, for example, or Richard Henry Dana) were lost in the crowd, or hid decency behind a mask of pretense. Almost none of those seafarers, except for an occasional captain like Cook, Vancouver, and Golovnin, wasted much thought on the welfare of Hawaiians. The journals of Don Francisco Marin and Stephen Reynolds reveal a Honolulu that is not described in history books.

Inevitably, in the manner of all naive peoples, Hawaiians too learned the wicked ways of foreigners much faster than they learned the good things the foreigners' world could have taught them. One of the most pernicious of the alien vices was the excessive indulgence in alcoholic beverages—or "alcohol abuse," as we label it today.

Hawaiians of old, unlike most others of the world's people, had not discovered the several fermentation processes by which crude alcoholic beverages can be made. The only comforting potion they knew before 1778 was the infusion prepared from the narcotic 'awa plant, *Piper methysticum,* but this was reserved almost exclusively for chiefs. Foreigners gave Hawaiians their first taste of beers, wines, and distilled "spirits" (all without benefit of ice, of course). To natives these were known collectively and indiscriminately as *wai wela,* hot water, or *lama,* rum. Until about 1809 (or thereabouts) all alcoholic beverages drunk in the islands were imported from Europe or America. In that year William Stevenson (an Englishman, according to Mouritz), who had "escaped" from Britain's penal colony at Botany Bay in New South Wales, "introduced . . . the mode of distilling a spirit from the tee-root." He became so fond of his product "that the king was obliged to deprive him of his still." Despite Stevenson's deplorable tendency, Archibald Campbell maintained that he was

> an industrious man, and conducted himself with great propriety. He had married a native, and had a family of several children. . . . When I knew him he had bound himself by an oath not to taste spirits except at the new year, at which time he indulged to the greatest excess. He chiefly employed himself in his garden, and had a large stock of European vegetables.[59]

Other folk in Honolulu hurried to take up the profession that Stevenson had been obliged to forgo. An abundance of ti roots, available for the very hard labor of digging them up, and an unquenchable thirst among natives as well as haoles, put a number of stills into action. Soon 'ōkolehao, Hawai'i's peculiar and potent contribution to the world's supply of hard liquors, gained both a name and a devoted following. Once made, 'ōkolehao came to stay. "It was wonderful how the ti root was converted into a strong liquid," wrote John I'i. "It was like the flowing of perspiration from a bud when heated on a stove. . . . [One day I'i] tried two glasses full and his senses became blank."[60]

Because they coveted foreign things, often just for the pleasure of owning them, Hawaiians felt the burnings of envy and the joys of acquiring foreigners' artifacts. They gladly became slaves to the wish to possess those objects from distant lands. The love of money for its own sake made few misers among Hawaiians, however. Mean-spirited and selfish folk had always been scorned even before haoles came. *"He pua na Pīpine,"* such a man or woman was called, "you are a descendant of Pīpine," "a notorious miser who lived long ago in Ka'ū."[61] On the other (and open) hand, the happy spendthrift (usually a drunkard) was much too familiar a figure.

But the need for money with which to buy the things they wanted did affect most town Hawaiians, and in doing so robbed them of the simplicity in living that they had enjoyed in the days of old. Where once they were servants only to chiefs, now they were slaves to money as well, and to the foreign articles they wanted to buy, while still owing service to the ali'i. In other words, without quite knowing what was happening, they became exactly what almost all of us are today: economic peons, held in bondage by fetters made of someone else's gold, chained to their jobs because those jobs helped them to get the tools and the gauds and the toys that clever foreigners dangled before their reaching hands. Just as we sign notes and contracts and applications for credit cards, mortgaging our lives to the future, so did they, chiefs and commoners alike, put their marks to pieces of paper.

Worst of all was their confusion when they compared themselves with the newcomer. The contrast was shattering. When they looked upon haoles, with all their strengths, Hawaiians forgot their own strengths, saw too many of their weaknesses. When they observed how haoles obeyed neither gods nor men, Hawaiians asked why they should continue to be so obedient. When, emboldened by haoles' impunity, Hawaiians broke the kapus and no longer respected their gods, they betrayed themselves more than they forsook their gods. When the kapus were broken so frequently, the whole structure of their society was weakened, was ready to collapse, like the beams of a house when the rot has got at its posts. In losing respect for the gods, they lost their trust in themselves, they lost their place in the ordered realm under the Eye of Kāne.

While Kamehameha lived, he was the strong anchor that held them fast to the sheltering shore. But when he died no one took his place. The people, high as well as low, were cast adrift on the sea of chaos.

இ௸௸௸

Honolulu's frenzy, noisy night after busy day, defeated the Conqueror. In 1812 Kamehameha retreated to Kailua on the island of Hawai'i, taking only a small part of the court with him. After that he ruled his kingdom through high chiefs he appointed as governors of the islands he would see no more. At quiet Kailua he died in peace, on 8 May 1819.

While he lived the old kapus were obeyed—in public at least—because he wanted them to be enforced, and the ancient gods were honored because he respected them. But even as he lay dying Ke'ō-puolani and Ka'ahumanu, who were his favorite wives, several of the high chiefs who were his closest counselors, the priests who served the gods of old: all knew that when the Great King died the old ways must die with him. For them, the gods had lost their mana and the kapus had become nothing more than hindrances laid upon chiefs as well as commoners, and always annoying to foreigners. Hawaiians had learned too much from foreigners during the forty-one years since Captain Cook and his men of the world arrived.

Much too soon, in November 1819, Ka'ahumanu and Ke'ōpuolani persuaded the new king to give the sign that the time had come to lift the heaviest burden from the backs of the people. At a great feast in Kailua, in the presence of many chiefs and commoners and foreigners, 'Iolani Liholiho, Kamehameha II, dared to break the law. Not without fear of the consequences, he sat down at the eating-mat, to share foods with Ke'ōpuolani, his mother, with Ka'ahumanu, his formidable "adviser," and with other women of the royal household.

But then, for many years, he had been steadying himself (in a manner of speaking) for this climactic change with libations of fortifying rum—or of whisky, or gin, or 'ōkolehao, or of anything else warming that might ease his fears of the unknown. During one of those accesses of false courage his companions heard him say: "Sooner let the Akua be destitute of his sacrifices and honors, than we of our pleasures."[62] Courage, then, whether false or true, accompanied him that day to the eating-mat. When this 'ai noa, this free eating, was done—without show of anger from the gods—the whole kapu system cracked open, like an aged kukui nut, revealing its emptiness. The rule of the gods was ended.

Hewahewa, highest priest in the kingdom, approved this break with the past. His orders went out, from Hawai'i to Ni'ihau, and consenting priests and rejoicing commoners set fire to temple buildings in heiaus throughout the land, throwing down the images of the gods from their high places, to burn them, or bury them, or cast them into the sea—or, in a few places, to hide them away, secretly and reverently, to await a later and less troubled time.

Hawai'i nei was a nation without a religion then, and almost without law. Only the profound respect of commoners for chiefs, and of chiefs for the mana of the new ruler, preserved the kingdom from sinking into disorder.

❧❧❧❧

Anticipating the change, some of the more canny high chiefs and chiefesses had already prepared themselves for this break with the past—and with the gods. Ka'ahumanu herself, a most willful woman and a frequent trial to her husband, Kamehameha I, broke many of the eating kapus even while he lived. And, on several occasions (according to gossip), she also broke the kapu against adultery, yet survived her husband's anger as well as priestly condemnation.

But younger ali'i, less powerful than Ka'ahumanu in rank and in mind, had to be more cautious at their experiments in disobedience. They tested the patience of the gods aboard foreign ships. There, in theory, commoners would not see them eating together, and the gods might be more lenient because they were being misled by haoles. Gavan Daws has described one of these essays in artful dodging:

> When the Russian Otto von Kotzebue visited Honolulu in 1816 he found a common woman's body floating in the harbor. She had been killed for breaking the eating kapu; but then male and female chiefs came on board Kotzebue's ship to eat together—a most irregular arrangement, although some other prohibitions still held. The chiefs arrived well dressed and well mannered, but as it turned out they did not eat much. The pig served by the Russians had not been consecrated, and it had contaminated all other food cooked at the same fire. So the Hawaiians watched while the Russians ate, and themselves merely nibbled at biscuits, cheese, and fruit. Toasts were drunk back and forth to the Emperor of Russia and Kamehameha, and all were the best of friends. The female chiefs were at table, where they really should not have been, and they drank heavily enough to become tipsy.[63]

Hawaiians' gentle declaration of independence, begun with the 'ai noa, was evidence of a rebellion of the mind, manifesting their need for freedom, not merely a protest of the body, demanding license for its passions. The 'ai noa is a testimony to the power of reason—even in men (and women) whom foreigners still considered to be "primitive." The orderliness with which it was achieved is a tribute to the character of the Hawaiian people—as it was also a portent of things to come.

Even so, as Daws has pointed out, this was an "incomplete revolution." The free eating, the overthrow of the kapu system, were achieved because of decisions

> taken by a handful of chiefs. The commoners, as usual, followed where their aliis led. Certainly the ordinary Hawaiians had good reason to be relieved when the life and death burden of religious observation was lifted, but just as certainly they did not abandon their old faith completely. Many images from the heiaus were hidden and worshipped secretly; the bones of dead chiefs in the mausoleum at Honaunau were venerated as before; the gods of fishing and planting continued to be given first fruits; Pele, the goddess of the volcano, had her devotees for decades after 1819; travelers' shrines were piled with offerings; and the spirit world of the Hawaiians was still filled with powerful supernatural beings.[64]

But, as Daws and others have explained, this revolution was incomplete in too many ways—most of all because it provided no system of thought and governance to replace the one it had rejected.

Britain's poet, Lord Byron, burbling about the upheavals in France 200 years ago, exclaimed: "Revolution alone can save the earth from hell's pollution." *Hélas!* Romantical poets are better at fancies than at prophecies. No revolution anywhere, before or since, has ever been that cleansing—least of all the bloody savage Terror that Frenchmen contrived for themselves in the 1790s.

The modest revolution in Hawai'i (about which neither Byron nor his contemporaries in Europe and America ever heard a word) only opened wider the gates of hell, to release all its assorted pollutions upon the hapless islanders.

In one of his works Freud included a quotation from Goethe. The thought applies as much to the progress of confused Hawaiians as to that of Europeans (or Americans): "From heaven through the world to hell."[65]

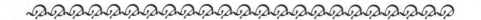

SEVEN

The Time of Troubles

Hawaiians received a few benefits and many woes in return for their hospitality to visitors from the great world beyond their horizons. Whereas they could have continued to live comfortably enough without the benefits, they were almost annihilated by the harmful effects of their association with foreigners.

Denis Diderot was not the only philosopher to worry about the fate of Polynesia's people as Europeans began to swarm into the South Pacific. His shouts of warning to the Tahitians—"Weep, wretched people of Tahiti, weep!"—were preceded and followed by squeaks of agitation from lesser prophets foretelling doom for the innocents of Oceania.[1]

George Forster's impossible hope was published nineteen years before Diderot's condemnation of Europeans appeared in print. Forster, the junior member of a noted father-and-son team of naturalists who accompanied Captain Cook during his second voyage to the Pacific Ocean, from 1772 to 1775, published a book in London in 1777. That was the year before Cook, on a third voyage to the Pacific, discovered the Hawaiian Islands. Forster "sincerely wished" that Europeans would stop all intercourse with Polynesians "before the corruption of manners which unhappily characterizes civilized regions, may reach that innocent race of men, who live fortunate in their ignorance and simplicity."[2]

Even as he composed that futile protest, he must have known that no one in Europe would heed him. And of course no one did.

ぐ・ぐ・ぐ・ぐ

In itself, a resident population of foreigners would not have been harmful to Hawaiians. Thoroughly evil haoles who contributed nothing of value or use to natives were soon recognized and ordered to leave the country by vigilant King Kamehameha or by the chiefs who governed the outlying islands in his name. Nonetheless, few of the haoles who were allowed to remain equaled in merit men like John Young, Isaac Davis, Don Francisco de Paula Marin, merchant James Hunnewell, Captain John Meek, Captain Alexander Adams, Captain George Beckley, and trader Stephen Reynolds (not all of whom were exactly paragons of virtue for Hawaiians to imitate). Kamehameha and his people were fortunate in gaining the services of such relatively good men as those. The unnamed others who stayed, although not wholly bad, were not distinguished for either upright-ness or contributions to local welfare.

Nevertheless, at the very least, all haoles, good or bad, would have been causes of disaffection for native people and sources of disruption to native mores. By their behavior, if not by actual persuasion, the newcomers would have induced natives to question and ultimately to forsake the kapus which regulated Hawaiians' thoughts and actions before the 'ai noa, "free eating," that clear break with the past. In sociological terms, natives questioned the old values they had respected for so long, and tried to replace them with new values (which usually were not any better than the old) or with no values at all. And when, as was so often the case, a few rebels among the natives accepted some of the new standards, while staunch conservatives insisted on retaining all of the old, further conflicts and confusions arose, to make even more difficult the complex process of transition. This transition would have occurred in any event as the natural consequence of occasional contacts with foreigners in ports or on beaches, even if haoles had not come to live in the islands. But resident foreigners hastened the rate of change, imposing a pace that proved to be too rapid for the native society to accommodate without stress and harm.

Samuel Hitchcock, that teenage entrepreneur and "troublemaker" on Kaua'i, of whom Captain Douglas complained in 1789, probably was the first haole who actually lived among Hawaiians for more than a few days' shore leave. Hitchcock's presence gave trader Douglas an idea: if the youth could survive the experience, then perhaps so could older white men. In 1790 Douglas—apparently the first foreigner to recognize that sandalwood grew in the Sandwich Islands—left two members of his crew on Kaua'i, with instructions to collect the precious wood for him. A year later, American trader John Kendrick, master of *Lady Washington,* assigned three of his men "to collect sanders wood and pearls."[3] The sailors and the sandalwood they had gathered, but only a disappointing harvest of pearls, were picked up when their ships returned for them after an absence of almost two years.

The largest island, Hawai'i, acquired its foreign colony at about the same time. By January 1794 eleven haoles were living at Kealakekua Bay. Edward Bell, clerk on HMS *Chatham,* a tender to Captain Vancouver's expedition, considered them "a motley set, a most curious collection . . . for among them were English, Irish, Portuguese, Genoaese, Americans, and Chinese."[4] Foreigners left the islands as casually as they arrived. Whatever reason a man may have given himself for jumping ship, a few months of "going native" did not necessarily convert him into a renegade who cut all ties with home—or with the sea.

๛๛๛๛

Whether they became transient or permanent residents, haoles who did live among Hawaiians influenced them in many ways. Archibald Campbell, writing about "the nearly sixty white people upon Wahoo alone" in 1809–1810, appraised them from a haole's point of view:

> Many inducements are held out to sailors to remain here. If they conduct themselves with propriety, they rank as chiefs, and are entitled to all the privileges of the order; at all events, they are certain of being maintained by some of the chiefs, who are always anxious to have white people about them.
>
> The king has a considerable number in his service, chiefly carpenters, joiners, masons, blacksmiths, and bricklayers; these he rewards liberally with grants of land. Some of these people are sober and industrious; but this is far from being their general character; on the contrary, many of them are idle and dissolute, getting drunk whenever an opportunity presents itself. They have introduced distillation into the island; and the evil consequences, both to the natives and whites, are incalculable.[5]

Campbell explained that the number of white people on O'ahu was "constantly varying." Of the sixty haoles there in 1809–1810, about a third were Americans, "the rest were almost all English . . . [and] six or eight were convicts who had made their escape from New South Wales."[6]

In 1818 Captain Vasilii M. Golovnin, possibly the most friendly commander to visit Hawai'i since Vancouver, and certainly the most charitable in the opinions he entertained toward everything native, qualified Campbell's observations from a more elevated position:

> The majority of [the Europeans] cannot boast of high morals, and they are all uneducated, lacking in scientific knowledge; such people can only teach the natives what they themselves know, and their knowledge consists merely of various crafts and trades, of sailing ships and using firearms.[7]

Looking ahead, Golovnin hoped for a happy ending to the Hawaiians' apprenticeship in the ways of the West:

> Were it possible to introduce the Christian faith and the art of writing among the Islanders, they would in one century reach a state of civilization unparalleled in history. But it is not easy to introduce an outside religion to a free and strong race.[8]

In 1868 Samuel M. Kamakau, in a sweeping summary that revealed as much about Hawaiians as about haoles, considered foreigners from his insider's point of view—which, we sense, came close to the truth:

> Some were red, some black, some white; some were educated while some were uneducated. Some had come to seek riches, by trade and commerce; while some came as laborers under certain people, and others as escaped sailors. . . . Some were received with open arms by the chiefs and the commoners and became favorites to the Hawaiians, and died under the care of the chiefs, leaving children who became heirs with the Hawaiian people. Some of these foreigners became good advisers to the government while others sought only for their own good, depriving the government of much wealth and property, and placed the Hawaiians under their feet, and many of these were of high notions, full of conceit, and had no use for the Hawaiians.
>
> Some of these people loved only money, and wished to place heavy burdens upon the people of the land. Then again there were those who had real love for the Hawaiian people, and by their deeds showed this love to the Hawaiians.[9]

ഔഔഔഔ

English and American captains engaged in the China trade soon discovered that Chinese men made good sailors—and even better cooks, cabin boys, and craftsmen. Some of John Papa I'i's memories from childhood related to "a house for the very first Chinese ever seen" in Honolulu. That house stood near the beach of Nihoa. The time would have been about 1815. The Chinese who lived there "prepared food for the ship-captains who took the sandalwood to China. . . . Because [their] faces . . . and their speech (which we now commonly hear) were unusual, they were observed by great numbers of [Hawaiian] people."[10]

Those first Chinese residents are significant in their own right as individuals contributing their parts to Hawai'i's social history. But they may have been important in another and less happy way. Many years later, when "the Oriental leprosy" was beginning to spread through the susceptible native population, persistent talk among islanders directed suspicion on "Chinese cooks" for having introduced the disease. This was said to be the reason why Hawaiians called the disease *ka ma'i Pākē*—the Chinese sickness.

Another explanation for the name *ma'i Pākē* blamed the appearance of the disease in Hawai'i upon George Nae'a, a lesser chief. The very few references to him in accounts after the late 1850s speak of Nae'a as "the husband of Queen Emma's mother," never as Queen Emma's father. Apparently he had spent some time in China and developed leprosy after returning to Honolulu. Because he was a chief, Hawaiians thereupon called leprosy *ka ma'i ali'i,* the chiefs' disease. Mouritz wrote that Nae'a "was a leper in 1838, and died in 1854," implying that during all those years he was a source of infection for vulnerable Hawaiians.[11]

When, a few years later, Peter Ka'eo, a high chief and a cousin to Queen Emma, consort of King Kamehameha IV, also developed leprosy, Hawaiians found further reason to call the disease ka ma'i ali'i.

ᏸᏸᏸᏸᏸ

In Hawai'i too, as in India, Africa, Latin America, and other islands of Oceania, white men thought that dark-skinned natives existed in order to serve white men from Europe and America. No one among those certitudinous haoles in Hawai'i doubted this dispensation, just as even the best of them did not doubt that, in employing natives, lordly foreigners helped to raise "kanakas" a step or two above the "ignorance" and the "barbarism" in which they had dwelled before haoles arrived to uplift them. Proud chiefs, who could trace their lineage through fifty or sixty generations, might have resented such patronizing, but they did not have to bear the consequences of it.

Once again the burden fell upon commoners. They had always served their domineering chiefs, out of devotion if not in actual fear; and officers from sailing ships would have been regarded as aliʻi of another color, albeit something less than descendants of gods. Chiefs, never questioning their right to command or to take, joined with visitors in exploiting commoners, often treating their people much more cruelly than foreigners did.

British trader John Turnbull, visiting in 1802–1803, saw this system in operation, and did not like it:

> In these islands . . . obedience is understood as well as tyranny, and the despotism and wantonness of command in the chiefs is only equalled by the correspondent timidity and submission of the people. Philosophers are much mistaken who build systems of natural liberty. Rousseau's savage, a being who roves the woods according to his own will, exists no where but in his writings.[12]

Golovnin too deplored "the miserable condition of the commoner people, whose life and property are entirely at the mercy of the chiefs."[13]

Obedient, "unmurmuring," always passive, commoners performed the tasks assigned to them. But as serfs everywhere have always done, they tried to even the score in little ways: they worked no harder than necessary, did nothing more than they must, and—with only a few strong exceptions—never gave up their utter dependence upon the chiefs who were responsible for "taking care" of them. Most commoners saw the uncertainties in independence and understood the futility of trying to amass possessions that the tax gatherers of their overlords could seize with a flick of a finger. Not until Christian missionaries from America came in 1820 to live among them would all Hawaiians have the chance to hear about the worth that some haoles placed on a single soul and the dignity they accorded an individual person. The self-serving haoles who preceded these missionaries withheld from Hawaiians any knowledge of such unsettling thoughts.

Many foreigners after John Turnbull remarked on the subservience of commoners to chiefs. As late as 1825 Robert Dampier, a young Englishman assigned as artist aboard HMS *Blonde*, noticed that, while the commoners "are blest with the most mild and tractable natures possible," the arrogant "chiefs possess unbounded sway over them; their will is a perfect law."[14] As one of the major consequences of this relationship, Dampier believed, "these islanders seem to have no idea of trade." Despite the "fertility and teeming richness of the soil," they did not bother to grow coffee, cotton, and sugarcane, "but simply attend to the only article of commerce which nature spontaneously has afforded them . . . the Sandal Wood."[15]

Nonetheless (and Dampier was not the first to notice this), neither chiefs nor commoners had failed to learn some basic lessons in economics or trade:

> The Chiefs having conceived (and I believe very justly) that the Americans have been constantly imposing upon them, by offering their goods at an exorbitant price, now demand themselves, at a ridiculously high price, not only for the Sandal Wood, but also for the necessaries for victualing the different ships, constantly arriving for this purpose. . . . The Americans . . . richly deserve this severe retaliation.[16]

With the confidence of an outsider who, after a week's sojourn in a foreign country, thinks himself sufficiently informed to write a book about it, Dampier (contradicting himself once again) declares:

> They begin now to understand the value of money, and are no longer willing to barter for beads or insignificant trinkets. We constantly had plenty of traffickers about the house . . . bringing Idols, Shells, Stone Axes, and other Curiosities, for which they invariably demanded a dollar.[17]

After having enjoyed forty-seven years of experience with foreign tourists, Hawaiians were catching on to the ways of commerce at a rate faster than Dampier allowed:

> Observing that several of us were eager to possess some of these ancient Idols they diligently set to work, and soon fabricated a great number of grim looking deities. To these they endeavored to give as ancient a look as possible hoping thus cunningly to impose upon our credulity.[18]

Such a crafty adaptation to souvenir hunters indicates that some Hawaiians had figured out systems for making a few fast kālās long before Dampier and his shipmates arrived. Moreover, in foreign coins of gold or silver or copper shrewder commoners had found at last a tax-free way to reward themselves for their labors. Those dollars, shillings, piastres, and reals were spent so fast in the fleshpots of Honolulu that very few of them were yielded up to the tax collectors of chiefs. Dutiful commoners still supported their liege-lords with days of labor, *kō'ele,* and payments in hogs, taro, poi, kapa, or other produce, but generally they kept or spent on themselves whatever cash they earned from foreigners. Under the circumstances, having no place to hide it, they were practically forced to spend it quickly. But the spending—and the earning too—gave them an incentive to work such as they had not known in the old days.

In effect, this discovery of the purchasing power of their labor led to the beginning of the economic emancipation of a few clever commoners who lived in the port towns, especially in Honolulu. Yet, as they demonstrated all too clearly, they did not know what to do with freedom, or how to save their money—as some haoles did. Salutary though it might be in principle, this kind of emancipation came too soon. Political freedom had to come first.

Naturally, the small sums in cash that a few Hawaiians received for their services eventually led to large consequences that no one expected. When they became acquainted with foreigners' coins, and accepted the ideas of exchange that they represented, Hawaiians dealt another strong blow to the foundations of their society. Fernand Braudel explained the effects of this change:

> The same processes can be observed everywhere: any society based on an ancient structure which opens the doors to money sooner or later loses its acquired equilibria and liberates forces that can never afterwards be adequately controlled. The new form of interchange disturbs the old order, benefits a few privileged individuals, and hurts everyone else. Every society has to turn over a new leaf under the impact.[19]

ʻʻʻʻ

Most commoners, however, not only in 1825 but also long after Dampier's visit, could not escape the commands of chiefs or the toils of foreigners.

In the beginning, commoners' duties with respect to foreigners were limited. Men supplied the labor for growing foodstuffs; for provisioning waiting ships with victuals, firewood, and water; for unloading and loading cargoes; and for other occasional jobs along the waterfront, such as towing vessels through the narrow entrance of Honolulu harbor into the anchorage within. Women offered their bodies, in the primary service that interested sailors, or waited upon them in grogshops and food stalls.

Yet within nine years of the discovery of the Sandwich Islands, ingenious visitors and obliging chiefs were putting commoners to other uses. In May 1787 the "child-wife" of Captain Charles W. Barkley, herself the first white woman to see Hawai'i (and to be seen by Hawaiians) took away with her as a lady's maid a young native named Winee, who therewith became the first identified Hawaiian woman to leave the islands for foreign parts. Before long many a captain who sailed without a wife either enticed or abducted a girl or two to console him during his months at sea. Rarely did those girls return to Hawai'i aboard the same ships that bore them away. Their maritime mates did not always abandon these pacific mistresses. Usually they turned them over to other captains, who promised to bring the girls home and often did so—richer in experience and trinkets, perhaps, but somewhat the worse for wear.

Some girls did not come home again. Winee herself was among the first of the sad casualties. Although the Barkleys treated her with every consideration, she contracted "a lingering illness." Much to their distress, for Mrs. Barkley "was so pleased with the amiable manners of poor Winee that she felt a desire to take her to Europe," they decided to leave the ailing girl, "already far advanced in her decline," with British friends in Canton, to await the time when some kind captain would take her back to Hawai'i. John Meares, master of *Felice,* offered her this courtesy, but poor Winee died on 2 February 1788, before his ship crossed the China Sea.

Hawaiian males, even more eager to see the world, must have wangled passage from sympathetic captains even before the Barkleys carried off Winee. Judging by contemporary accounts, quite a few "Sandwichers" appeared in one foreign port or another, not always as sailors signed on for a voyage. Sometimes they sort of went along for the ride, as friends of the crews who later deposited them in Canton or Macao or Manila.

When Captain Meares sailed from Taipa Bay near Macao in January 1788, he took as guests aboard *Felice,* in addition to Winee, an American Indian from King George's Sound in Alaska and three Hawaiian males. Two of these were commoners: "a stout man and a boy from the island of Mowee . . . who had been brought to China, by different ships, rather as objects of curiosity than for the better motives of instruction to them, or advantage to commerce."

The third Hawaiian was Ka'iana 'Ahu'ula, "a prince of Kauai," whom Meares himself had taken to China aboard *Nootka* in September 1787, with the laudable intention of instructing that elegant chief in the ways of the world. Ka'iana was very much "an object of curiosity" to the Chinese as well as to Europeans living in Canton and Macao. About thirty-two years old at the time, "he was near six feet five inches in stature, and the muscular form of his limbs was of an Herculean appearance. His carriage was replete with dignity . . . and he possessed an air of distinction."[20] As a portrait of him shows, Ka'iana happened to be one of the handsomest men who ever lived in any country, and that won him admiring attention wherever he went —outside of Hawai'i. The Chinese "appeared to regard him with awe, and . . . the timid crowd never failed to open him a ready passage." They called him "The Great Stranger."[21]

That voyage aboard *Felice* was almost as calamitous for Ka'iana as it was for Winee. He attended her with great solicitude until she died, and "caught a fever which with the humane anxiety he felt on her account, confined him for some time to his bed." After a short stay at Zamboanga in the Philippines, Ka'iana recovered, to live seven years longer, until a more spectacular death could claim him. But Kane, the man from Maui who took care of Ka'iana during his illness, contracted the fever and died at sea on 23 March. The vulnerability of their race to foreigners' diseases marked Hawaiians abroad as it did at home.

Ka'iana's sickness, which also affected several of *Felice*'s crew, probably was a food-borne or water-borne intestinal infection, called "bowel fever" in those days, now known as a salmonellosis or a shigellosis or an amoebiasis. Winee's complaint is more difficult to identify: it could have been tuberculosis, or an intractable pneumonitis, even a chronic intestinal infection acquired somewhere during her travels with the Barkleys. The possibility of a venereal disease cannot be dismissed, although, in charity, it should be discounted because Winee does not seem to have been that sort of girl. Ka'iana need not have caught his ailment from her. The fact that several members of *Felice*'s company were ill at the same time suggests that they, Ka'iana, and Kane became infected while still ashore at Taipa or Macao.

At long last, on 10 December 1788, Ka'iana and the boy from Maui reached Kealakekua Bay. Kamehameha, impressed less by Ka'iana's person than by his wealth in firearms, ammunition, and souvenirs of China (and perhaps also by his knowledge of foreign ways and haole speech), invited the traveler to settle in his domain.

Flattered by this interest, and having learned that he and his family were no longer safe from the enmity of Ka'eo, king of Kaua'i, Ka'iana accepted Kamehameha's offer.

For all his splendid figure, Ka'iana seems to have been a man of little common sense and less loyalty. The first mistake he made (although he could not have known this) was the indulging of his wish to go a-traveling: by leaving home, he became the first Hawaiian of rank to be uprooted and distinguished and displaced, to be educated beyond all possibility of contentment on his return. The second mistake, which he would rue, was the decision to stay with Kamehameha: his possessions, and probably his self-esteem, aroused dislike in Kamehameha's ally-chiefs. "Rendered desperate by his haughtiness of spirit," as Captain Charles Bishop wrote in 1795,[22] he who was accustomed to being the object of admiration among foreigners could not accept with grace the role of a vassal who received no respect at all from the even haughtier supporters of Kamehameha.

The third, and the worst, of his errors in judgment was yet to come. And when it came, his life would be the forfeit: he was killed in the Battle of Nu'uanu in 1795, when Kamehameha added O'ahu to his kingdom—and Ka'iana fought on the losing side.

ぐびびび

By 1790 or 1791 Hawaiian men were being employed as sailors aboard merchant ships plying between northwestern America and China. They proved to be such excellent crewmen that thereafter captains recruited "Sandwichers" at Hawaiian ports as regularly as they took on food and water. Hawaiians had much to commend them: they were able-bodied, strong, and skillful; they worked cheerfully for lower wages; and, because they did not have to be paid for the entire round trip from a vessel's home port in Europe or in America, they reduced the total expense for a ship's cruise.

If they did return to their homes in Hawai'i, a number of native sailors became useful intermediaries between their people and visiting mariners. As they neared a Hawaiian shore many a ship's company were surprised to be met by an outrigger canoe carrying several "dark-skinned, naked savages," at least one of whom hailed them in fluent colloquial English. The rest of his conversation, a mixture of sailors' oaths and pidgin English learned during his service at sea, was rather more comprehensible than the purest of Hawaiian would have been. The cheerful greeter, whose name as often as not would be "Jack" or "Tom" or "George," in remembrance of the haole ship-mate who had befriended him, would guide the vessel to anchorage and serve her officers as interpreter, often as intercessor, in negotiations for food, water, and labor. Almost invariably such native agents were both efficient and honest. Their helpfulness commended not only themselves but also the shipmates with whom they had sailed.

Hawaiian men, being good sailors, might have been safe at sea, but they were in danger from the moment they reached a foreign port. Many promptly succumbed to acute infectious diseases, especially to smallpox and the "bowel fevers," while others contracted slower ways of dying, such as tuberculosis, "lung fevers," and the venereal diseases. Although their susceptibility was well known by 1800, it did not deter captains from signing them on as seamen. If they died, captains shrugged: they could always be replaced. Every port had its jetsam of derelict Europeans or Americans looking for a berth, as well as its crowds of excitable Chinese and ferocious Muslim lascars, or inscrutable American Indians, as ready to see the world as Hawaiians were.

One captain, however, brought a Christian's conscience with him around the Horn. He was Amasa Delano (who in time would become the maternal grandfather of President Franklin Delano Roosevelt of the United States). In 1801, as captain of *Perseverance*, out of Boston, he recruited five Hawaiian seamen at Honolulu. "When I arrived at Canton," he wrote later, "my first concern for these people was to have them inoculated for the smallpox. I had in my previous voyages seen many of these poor creatures die with that loathsome and fatal disorder in that place."[23]

Delano, much better informed than the average merchant-captain of his time, had learned about Jenner's method of vaccination, which American physician Benjamin Waterhouse introduced to New England in 1800. Although Delano knew that Chinese physicians used as their inoculum the more dangerous (if attenuated) "matter" taken from actual convalescent cases of smallpox, rather than the safer "kinepox" recommended by Jenner, he had no choice in Canton. Fortunately for his five Hawaiian charges, they survived both the inoculation and their subsequent exposure to Canton's carriers of the fully virulent smallpox virus.

Sometimes, too, a considerate captain would delay his ship's arrival at a Hawaiian port when a serious disease broke out among her crew. Captain George Anson (the Lord Byron who succeeded Britain's famed poet to that title) made such a decision in mid-February 1825. At the time he was commanding HMS *Blonde,* dispatched by the British government to bring to Hawai'i the bodies of King Kamehameha II and Queen Kamāmalu, who in 1824 had died of the measles in London.

After *Blonde* returned to Valparaiso, Chile, from a visit to the port near Santiago, Robert Dampier wrote:

> We found out, that the Small Pox had spread itself on board our ship. This unseasonable visitation caused Lord Byron the utmost anxiety and distress, as it would be utterly impossible to proceed in this state to the Sandwich Islands, incurring the hazard of depopulating and exterminating the whole race of Sandwichers.

Lord Byron, accordingly, sent his sick sailors to a hospital in Valparaiso, and then gave "all hands the benefit of a short cruise of a week or ten days," until he was sure that "the disorder had departed with those infected."[24]

In truth, the ocean's great distances, more than the thoughtfulness of captains, spared Hawaiians the horrors of smallpox until 1853. The reason was entirely mechanical: all sailing vessels, before the era of the fast "China Clippers," moved too slowly to carry the smallpox virus across the sea to Hawai'i. But in March or April 1853 (no one quite knew when) a ship (no one quite knew which, but probably a clipper) reached Honolulu, carrying at least one person still showing symptoms of smallpox. Police officials duly isolated him, according to regulations—but in a hut on shore, not quarantined aboard ship, as he and all other people on that vessel should have been detained.

From him the smallpox virus spread to contacts—most of whom were susceptible, of course. By May a full epidemic was in progress in Honolulu. It did not end until January 1854. The populations on all islands were affected. No one ever knew how many people sickened, how many died. Official government figures released in 1854 declared "between 5,000 and 6,000 fatalities," in a total population of about 84,000. Comparison of census counts taken in 1850 and 1855 indicates much greater losses. Estimates range from 10,000 to 15,000.[25] "Nearly all the victims were Hawaiians," wrote Richard Greer, in his fine account of this epidemic.[26]

⟨ʃ⟩~⟨ʃ⟩~⟨ʃ⟩~⟨ʃ⟩

Between 1800 and 1820 several hundred Hawaiian men, possibly as many as a thousand, went to sea in foreign ships. Many went away in hope, only to die; others managed to return when adventure no longer beckoned. In itself the absence of this modest number of males during those years would not have had much effect on the future of the Hawaiian people. But the recruiting of Hawaiian sailors during this early period did establish a pattern that eventually affected the nation very seriously indeed.

By 1850, when the native population was severely reduced and in increasing peril, more than 4,000 of its men were employed on merchant vessels or whaleships sailing on all the seven seas. The absence of so many young virile males in the prime of life represented a loss which the nation could not afford. Many of those sailors never returned, having succumbed to hardships at sea or to infectious diseases contracted from shipmates or from people in foreign countries, or having submitted to the varied attractions of alien lands. Whether or not they returned, their prolonged absence deprived the kingdom of workers and fathers at a time when they were most needed at home.

Thus, owners of newly founded sugarcane plantations, unable to recruit enough field workers in the islands, turned to foreign countries for laborers. Encouraged by the Hawaiian government, in 1852 they imported the first contingent of contract laborers, bringing them from southern China. This was the beginning of the planned introduction of workers from many nations and ethnic groups. Their importation changed forever the racial composition of the population of Hawai'i.

Worst of all, in part because of this prolonged gene drain, the birth rate among Hawaiians declined alarmingly. The young men who should have been at home, making more Hawaiian babies (at least some of whom would have survived), were gallivanting around the world, squandering their wages, genes, and lives in foreign lands—or, even sadder, like those forlorn bachelor "kanakas" whom Richard Henry Dana found living in an abandoned oven at San Pedro, California, in the 1830s, earning little money and making no babies at all.[27]

෮෮෮෮

The discovery that sandalwood grew plentifully in these islands turned Hawai'i from a resting place, where haoles spent for-

eign forms of money, into an extensive plantation, where money figuratively grew in trees. After little more than the length of time that
Captain William Douglas needed to transport the first shipload of
sandalwood to China and to return with the exciting news that it was
worth good money, the islands' primary businesses—provisioning
and prostitution—faded into supporting services, as the sandalwood
trade took preeminence. Merchant captains, China's middlemen,
King Kamehameha I and his ally chiefs, all rejoiced in this new
source of income. Everyone profited except the commoners. They
learned the dreary lesson that discovery happens only once, while
exploitation goes on forever.

After Douglas's hunch was confirmed by the eagerness of Canton's
merchants to pay "an exhorbitant price" for specimens of sandalwood he brought them, trading ships carried the novel cargo to China's ports. There, as in many others of Asia's cities, the sweet-
scented, golden yellow wood was fashioned into costly furnishings
and carvings, or heated to yield aromatic oils, or powdered to make
an important component of incense. The midocean country from
which came this new supply of sandalwood was known to Chinese as
"Tan Heong San, Sandalwood Land," or as "the Fragrant Isles."[28]

Until 1819 most of the profit gained in Hawai'i from this trade
went to the king: Kamehameha I kept the resource under control,
making it a royal monopoly. Kamehameha II, neither as smart nor as
strong as his father, permitted the high chiefs to cut down for their
profit the trees growing on the lands he had allotted them.

No one has ever been able to reckon how many thousands of
piculs of sandalwood were exported, or what they were worth in
terms of money or merchandise. (The picul, a Chinese measure,
weighed 133⅓ pounds.) In 1821, when the trade was reaching its
height (and in Hawai'i one picul of sandalwood was worth ten American dollars), a merchant in Honolulu estimated that 30,000 piculs
of the valuable wood were shipped to China during that year alone.
By 1844, as the trade faltered to an end, the chiefs of Hawai'i had
received in return more than a million dollars in goods or in gold.

During those fifty years, exploitation had done its worst. No
longer fragrant, the islands had been stripped of almost their last
seedling of sandalwood. The native population had declined to fewer
than 100,000, although this great mortality cannot be attributed to
sandalwood harvesting alone. On more than one occasion, in order
to satisfy the demands of traders and the avarice of chiefs, hundreds

of commoners at a time were ordered to gather the wood in the mountains and to carry it down to the shore. Thus, in the spring or summer of 1822, Daniel Tyerman and George Bennet, British missionaries visiting on Oʻahu, saw "two thousand persons, laden with faggots of sandalwood, coming down from the mountains to deposit their burthens in the royal store-houses, and then depart to their homes, wearied with their unpaid labours, yet unmurmuring at their bondage."[29]

In April 1830, on Kauaʻi, resident American missionary Peter Gulick wrote that he

> felt distressed and grieved for the people who collect sandalwood. They are often driven by hunger to eat wild and bitter herbs, moss, &c. and though the weather is so cold on the hills that my winter clothes will scarcely keep me comfortable, I frequently see men with no clothing except the maro. Were they not remarkably hardy, many of them would certainly perish.[30]

The Reverend Mr. Gulick did not yet know that the people were not remarkably hardy. They were perishing in great numbers because of those enforced expeditions into the mountains. Exposure to rain and cold on the higher slopes where sandalwood trees grow, famine caused by neglect of agriculture, and wave after wave of epidemic diseases killed those docile commoners as relentlessly as they were killing the sandalwood trees. Some seedlings would spring up again, in time, in some places. But the people never recovered.

"While the people hungered and went naked," their lords accumulated more possessions than they could possibly use. They filled homes and storehouses with awkward uncomfortable pieces of Western or Chinese furniture, tarnishing mirrors, dusty chandeliers; with chests full of mildewed haole clothing and foreign fabrics by the bale; with saddles, cutlasses, teapots, cooking pots, and chamberpots; with crates of glass beads, boxes of sugared sweets, and bottles of spirits; with armories of pistols, muskets, and rifles, most of them too ancient and too rusty to be fired. Conspicuous consumption at its flagrant worst was compounded by islanders' innocence and traders' guile: chiefs who were just learning to write happily scrawled their names (or made their marks) on promissory notes thoughtfully prepared for them, in English they could not read, by Honolulu's cordial shopkeepers.

To unmurmuring commoners and protesting missionaries, these

hoards of loot were not made any more acceptable when much of the stuff rusted or rotted away before it was ever used. The Reverend Artemas Bishop, an American missionary who arrived in 1823, was racked to his Calvinist core when at Kailua he saw "one of [high chief] Kuakini's large double canoes loaded deep with bales of broad cloth and Chinese silks and satins which had been damaged by long storage" put out from shore to dump its cargo in the ocean.[31]

Despite their ample incomes, those feckless chiefs, who took more pleasure in buying things than in paying for them, sank as deep into debt as they did into self-indulgence. By 1829 the lot of them owed about $100,000 to Honolulu's worrying merchants. Long before then, these mechant gentlemen, no longer friendly, bleeding through their very pockets, began to scream for help from their home governments. After 1826, Britain, France, and the United States, seeing their duty to hardworking citizens suffering in the reprobate Sandwich Isles, sent ships-of-war commanded by arrogant officers to impress upon the derelict chiefs the sanctity of haole writs. As an added safeguard to foreign investments, the Great Powers installed in Honolulu a line of litigious consuls who, for more than thirty years, were devilishly clever at contriving ways to plague the native government while protecting the interests of their countrymen—and of their plotting devious selves.

Even with such relentless persuaders, some chiefs never got around to redeeming their yellowing promissory notes. By 1843 these added up to a burdensome $120,000. That year, to save the surviving chiefs and himself from incessant dunning, Kamehameha III decided to consider their debits as "the national debt" and, amid sighs of relief from all parties, paid the creditors with money from his government's all but empty treasury.

☙☙☙☙☙

For Hawaiians in general, their initial experiences with haole traders, so concerned with reckoning up profits and losses, were little more than a perpetual annoyance, like being pursued by fleas hopping out from the thatch of a grass hut. Commoners were slow to understand that, whether they liked it or not, they were being schooled in a new way of life as they were being taken over by a novel system of economics. Ready or not, they were being civilized according to the standards of English and American shopkeepers— who never doubted that their brand of civilization was the only possible one for every novice nation to adopt.

These merchants, whether they lived in London, Boston, Canton, or Honolulu, or sailed in ships across the waters of the Pacific Ocean, did not consciously set out to convert Hawaiians to the Anglo-American ethos. Nothing was further from their minds. The only conversions that interested them were those that transmuted pieces of merchandise into ounces of gold. Simply by being themselves, seaborne sellers of textiles woven in England, traders of Virginia's tobacco for island victuals, peddlers of needles, pins, scissors, fishhooks, knives, and hatchets made of shining steel, dangled before entranced Hawaiians all the things their countries produced so lavishly. Things, not ideas, not philosophies, captivated Hawaiians. And those captive innocents submitted willingly to the civilization of which such wonderful, useful articles were both the advertisement and the trap. Before ever Kamehameha I ceded his island to Britain's distant king, he and his people were caught in the Westerners' golden web.

Because American and English traders outnumbered those from other nations, they dominated the Hawaiian people during the impressionable period when they stepped out of the neolithic past into the capitalist present. Hawai'i would not be an American state today, and its history would be entirely different, if Spanish, French, German, or Russian merchants had established their forms of economic and social dominion over Sandwich islanders in that critical first quarter of the nineteenth century.

Money-minded as they were, American and British traders, like their governments at home, took no interest in annexing the Sandwich Islands. These entrepreneurs may not have been the best examples of democrats, or forthright proponents of the Rights of Man. But, because they had been free men in the lands from which they came, in Hawai'i they did not wish to own a man or aspire to enslave a nation. They merely wanted Hawaiians, and visiting foreigners also, to buy the commodities they offered for sale—and, naturally, to pay for those articles in kind or in cash. In the social as well as in the business sense, they practiced free enterprise. With their laissez-faire attitude in all matters, they offered no threat to the political establishment in Hawai'i. As a result, that indigenous system not only endured, but was actually strengthened, during the decades when Hawaiians were most defenseless against foreign aggrandizement. And for a while, for a longer time than their relatives in other parts of Polynesia were granted, Hawaiians did not have to submit to being conquered as well as to being civilized.

ᘓᘓᘓᘓ

In the course of being converted to the joys of civilization—
"in being snivellized," as Herman Melville jeered—Hawaiians were
exposed to the inevitable mixture of banes and benisons.

Melville, ungenerous toward events and people he disliked (missionaries foremost among them), dismissed the processes of civilization much too brusquely, because during his years as a sailor aboard
ships in the Pacific he had seen the adverse effects that all foreigners
were having on Polynesians. He did not see far enough into the
future, however, and refused to understand that, despite its inexorable cruelties to individuals, civilization also confers rewards upon
societies that otherwise they would never attain. Braudel has pointed
this out: "Civilizations do indeed create bonds, that is to say an
order, bringing [together] thousands of cultural possessions effectively different from, and at first sight even foreign to, each other—
goods that range from those of the spirit and the intellect to the tools
and objects of everyday life."[32]

The blessings of civilization cannot be denied—by those who manage to live long enough to gain them. Yet the first generations of a
society being exposed to the juggernaut are subjected to almost intolerable pressures and tensions and dangers, both psychological and
physical. Among Hawaiians, for example, in the new era they
entered in 1778, every thing and every thought and every relationship suddenly became more complex, more charged with uncertainty, more fraught with unpredictability. For most Hawaiians, the
gifts that civilization brought in its Pandora's box must have been
confounding, maddening, shattering. But for the strong few, who
found Hope too at the bottom of the box, those gifts must have been
exciting, stimulating, liberating.

ᘓᘓᘓᘓ

With the growth of Honolulu, as seaport and center of commerce, the islands became in fact, if not yet in name, "the Crossroads
of the Pacific." Honolulu may have started as a sleepy little village,
dozing under a hot sun, waiting for its next ship to come in, but it did
not stay that way for long. By 1800 the position of "Brown's Harbor"
was well known to mariners, and the safety of its anchorage had
been widely recognized. Thereafter the number of vessels and seafarers seeking its conveniences increased rapidly. Although official

records of arrivals and departures were not begun until 1824, entries in journals kept by residents such as Don Marin and James Hunnewell show that during almost every week of 1818 and 1819 at least one ship entered the harbor. Inasmuch as, on the average, a ship's complement of officers and crew numbered about twenty-five men, the town welcomed a considerable flow of visitors, and money, during the course of a year.

Most vessels were American or British merchantmen engaged in the China trade, or, infrequently, a British whaling ship on her way to the southern grounds near Australia. But Russian, French, and Spanish vessels, and one flying the flag of the new Republic of Argentina, also put in at Honolulu for provisions and refreshment. Other island ports of call too, especially Lahaina on Maui and Kealakekua Bay on Hawai'i, drew their shares of visitors, although they were by no means as busy as Honolulu. Then, in 1819, a whole new chapter in Hawai'i's history began when *Balena* out of New Bedford and *Equator* from Nantucket arrived at Kealakekua Bay, the first American whaling ships to venture this far into the Pacific Ocean.

Eighty years later, Dr. E. S. Goodhue, an incorrigibly pessimistic Victorian settled in Honolulu, sniffed: "This meant the beginning of a foreign influence which has had to be met, in all its pernicious forms, from that day to this."[33] Even earlier, in the 1840s, the Reverend Sheldon Dibble extended the indictment to almost everyone other than American missionaries:

> The vice of licentiousness was not diminished but rather, if possible, increased by the intercourse of early visitors from foreign lands. Many ships, indeed, that visited the islands were no better than floating exhibitions of Sodom and Gomorrah; and the crime in their case being attended with that awful curse which God annexes to it in civilized lands, made tremendous havoc among the unwary people. . . . The desolating curse knew no barrier, but like a raging fire, driven by a strong wind through a dry forest, spread at once to the very extreme parts of the islands, and there is much to fear that its ravages cannot be entirely arrested before it shall even exterminate the race.[34]

ಶ೭ಶ೭ಶ೭

Although King Kamehameha I had avoided Honolulu since 1812, the Council of Chiefs who tried to advise his son and successor could not ignore the fact that its harbor was the most important place in the nation. In September 1820 they persuaded 'Iolani Liholiho, King Kamehameha II, to transfer his residence from Kailua on Hawai'i to Honolulu. The young king liked O'ahu's dingy noisy port no better than his father had, but he realized its significance and finally established his official residence there in February 1821. With that Honolulu became (for a while) the capital of the kingdom, even though Liholiho still flitted about "from place to place, and island to island, as humor prompts." During his frequent absences the powerful high chiefs who supported him as loyally as they had served his father remained in Honolulu to manage the nation for him.

As the town grew in size it added to the kinds of services it could offer foreign ships and sailors. By 1812 several merchant companies in New England had set up agencies, operated by American residents, to look after their ships, cargoes, and crews. In 1820 John C. Jones, the local representative of Marshall & Wildes, a Boston firm, was appointed "Agent of the United States for Commerce and Seamen," an office something lower than that of consul, which nonetheless authorized him to protect the property and the interests of American citizens. Following this lead, in 1824 Great Britain sent Captain Richard Charlton, the most rancorous "diplomat" ever to afflict the Hawaiian kingdom, to live in Honolulu as London's mobile "Consul for the Sandwich, the Society, and the Friendly Islands."[35]

By 1823 the town supported four general stores, "abundantly furnished with most articles contained in common retail shops and groceries in America." The four stores had "an aggregate trade of $100,000 per year."[36] And in 1825 Honolulu acquired "two public houses for the accommodations of strangers."[37] Presumably these served as inns, rather than as brothels.

In 1820 about 2,000 people, more or less permanent residents, inhabited the sprawl of thatched huts, flimsy sheds, and occasional adobe houses that dotted the narrow plain between Nu'uanu stream to the west and Kaka'ako to the east. The number of foreigners could not have exceeded 200. With their native wives or concubines and half-breed children, they lived little better than did commoners.

The king and the chiefs of his court, with their families, retainers, and servants, dwelled in slightly more pleasant compounds along the harbor's shore. Except for the few coconut palms and kou trees remaining from the time before Honolulu began, and the fruit trees that Don Marin guarded in his vineyard farther inland, the town was as unshaded and hot as a lava flow in desert Ka'ū, as "wicked" as Sodom and Gomorrah combined. From one end to the other, amid the thatched huts, the four general stores with their warehouses, the two inns, the seventeen grogshops, scattered greasy-food booths, and uncounted brothels, no civic improvements for the benefit of the populace brightened the scene. Nor did the town possess a government building other than Ke Kua Nohu, the fort of Honolulu, started by Dr. Georg Scheffer and his Russians in 1816 and, on orders from Kamehameha I, completed by his prime minister Kalanimoku in 1817.

The king's "palace," when Liholiho deigned to be in residence, was the seat of government. When he fled the town, Kalanimoku and Kaʻahumanu (the most imperious of the several widows left by Kamehameha I) ruled in his stead. Inasmuch as they ruled Liholiho too, the affairs of the kingdom did not suffer much in his absence.

For a time after the court moved back to Honolulu from Kailua, Kalanimoku lived in the fort, "near the House of the Gods, close to the edge of the sea." Late in 1822 he caused to be built a large stone residence, the first of its kind in the islands, at the eastern edge of town (about where the Library of Hawaiʻi now stands). In 1824 the big high-ridged thatched houses of the king, the relict queens, and other members of the royal family were raised in a spacious level field adjoining the western side of the yard around Kalanimoku's stone mansion. Those households of the greatest nobles in the land "were surrounded by a very large wooden fence, and the enclosure was called Pohukaina."[38] Thenceforth, the successive palaces of the kings of Hawaiʻi would stand within the sacred precincts of Pohukaʻina, the Place of Ordered Calm.

☙☙☙☙

As Honolulu and its population increased in size, so too did the material wealth of the common people. For them wealth was measured in many forms, from haole tools and utensils to coins of gold, silver, or copper minted in alien lands. The great variety of trade goods brought in by foreigners allowed both chiefs and commoners to acquire luxuries before they felt the need to employ humbler articles in easing their labors. According to Stephen Reynolds (who may not have remembered correctly), implements for farming "were not in use until about 1825–1826," and "household utensils were but very little used" until the 1840s.[39] Captain Vancouver presented Kamehameha I with kitchen and table utensils which the king used only when haoles came to call; and in 1801 Captain Benjamin

Worth, master of *Catherine* out of Boston, gave Ka'ahumanu some white plates, for which "he was ever known by the name of Pa-Keokeo (white plate)."[40]

As they accumulated foreign things, and small sums in currency, Hawaiians also acquired the concept of being paid in coins for labor or for goods they brought to market. Slowly and surely, during the course of two generations, the economy of the port towns and their environs changed from one of barter to one based upon money, from a system founded entirely upon subsistence farming to one of nascent capitalism based on the values of goods and services.

The social system did not change as rapidly: chiefs still kept commoners in thrall; high chiefs still ruled over lesser chiefs; and everyone, high or low, native or foreigner, depended for land and life on the pleasure of the king.

Whatever their rank, only a few Hawaiians recognized the dangers in this precarious (and incongruous) relationship between economics and ethics. The smart ones moved to the towns, where they could be relatively free from the control of local lesser chiefs, but not from the reach of the king or the highest chiefs. In rural areas, however, the old system continued in full force for many more years. Some chiefs, especially those on islands other than O'ahu, strenuously opposed the haoles' casual way of employing—and rewarding—commoners as laborers available for hire. Those reactionary chiefs, become very astute middlemen, preferred to assign commoners under their command to do the tasks that haoles wished to have performed, and to deposit in their own money chests the payments for services rendered. In terms of payment for labor, this arrangement, so nice for the chiefs, lasted until after the Mahele, the Dividing of Lands, in 1848. In terms of political control, the chiefs continued to dominate commoners until long after the end of the monarchy in 1893.

Political evolution did not keep pace with economics. Despite the fact that many individual Hawaiians received a considerable income each year from visitors, the nation as such received none—for the simple reason that the kingdom had no organized bureaucracy with functioning ministries and a corps of civil servants. The king and his advisers, the Council of Chiefs who served him personally, not the nation as a whole, governed the kingdom in one sense. But they ran it for their benefit, not for the sake of the people in general. The king and the chiefs might be relatively rich as individuals, but the nation was penniless.

Until 1843 commoners and vassal chiefs paid taxes in foodstuffs, fishnets, lengths of kapa, and similar articles suitable for barter, or in the kō'ele, "landlord days" of labor. Taxes paid in kind were consumed or stolen almost as fast as they were tendered. And few days of labor were devoted to public works, such as roads, walls around pastures, or port facilities. Usually those landlord days were spent in tilling fields owned by chiefs or, later, on trips into the mountains to collect sandalwood.

While all this expenditure of labor involved commoners in the old way, the need for the ruling chiefs to adapt to the new times was not met. The king and his councilors, having little knowledge about other modes of governing, could not create a stable centralized oligarchy, or enact laws for controlling foreigners and natives, or devise means for acquiring a regular income in cash, or even establish a treasury into which to deposit the king's personal income. As long as Kamehameha I lived, keeping control over the nation, the old system functioned remarkably well. But when the Conqueror died the strength of his hold departed. Liholiho, spoiled and self-indulgent, "soaked in rum," as the Reverend Hiram Bingham scolded, had little interest and less ability in the business of government. As a result, the chiefs high and low did very much as they pleased. Kalanimoku, who had been the Conqueror's prime minister, was the only chief in the land who put the nation's interests before his own, who dedicated his energies and his power to serving not only the new king but also the kingdom as well. Yet Kalanimoku was only one ali'i among many; he was perennially ill with the dropsy; and, most regrettably, he knew little about the craft of government practiced by the great nations of the West. The other chiefs, almost as selfish and irresponsible as the young king, followed his example, not Kalanimoku's. This lack of leaders was another persisting effect of the ma'i 'ōku'u epidemic in 1804.

Liholiho, as unpredictable as Kīlauea's volcano, as shifting as smoke, baffled everyone. Under him resident foreigners found life very precarious indeed: the lands on which they dwelled, the privilege to do business in the islands, in some cases even the foods they ate, were his to give and his to take away. His word, too, was written in smoke.

Foreigners lived and labored—and hoped—from day to day, always uncertain of their tenure. The first company of American missionaries, who arrived in April 1820, were admitted to Liholiho's

realm for one year—on probation. Before the year ended one of them
wrote home:

> Should [the king] be displeased, the land [allotted to the Mission] may
> be taken away tomorrow. White men, who hold extensive lands,
> derive little benefit from them, unless they cultivate their ground them-
> selves. A fare, precarious and coarse, is the portion of most foreigners,
> who reside here: yet none, who have any sobriety or industry, are in
> danger of starving.[41]

Even Don Marin, settled in Honolulu since the mid-1790s, was
not safe from Liholiho's flickering displeasure. On 22 September
1823 Levi Chamberlain, superintendant of secular affairs for the
American Mission, wrote in his journal:

> Notice has been received today that [Kalanimoku and Boki], com-
> manded by the king, then at Lahaina, have ordered Marine, Mr. War-
> ren, Mr. Navarro, and Mr. Temple to be stripped of their property. A
> large number of kanakas entered Mr. Marine's house this morning to
> put the order into effect.[42]

And yet those egocentric aristocrats, the self-indulgent king, the
lack of a central government, could not stop the processes of change.
Foreigners were like a swollen river impounded by a dam of earth:
their presence wore away both the resistance of chiefs and the inertia
of commoners. Whether they liked it or not, Hawaiians were forced
to change their ways.

☙☙☙☙

They adopted not only foreigners' tools and utensils, the
most practical and accessible of things, but also their clothes and
essential parts of their languages, their habits and diversions, many
of their little vanities—and all their vices.

At first the wearing of haole clothing was haphazard and inadequate to a degree that foreigners considered ludicrous: as when a
man might stroll about Honolulu clad only in a loincloth and a sea-
man's battered cap, or in a cast-off woolen shirt without the *malo*.
Yet even that small sampling conferred status upon the wearer, the
while it announced his intention to don the entire haole costume
(except for shoes!) as soon as he could afford to buy it.

These reachings for elegance in attire could not have improved
much "the usual costume of the early Hawaiian—a smile, a malo,

and a scaly cutaneous eruption," as some overdressed haole snob, fresh off a boat, described him.[43] But at least they helped, a little, to cover the nakedness that so scandalized puritanical folk, especially the ones who came from New England.

Naturally, the chiefs led the way in this fashion parade. Kamehameha himself was the first to acquire the complete wardrobe of an English gentleman, although he had little liking for it and wore it as seldom as possible. Lesser folk, not so affluent or so confident as their chiefs, displayed themselves in finery whenever they could, in the endless game of one-upmanship. As usual, the ladies challenged each other with greater devotion than the men: whereas a male would be happy with only a shirt, a woman must deck herself from crown to instep in haole apparel, the more the better. The high chiefesses, in their public appearances, were especially grand.

ლ-ლ-ლ-ლ

Inasmuch as few haoles bothered to learn the "*kanaka* gabble," that fluent rush of vowels which consonants try in vain to stem, Hawaiians perforce had to learn something of the foreign tongues. They soon picked up the basic words in English, French, Spanish, Russian, or Chinese, softened them by dropping the harsh Rs and ugly Gs, and gave them back, more or less recognizably, to converse with foreigners in the assorted dialects of "business" speech—or "pidgin," as Canton's merchants pronounced the word—to everyone's satisfaction. In the course of time, foreigners perforce added to their vocabularies the gestures of mimicry and the few absolutely essential Hawaiian words—like *pau, mauka, makai, hana, hula, 'Ewa, Waikīkī, panipani, kaukau,* and *aloha*—without which communication would have been impossibly slow.

ლ-ლ-ლ-ლ

Hawaiians acquired new skills and crafts, or adapted old approaches to new materials, thereby helping themselves as well as foreigners. Because natives admired and wanted sailing vessels above all other foreign things they had the means to make, they asked first to be taught how to build a ship. Captain Vancouver, in February 1794, understanding their interest, and finding it much more agreeable to his conscience than satisfying their requests for armaments, assigned his ships' carpenters the pleasant task of teaching Kamehameha's canoe makers. They learned quickly. By 1803, as Turnbull noted, they had built for the king "more than 20 ships," ranging in size from twenty-five to seventy tons.[44]

While some Hawaiians fashioned ships, others studied how to rig them. By 1802 native and haole sailmakers, ropemakers, blacksmiths, and carpenters labored for the king and for visitors at Kailua, Lahaina, and Honolulu.

Hawaiian ability in shaping woods and in building structures with unmortared stones did not find much employment during this period, except in the construction or restoration of temples, an important concern to Kamehameha I. Foreigners taught native laborers how to make the adobes and to mortar the stones that formed Honolulu's few storehouses with any claim to being reasonably fire-proof or thief-proof. And the "two foreigners residing in Lahaina [who] built for the king a two-story brick house in 1796,"[45] even if they were the ablest of bricklayers, could not have done all that work by themselves. They must have taught native apprentices the methods for baking bricks shaped from Lahaina's mud and dried grasses for straw, as well as the techniques for burning reef coral in order to obtain the lime needed for mortar.

In skilled workers such as these, not to mention entrepreneurs with more individualized occupations, such as prostitutes and thieves and image-makers, Hawai'i acquired something absolutely new: the first members of an authentic middle class, dependent for a livelihood on no one but themselves. Although this incipient middle class represented only a small percentage of the whole population, eventually they and their children became important contributors to the economic, political, and cultural growth of the kingdom.

Furthermore, because their economic and intellectual levels were higher than those of prostitutes, pimps, and habitués of waterfront grogshops, they tended to avoid the company of those debased folk who shared diseases along with their lewdness. The members of this rising middle class, accordingly, were more likely to escape the blighting venereal diseases, although they could never escape entirely the claims of the other epidemic contagions. From this burgeoning middle class came most of the upright, clean, hardworking townsfolk who supported preachers and priests of the several Christian denominations when they arrived, and who lived long enough to provide the towns' reliable craftsmen—and, most important of all, to produce the healthy children who kept the race alive in spite of all the assaults upon it.

ଓଓଓଓ

Hawaiians also learned the meaning of time—as haoles reckoned it. They themselves measured time by the cycle of the lunar months, which before 1778 had been accurate enough (with help from occasional intercalations) for marking the seasons of their years. But now they were made acquainted with the tyranny of the chronometer, ticking out its little hours, minutes, and seconds. Because haoles aboard their sailing ships lived and worked according to schedules ordained by tides and winds, by the desperate need to round Cape Horn before winter's storms beat in or to cross the Tropics before the Dog Days' calms, foreigners arrived and departed on the flow and ebb of these planetary forces. And, once in port, still mindful of the perils of the sea, they called for services imposed upon them by the turnings of the cosmic clock. "Hawaiian time" did not come to an end in natives' affairs, but they did have to submit to civil time in order to fulfill their promises to anxious captains, studying their chronometers, and to nervous merchants, fingering their pocket watches.

ଓଓଓଓ

Because American storekeepers "opened early and closed late," the business day for everybody began at eight o'clock in the morning and ended at eight o'clock in the evening—or later, if customers kept coming in. Sunday as a time of rest was not observed in this godless place. No one, foreign or native, ever had the chance to adopt the leisurely customs of folk in Spanish American colonies. The Yankee pace, uninterrupted by siestas, runs Hawai'i still.

ଓଓଓଓ

Ambitious Hawaiians gained some sense of enterprise—not merely of bartering for the moment, but rather of managing a business at a sustained level over a period of time. Foremost among these enterprises would have been the growing of fruits and vegetables (almost anything fresh and tasty, not only those delectable melons that John Boit praised); the raising of pigs and chickens (but not of dogs, which haoles spurned vehemently); the gathering of firewood for ships' galleys—all to be set forth in bartering with sailors eager to taste foods other than weevily hardtack and salted pork. Despite the fact that all these things, and the very soil that produced them, belonged to the paramount chief of a district, even the most alert of his subordinate officials could not account for every muskmelon, or cockerel, or billet of wood those fields and forests yielded. A daring farmer, or his sons, could move such marketable goods beyond the vigilance of an official (even sometimes with his collusion), especially if the farmer lived near a port town.

In the ports themselves, enterprising men and women served an obvious function: as providers of comforts to common haoles that lofty chiefs and their snobbish subordinates would not dream of offering. Women (and brothels) were the first of these services, of course, but soon after them came the dusty fly-blown lānais where sailors could buy things to eat and get a cup of apparently clean water to drink. Or something stronger perhaps, after 1809 or thereabouts, by which time those expert convicts who said they had escaped from Britain's penal colony in Australia managed to set up their stills in Honolulu.

Another kind of convert to the system of free enterprise was the 'aihue, the thief. Like all Polynesians, Hawaiians too, from the beginning of their association with haoles, proved themselves "prodigious expert in thievery," as Captain Cook observed. They took, or tried to take, everything that was not nailed down, and sometimes they made off with those things too, and with the nails as well.

By 1818, however, having become better acquainted with the world's portable wonders, 'aihue were rather selective in their pilfering. Captain Golovnin, one of their prominent victims, came near to complimenting them: "Along with the other European 'arts,' [Hawaiians] have learned to steal like civilized people." While his ship Kamchatka lay moored in Honolulu harbor, and under guard, a team of 'aihue, "by reaching in the stern window from their canoes," plucked out of his own cabin "my small travel celleret and a leather covering for a chest."[46] Disposing of these elegant articles would have presented no problem to the thieves, who undoubtedly were well connected with the fences of Honolulu.

In becoming entrepreneurs and, naturally, in keeping some of the rewards for their labors, assorted self-employed individuals acquired the incentive to work for themselves which they had not been given in the days of old, when all too frequently overlords and tax gatherers took away more than a fair share of commoners' products. In the new times, coins and other small foreign articles were more easily hidden than pigs, chickens, and bundles of taro had been. As they accreted these private treasures, commoners became more acquisitive, more aware of the rights of privacy and the comforts of property. This new ferment of possessiveness eroded the feudal structure even more rapidly than did the doubting of the kapus. A man who must bow down before chiefs and priests could pretend to respect them and their gods. But how could he be expected even to pretend to respect chiefs who took away his very personal possessions, earned by diligent labor for his own sake?

At least a few Hawaiians, commoners as well as chiefs, who associated with foreigners in the port towns realized that haoles were showing them other ways to live—and to think—than the one into which they had been born. In what for them must have been the most difficult feat of all, some Hawaiians began to think as haoles did, to plan ahead as they looked ahead, to a future instead of only to the immediate present. In doing so, these thinkers came again, by another route, to questions burning in them about the ways of old: by what right do the chiefs own every moment in our lives, every one of our possessions, our very bodies? Where are the gods, about whom we hear so much but see nothing at all? Why should we respect those remote and unseen gods, who permit us to be used, despoiled, destroyed?

Such thoughts about freedom, however much we today may take them for granted, are not ingrained in members of a primitive society. Such thoughts, and the consequences they imply, are nothing less than revolutionary. In acquiring these rudiments of the intellect in a modern society, regulated though it is by the clockwork machine and the esteem for private property, some Hawaiians emerged from the jungle of the neolithic age into the modern world.

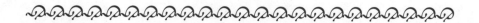

EIGHT

The Time of Dying

Hawaiians learned also the baser aspects of civilization. Where once they had been so careful about keeping households neat and clean, if only because the kapus commanded such respect, now too many of them sank into squalor, amid accumulations of rubbish that scavenging animals could not eat and shiftless people did not bother to remove.

Hawaiians learned also the pleasures of getting drunk on homemade "swipes" and 'ōkolehao, or on costly imported "spirits." The usual unhappy consequences of squandering money and time followed, where everyone in a family suffered. Gambling in the novel haole modes became a new passion, as Golovnin noticed in 1818.[1] A commoner who had no coins to hazard could always find the stake in a wife, a sister, or in himself. The winner of such a prize could bed it, or exchange it easily enough for cash offered by a cruising sailor.

In and out of grogshops, Hawaiians learned the obscenities mouthed by sailors, in several languages. Swearing helped to relieve the miseries of hangovers or frustrations, as a man beat his wife or children or neighbors when the rage of despair seized him.

As Hawaiians themselves said, in later years, these were *wā na'au pō,* "dark and sinful times."

The Reverend Artemas Bishop, having studied Hawaiians since he arrived among them in 1823, expressed his deep concern in an article entitled "An Inquiry into the Causes of Decrease in the Population of the Sandwich Islands," which he prepared for *The Hawaiian Spectator* in 1838. "It is not civilization, but civilized vices that wither the savage," he wrote. "He drinks into them like water, without knowing that their attendant diseases are cutting the tendrils of his heart, and drawing away his life's blood." As did other observers, Bishop be-

228

lieved that alcoholic beverages and "licentiousness" (by which he meant prostitution and the venereal diseases so readily shared among promiscuous people) were the major vices leading to destruction of the Hawaiian populace.[2]

Petrarch had observed all this long before (as Robert Burton observed in *The Anatomy of Melancholy*): "We change language, habits, laws, customs, manners, but not vices, not diseases, not the symptoms of folly and madness—they are still the same."

朇朇朇朇

The one lesson that Hawaiians did not learn from the new way of life was the fact of their dying. Some among their elders may have suspected this truth, because they were the ones who must "care for the bones" of the dead. For the people were dying—not only from obvious epidemics like the squatting sickness of 1804, which killed many men, women, and children within a few weeks and then seemed to fade away to an end. No, this rate of dying was slower, more insidious, scarcely noticeable. This kind of dying carried off a few people here, a few more there, week after week, year after year. Until suddenly, one day, a man looks around and sees at last what is happening. High Chief Kuakini was such a man. "*Auwē!*" he exclaimed. "*Pau i ka make. . . .* All are dead . . ."[3]

Certain elders may have guessed that the race was dying. But how could they have known the magnitude of this loss, without actual counts of numbers living and numbers dead to instruct them? Without newspapers to print obituary notices by the score and alarming editorials by the yard? Without preachers to warn them, in mournful sermons, about the nearness of Death?

Except for the disappearance of members within a family or of people in a small neighborhood, these elders could not have known about losses among folk in districts far from home. Because no Hawaiians could write or read, they exchanged no letters with people in distant places. Only mouths brought messages, only mouths told truths—or lies. And who can be sure that he hears the truth when a man speaks? A talking mouth commits many an error. The elders might have heard hints about the passing of the race, in the talk of travelers wandering toward the towns, who told of deserted homes and villages along the way, of abandoned taro patches, of fields growing only weeds—alien weeds.

About this time, according to David Malo, Hawaiians in Honolulu took to believing that syphilis and gonorrhea, and all the many horrible symptoms they displayed, were caused by the vengeful spirit of Captain Cook, seeking retribution from the nation whose warriors had killed him at Kaʻawaloa. His unforgiving spirit, the believers said, dwelled in *Ka Mū nui ʻeleʻele,* the Great Black Ghoul, which hid by day in the Koʻolau Mountains of Oʻahu, "then in the darkness of night flew over the houses of the people, scattering his poisonous pestilence."

This explanation can be found in none of Malo's works that have been translated into English. But Dr. Arthur Mouritz, who collected odds and ends of medical lore like this, maintained that it appeared in an "uncensored" Hawaiian edition of Malo's history, the approved English translation of which, entitled *Hawaiian Antiquities,* appeared only in 1903. Needless to say, said Mouritz, most copies of the Hawaiian version were "destroyed" before puritanical (or prurient) haoles could acquire them. No matter. The Great Black Ghoul makes for a good story. It would be a better one if it did not resemble so closely a number of similar tales from the folklore of China and Japan.

Whether or not "the Curse of Cook," as jesting haoles referred to the venereal diseases, was an important reason for mortality among Hawaiians, Malo certainly believed that it was. Without identifying the source for his figures, he asserted that, during the twenty years from 1778 to 1798, "at least 10,000 persons had died in this Koolau district [of Oʻahu] from the effects of the venereal diseases, a legacy left by the diseased crews of Cook's ships."[4]

Although he published his *Ka Moolelo* in 1858, the Reverend John F. Pogue joined the American mission in 1844 and knew very well the subjects about which he wrote in that *History.* His paragraph summing up the effects of the venereal diseases upon Hawaiians presented what must have been the standard point of view among both missionaries and concerned haoles long before 1844:

> The chief reason however for the great depopulation was the sickness procured by the women in their relations with white seamen. It is the cause for the rapid dwindling of the race, the death-knell of Hawaii! It is the cause of bodily disfigurement, of weakness in the children; it is the cause for the deserted roads; the causes are too numerous to enumerate. The entire head is attacked by this disease; the innards are weakened, and the entire system from the instep to the head becomes

victimized. If parents have it, it will be passed on to the children and grandchildren, in a continuing descent among those who practice adultery and fornication. This is Hawaii's greatest enemy, destroying the body and the soul of the people.[5]

Many ship captains, when they wrote their books about voyages they had made around the world or in the Pacific Ocean, gave some attention to the diseases (as well as to the attractions) they observed among natives seen along the way. Freycinet, who visited Hawai'i in 1819, was unusual in that he and his physicians devoted ten printed pages to a factual account of this dismal subject among the Sandwich Islanders. "Of these afflictions," he wrote,

"the itch" or scabies was the most widespread . . . the body [was] more or less covered with large scabies pimples, of which many were festering on the top; it is seen especially in the joints, and notably on the hands . . . men, women, children, from the poorest to the most sovereign chiefs, none seemed to be exempt; and pestilence of the same nature even sullied the skin of several Europeans who had been living for a long time among them. . . . I do not believe it to be contagious, and it does not seem to be caught except through prolonged cohabitation with an infected person.[6]

Despite Freycinet's disclaimer, scabies *is* a very contagious infestation. Many haoles knew that only too well—and did their frantic best to avoid contact with people suffering from the itch, even to the point of refusing to shake hands with high chiefs. Hawaiians of all ranks loved to shake hands, to rub noses or touch cheeks in aloha. The Reverend C. S. Stewart and Robert Dampier performed many an agile dance to escape the embrace of good-natured but itching greeters. Dampier was tormented almost out of his skin by playful young Kauikeaouli, ten-year-old King Kamehameha III, while he tried to paint the lad's portrait: "It required therefore my utmost ingenuity to keep him at arm's length without betraying my disgust at his amiable approaches."[7] (And yet, as we can see today in the Honolulu Academy of Arts, Dampier's portrait of the stalwart boy is beguiling as well as properly royal. It reveals none of the nervousness that troubled the artist, and none of the lesions that marred the young king's body.)

Freycinet did not observe as many signs of the venereal diseases as he expected. After the usual discussion about whether Captain Cook's sailors had introduced them, or "the Spaniards who had preceded him" in Tahiti, he did write about syphilis, but not about gonorrhea (which most Western physicians would not recognize as a different disease until after 1838). He was quite matter of fact in describing the cases he saw, using none of the graphic detail that later writers would employ:

> An ophthalmia which I observed, humors and lachrymous and salivary fistulas, could, however, very well have been [caused by syphilis], some scars, and an ichorous ulceration of the conjunctivae would also perhaps belong to this category.
>
> I learned from a European living on Mowi that on that island the venereal disease manifested itself frequently by buboes in the groin and the armpits and by chancres.[8]

In short, neither Freycinet nor his surgeons, Messieurs Quoy and Gaimard, saw many walking cases of advanced syphilis, and therefore did not consider it an important disease. In drawing this casual conclusion, they missed the important point: its very presence among even a few of Honolulu's residents meant that inevitably syphilis was spreading to other people, native and European—and, just as significant, to sailors from visiting ships as well as to people living in country districts or on other islands. In the rest of their report the French explorers mentioned a few other ailments, none very important, they said, judging by the small number of sick people they noticed. The worst of these conditions they called "leprosy."

Even though Freycinet, Quoy, and Gaimard did not depict the gory horrors that cases of advanced syphilis do show, those symptoms were definitely present in some of Honolulu's afflicted people in 1819. The best description of such unfortunates appeared in 1837. It was written by Dr. Alonzo Chapin, a member of the Fourth Company of American missionaries, who arrived in Hawai'i in 1832 and returned to New England in 1835. There, relying on memory, he wrote the article from which these quotations are taken. The signs and symptoms he described applied just as certainly to people in 1800, or 1819, or 1900, as to syphilitics in 1835. In fact, we would see them today in patients who have not been treated with modern miracle drugs, such as the recent antibiotics. In the 1990s penicillin is still the drug of choice. The early stages of syphilis can be cured with injections of penicillin that will maintain adequate blood levels of the drug for seven to ten days. Patients in the third and fourth stages of the disease, in order to be cured, should receive adequate dosages of penicillin for at least twenty-one days.[9]

Here is the gruesome account that Dr. Chapin presented to fellow physicians in the United States, using the jargon that identified him as one of the fraternity:

> The venereal disease has for the past fifty-seven years continued to spread and increase, perpetuated and extended too by almost every vessel which touches at the islands, till words would fail to express the wretchedness and woe which have been the result. Foul ulcers, of many years standing, both indolent and phagedenic [spreading], every where abound, and visages horribly deformed—eyes rendered blind— noses entirely destroyed—mouths monstrously drawn aside from their natural position, ulcerating palates and almost useless arms and legs, mark most clearly the state and progress of the disease among that injured and helpless people.
>
> I have seen more than one case of marasmus [wasting, starvation] induced by the difficulty of deglutition [chewing and swallowing]. The mouths of these patients were almost closed in the process of cicatrization [scarring], and the gums and fauces were destroyed by ulceration. In one of my patients . . . the external nose had entirely disappeared, and its place was occupied by a concavity and a foramen [hole] of an irregularly oblong form. The left eye was totally blind, and both [were] so disfigured by ulceration as almost to lose their identity. The mouth was shockingly deformed; the lips and alveolar processes mostly removed by absorption, and the teeth, having their necks and a portion of their roots divested of integuments, were irregular in their distances and positions, pointed in every direction, and but slenderly adapted to the purpose of utility. The whole countenance was much disfigured by deep eschars [scar tissue], and the body greatly emaciated; no food could be masticated by him, so bad was the condition of his mouth.
>
> The reflection is melancholy, that there is no prospect of this disease, so disgusting in its effects and destructive in its course, being soon eradicated. The natives possess, among themselves, no curative means which will control it. [Only] a small portion have ready access to foreign physicians, and many within reach appear too indifferent to their condition to make application, while most permit the disease to go on till secondary symptoms appear before they seek assistance. These circumstances, together with their prevailing and inveterate habits of promiscuous sexual intercourse, will serve still, to perpetuate and extend the disease.[10]

Such, such were the beauties of Honolulu—as well as of Hilo, Lahaina, of every other port town in Hawai'i—or, for that matter, throughout the Pacific and the whole world. In Rio de Janeiro at that time, to take only one foreign seaport for an example, "syphilis raged in an endemic state (as in all Hispanic America) and putrefied its victims 'down to the bone.' "[11]

Nowadays, we who are sheltered in so many ways from seeing the signs and symptoms of almost all disfiguring diseases can hardly believe that all these evidences of distress in a syphilitic can be caused by one kind of microbe while it is in the course of destroying only one vulnerable human body. Western physicians have called syphilis "The Great Imitator" or "The Great Impostor," because all too often its ravages resemble those caused by many other agents, both infectious and noninfectious.

If we multiply that one suffering person by hundreds, we shall have a better idea of the ordeal to which O'ahu's people were being subjected by syphilis alone. Multiply that number by at least two or three—for those other widespread contagions, notably tuberculosis, the intestinal infections, and the perpetual miseries of "the universal itch"—and we begin to understand how many people were being drawn into this process of wholesale destruction.

Small wonder, then, that the people of Hawai'i despaired and died. Small wonder that men like sour David Malo and bitter Samuel Kamakau raged against "heedless" haoles who had brought in all these afflictions to assail helpless Hawaiians. Unthinking and uninformed Hawaiians, then as now, unable to concede that haoles in those days did not know any better, began to hate *all* unthinking haoles for their "crimes." The man they blamed most for the killing of their race was the one who least deserved that hatred: Captain James Cook. They gave him no credit for having tried to prevent the introduction of "the venereal distemper." Nor do their descendants today, who, in their rage, have not bothered to study history. Hearing their accusations today, one would be led to believe that Captain Cook, personally and all by himself, presented the syphilis spirochetes, the gonococci, the tubercle bacilli, and a score of other pathogenic microbes, to the healthy happy Hawaiians who rushed out to greet him with such aloha. No one today remembers Will Bradley or all the other impatient sailors aboard his ships, and their determination to ignore the rules and regulations their commander had imposed on them. And no one today remembers the women of 1778, either, so eager to give hospitality to those white gods. Or the men of 1778, so happy to make their women available to those all-too-human haoles—out of aloha, of course, but also for a price.

When, a few years after 1778, other shiploads of whooping happy horny haole sailors rushed ashore, to throw themselves atop the local whores, they did not see the hideous warnings that signaled dangers ahead. Most disfigured women were too sick to leave their sleeping-mats, possibly even too ashamed to allow foreigners to see their foul phagedenic ulcers, eroded noses, scarred unkissable lips. Only relatively presentable prostitutes, still in the first or second stages of syphilis (when the ghastly mutilations are not yet apparent, although the spirochetes are being shed in their most infectious teeming millions), would have sallied forth to greet with cheerful alohas the eager sailors.

Those happy-go-lucky fellows would have gone off to other ports of call before the chancres appeared, the primary ulcers of syphilis, those flowers of evil, to tell them they were taking home some unwanted souvenirs of Hawai'i. Unworldly Hawaiian prostitutes never realized the one comfort they could draw from their syphilization: how generously they were sharing the insidious spirochetes with the wives, and lovers, and harlots of those sailors—and also, ultimately, with the sailors' offspring, yea, even unto the second and the third generations. As people have said, the world around, "syphilis is the vengeance of the vanquished."[12] As Lieutenant King recognized in 1778, it is "the saddest disease that ever heaven in its wrath plagued mankind with. . . ."[13]

And what can be said about all those Bestial Haole Males, beardless youths and full-grown men and grizzled patriarchs alike, whooping and hollering as they rushed ashore, intent upon bestowing all their terrible haole germs upon shy Hawaiian maidens, all cowering in the lush tropical foliage, desperate to escape A Fate Worse Than Death?

Well, to begin with, such a picture of rampaging lust is conceived only in the minds of writers for Hollywood's films and in the febrile imaginations of certain kinds of novelists and of the artists who create illustrations for the dust jackets of their books. Few accounts exist that describe occasions when those bawdy sailors pulled into a Hawaiian port. Apparently all arrivals, after 1800, were so ordinary and unexciting as to call for nothing more than a casual mention, if that much. Sailors in their troops set foot on a beach to be greeted warmly by troupes of local houris—or, according to desires, of aikānes and māhūs, the homosexual males. And then everybody went off to places where they could relax in comfort and enjoy the whole assortment of shoreside refreshments they all had in mind. The process was orderly enough, not because it was regulated by any authority, but because both visitors and hosts knew exactly what they were meeting for, and saw no reason to spoil the occasion in any way.

Indeed, some very cooperative chiefs helped to organize the occasions to everyone's advantage, especially theirs. Ebenezer Townsend, in 1798, described how this was done: "Tidi Miti [Keli'imaikai, a chief] first took me . . . into a circle of about sixty girls, who partially rested themselves with their elbows on their knees, and by their expressive signs told me . . . I could take who I pleased."[14] Naturally, those provident chiefs received a share of the revenue their girls earned.

Only later, in the 1820s, after American missionaries began to impose their single standard of morality on the ruling chiefs (and therefore on the commoners) did violence attend the arrival of some bands of sailors. Those free spirits, rudely disappointed in their expectations for partaking in the pleasures of the port, expressed their annoyance in riotings, in concerted masculine bawlings emitted in front of the residences of chiefs and the dwellings of mission families, and even in attacks upon the angular persons of certain unfortunate missionary preachers whom the sailors managed to rout out in Honolulu and Lahaina.

But before the missionaries came to change the order of things, sailors ashore had few troubles with natives. Such difficulties as sailors did encounter were aroused by brawls among themselves, either in confrontations with seamen from other ships or, sometimes, in conflicts among men or officers from their own vessels.

Captain Abel Duhaut-Cilly, master of *Héros,* a French trading vessel moored in Honolulu harbor from 17 September to 15 November 1828, made this clear in his amused account of a night in the town (in which, of course, decorous Frenchmen took no part):

Once arrived at the Sandwich Islands all compete in their inclination to debauchery. Englishmen or Americans, officers or sailors, all have the same habits. As soon as they set foot on land, one sees no longer in the streets any but drunken men; one hears only quarrels and disputes. It is a spectacle for the Sandwich Islanders; you see them running, as they shout, toward the places where the Yankees and the John Bulls are settling their disputes. The captains, often more intoxicated than their sailors, appear unexpectedly; they wish to send them back to the ship; the latter resist; the captains strike; sometimes the sailors reply; all scold at once; the "God damns" and "damnations" are the thunder; the kicks and fisticuffs are the hail; the black eyes are the havoc of the thunderbolt. It is only far into the night that this storm dies down, to begin again the next day.[15]

David Malo, never missing a chance to attack Captain Cook, described wild sailors' orgies that no Hawaiian could have seen because they could not have happened. Referring to the time when Cook's ships lay at anchor in Kealakekua Bay in 1779, Malo wrote (in that "suppressed" edition mentioned by Mouritz):

Our people looked upon a number of naked sailors running up and down the beach at Kaawaloa and Napoopoo, screaming, shouting, making indecent gestures, and chasing the nearby women and girls with the intent of herding them into their grass houses, when their husbands and brothers were absent inland at work, or out on the ocean fishing—this pastime of lewdness continued daily, and went unrebuked by the officers of the ships who were present and viewed the shameful spectacle.[16]

A careful reading of the score or so of logs, journals, and diaries, both published and unpublished, written by officers, petty officers, and midshipmen aboard HMS *Resolution* and HMS *Discovery,* reveals not a hint about even one such orgy as Malo invented for his history. Britain's sailors may well have enjoyed their saturnalias, but certainly would have arranged to hold them in settings more secluded, rather than on Nāpōʻopoʻo's rocky ankle-twisting strand, in full view of their disapproving captain.

Haoles taught Hawaiians how to kiss in the exciting way that today the lascivious French are credited with having devised, although in fact it must have aroused salacious folk long before France and Frenchmen existed. Until those innovative sailors arrived, Hawaiians greeted each other with very hygienic expressions of aloha, by touching cheek to cheek or, in excesses of fondness, by rubbing nose against nose. Haole sailors held decidedly different notions about kissing. Not for them this primitive rubbing of noses, or the chaste pressing of lips upon closed lips, such as young Puritan couples might permit themselves in moments of felicity.

Those haole sailors, voracious in sex as in everything else, behaved like veritable cannibals when they hit the sleeping-mats. Lips, mouths, teeth, tongues, tonsils, throats, and torrents of spit: all were put into the service of lust. Such juicy "exchange of body fluids" (as we say nowadays in the Age of AIDS) would have been relatively harmless if the lovers' mouths harbored no dangerous germs. But what if Peter had not been clean, what if this happily rutting sailor had caught syphilis in some distant port, and now, in Honolulu, the mucous membranes lining his mouth and throat were shedding myriads of spirochetes? Or what if, during fits of coughing, his rotten lungs raised bloody sputum and tubercle bacilli into his mouth? Or if the viruses that cause influenza, smallpox, mumps, measles, chicken pox, or even the common cold lurked there? Or if the crypts of his tonsils harbored the bacteria that cause diphtheria, whooping cough, streptococcic sore throat, not to mention half a dozen other serious infections?

The mouth, alas, even at the best of times and even in the cleanest of people, can be the most perilously befouled of all the body's orifices. "A person's mouth is not like the hoof of Attila's horse, that made sterile the soil on which it trod; just the contrary," as a sardonic Brazilian novelist wrote long ago. Of all the many arrangements for the direct transfer of dangerous germs from person to person, "French kissing" is the worst. Compared with this deep kiss he taught her, a sailor boy who snatched a bite from his dusky Iwa's mountain apple presented little threat to her health. And her family's poi bowl, into which he too dipped his fingers when he joined them at the eating-mat, would have been only a minor threat to his health. But for Hawaiians who shared in this novel kind of connection, the French kiss could be, literally, the Kiss of Death.

And when they fed their babies in the *ho'opū'ā* way, dribbling chewed morsels and saliva into an infant's mouth—

༄་༄་༄་༄་

As we might expect, the first missionaries from America to settle in Hawai'i were much disturbed by what they saw. "The people are in a distressing state in this place," wrote the Reverend Lowell Smith from Honolulu. "Backward in everything but Sin. I do long to be able to do something for them."[17]

In Lahaina, the Reverend C. S. Stewart noted: "We seldom walk out without meeting many, whose appearance of disease and misery is appalling, and some so remediless and disgusting, that we are compelled to close our eyes against a sight that fills me with horror. Cases of ophthalmia, scrofula, and elephantiasis are very common."[18]

Two members of the London Missionary Society, returning to England after visiting the society's stations in Tahiti, stayed in Hawai'i for several months in 1822. Their observations of Tahitians, being subjected to the same trials that were testing Hawaiians, combined with their trust in the Lord, enabled the Reverend Daniel Tyerman and Mr. George Bennet to be both generous and hopeful about the future of Hawaiians:

> These islanders are, indeed, in a state of nature, but not of innocence, and the truth is that they are miserable, not happy, under it, for theirs is *a state of nature fallen from innocence,* without the possibility of recovery, except by the faith of Christ, and redemption through his blood.[19]

But the missionary who expressed most clearly the plight of Hawaiians was the Reverend William P. Alexander. From his remote station in the isolated district of Hanalei on Kaua'i he sent this message of alarm: "What we do for this nation, we must do quickly—they are melting away."[20]

ʻʻʻʻʻ

Of small comfort to Hawaiians, or to Polynesians everywhere, would have been the news from Tahiti. The *Missionary Herald* for April 1823, published in Boston, noted the fate of Tahitians since 1774. In that year, Captain Cook (during his second expedition to the Pacific Ocean) estimated that 200,000 people lived on the single island of Tahiti. The *Missionary Herald* declared, basing this summary account on reports sent home from Tahiti by members of the London Missionary Society,

> From that time till the landing of the [British] missionaries in 1797 there were many destructive wars . . . private murders and assassinations. . . . The great majority of infants were killed by their own mothers, as soon as they were born. . . . Pomare [the "king" of Tahiti] offered 2,000 human sacrifices during the 30 years of his reign. But the greatest cause of depopulation was the universal licentiousness of morals . . . aggravated by the visits of Europeans . . . [that is, prostitution and the venereal diseases].

The London missionaries' first census, taken in 1800, counted "only 16,000 souls in Tahiti. . . . Pomare told the missionaries that they had come to the *remnant* of his people."[21]

This is a good example of the unreliability of reports about populations for any of the islands in Polynesia during the years before 1850, or even later for some places. Historians today think that Cook's estimate for Tahiti's population was much too high, just as they believe that his estimates for numbers of Hawaiians in 1778–1779 were too generous. Douglas Oliver, the foremost modern authority on Tahiti, collated all figures about the island's population that were published by observers from 1767 until 1800 and correlated these estimates with Tahitians' own accounts as well as with archaeological evidence. He concluded that Tahiti's population in the period from 1767 to 1774 was about 35,000.[22]

A decline in the number of Tahitians from about 35,000 to 16,000, during the course of twenty-six years, is dismaying enough, to be sure. That decline, however, was not as devastating as the report circulated by misinformed missionaries in Tahiti, London, and Boston. Nonetheless, the *Missionary Herald*'s erroneous account gave cause for great concern to Christians everywhere, especially in Hawai'i. (One notes that London's missionaries in Tahiti gave the same reasons for the decline in Tahiti's population as visitors to Hawai'i—and, after 1820, American missionaries there—gave for the "destruction" of native Hawaiians.)

ଔଔଔଔଔ

Some foreigners could see that the Hawaiian people were wasting away. Year after year, beginning with Portlock and Dixon, who visited the islands in 1786, an observant captain, or a naturalist-surgeon, or an artist would notice that many individuals were obviously ill, and that the total number of people was being reduced. All of these foreigners, in the books they wrote after returning to their home countries, repeated in a kind of somber litany the same catalog of reasons for this declining population:

• The frequent wars among ruling chiefs and the famines that followed these conflicts. This reason may have been acceptable in the years before 1804, when the ma'i 'oku'u epidemic prevented Kamehameha's invasion of Kaua'i. But following that disaster chiefs fought no more wars until after Kamehameha died in 1819. And then the two minor rebellions that did occur involved few warriors and their effects on the populace of the entire kingdom would not have been significant.

• "The venereal disease" and its concomitant, prostitution, as the primary means by which this disease was spread.

• Several other serious contagious diseases, especially tuberculosis, "bowel fever," and "the itch," or scabies. Other epidemic diseases too may well have struck, such as influenza, measles, and hepatitis, but no one identified them by name or symptoms. Don Marin's journal, for example, is full of passing references to "a new sickness," or "a new kind of fever," but these entries tell us only that Honolulu's residents were affected frequently by microorganisms they had not encountered before.

• "Universal" licentiousness and drunkenness—not only among commoners—with their attendant evils of laziness, filthiness, infanticide, abortion, poverty, and neglect of children. In such a setting infants who succeeded in being born did not live for long, and small children seldom grew to maturity.

All these explanations about causes of mortality were offered so consistently that, to some extent, they must have been founded on truth. But how reliable are the grand generalizations that those foreign observers expressed? Here, too, we are forced to wonder if, during their short sojourns in the islands, they did not hear the same old tales from the same old sources—informants who had made up their minds years before about almost everything that happened in Hawai'i nei, and who, settling in to become the local authorities, saw no reason ever to revise their opinions. In fact, Captain Golovnin said as much when, in 1818, he "enquired among the Europeans who have lived here for a long time," as he sought information about the "vice" of prostitution and its part in the spread of venereal disease. Those informants, almost necessarily resident haoles, could have enjoyed playing the parts of old hands, relaying the same old misinformation to naive newcomers. This kind of fabrication, composed of gossip, lies, ignorance, imagination, prejudice, and malice, all more or less stitched together by a very few flexible facts, is still being created today, and not only in Hawai'i.

Nonetheless, even though visitors could not have known with certainty about the actual numbers of natives who were supposed to have died of foreigners' diseases, they could see for themselves the signs of moral deterioration in licentiousness, prostitution, drunkenness, filth, and poverty. More than likely, therefore, the tragedy of misery, destruction, and death was too evident to be mistaken.

But none of the more observant visitors was prepared as yet, by the culture of his time, to notice the sickness of spirit that was ravaging Hawaiians' psyches as surely as those physical afflictions were claiming their bodies.

ᘐᘐᘐᘐᘐ

Hawaiians needed help because their society too was dying. When the temporal and spiritual rulers of the kingdom—Queen Ka'ahumanu, Queen Ke'ōpūolani, High Chief Kalanimoku, and High Priest Hewahewa—abolished the kapu system in 1819, and thus ended the rule of gods over men, they acted intuitively perhaps, but also selfishly and rashly, thinking that they were choosing the best course into the future for themselves, if not for the nation.

In ending the kapus they did gain some small freedom from irksome rules and invisible deities. Yet when they cast off the discipline of the law, the ruling chiefs put themselves and their people in double jeopardy. They lost much more than they gained. As is so often the case with reformers and revolutionaries, they set up nothing better in place of the system they had overthrown. What they thought would be the right way into the future proved to be a treacherous maze leading them into a wilderness of confusion and tribulation. They were not so learned in the wiles of foreigners, or so experienced in the conduct of nations, that they could contend successfully with problems thrust upon them almost daily by intruding haoles. In rejecting both gods and kapus, the chiefs lost the stability of custom and the certainty of social relationships prescribed for them in the moral code that had regulated the behavior of all Hawaiians, high and low, since the beginning of their history. With the 'ai noa, the "free eating," they shattered the religion and the mythos that gave meaning to life. In doing so, they brought down upon their nation nothing less than catastrophe.

Moreover, when they jettisoned these controlling forces, the ruling chiefs threw away the sources of their own great mana, and thereby cut off the flow of spirit power that gave life to the land and its people. In return, they offered nothing to fill the emptiness within. Because of that loss, both chiefs and commoners became like voyagers adrift on the trackless sea, without sight of the stars above to guide them.

The ruling chiefs in 1819, and the commoners they governed thereafter only in part, did not know about this impoverishment of the spirit. That knowledge would come only later. And then, for most Hawaiians, it would come too late.

ひひひひ

To understand the direct relationship between the decaying of a society and the physical destruction of its people requires instruction as well as perception. Few thinkers in any part of the world, before the second half of the nineteenth century, were prepared to recognize this interdependence.

Europe's great psychologists, during the last quarter of that century and the first decades of the twentieth, began to perceive what happened to individual Europeans who were breaking under the pressures imposed on their psyches by the taboos of the societies to which they belonged. These pioneering investigators discovered the principles by which they could relate the fates of individuals to the demands of the cultures in which they lived and strove—and, all too often, became neurotic, or psychotic, or even irremediably mad.

Thus, Sigmund Freud described the two major influences that, he thought, at all times contend for dominance in the psyche of each human being. He called these dual forces Eros and Thanatos: the instinct for Love, and the instinct for Death. Carl Gustav Jung, enlarging the province of the psyche, added to the consciousness of the individual the influence that he called the collective unconscious of all humankind. And, extending these basic concepts from the individual to the society, he declared: "A tribe's mythology is its living religion, whose loss is always and everywhere, even among the civilized, a moral catastrophe. But religion is a vital link with psychic processes independent of and beyond consciousness, in the dark hinterland of the psyche.[23]

A few European historians and ethnologists also, working among "primitive peoples" in Southeast Asia and certain islands of the Pacific, came to similar conclusions about members of non-European societies. Stephen H. Roberts, "MA, formerly Lecturer in Modern History, University of Melbourne," published in 1927 an interesting study entitled *Population Problems in the Pacific*. In it he presented opinions and conclusions that appear to have been founded upon his reading of publications by other investigators rather than upon fieldwork of his own. He attributed depopulation among Pacific islanders to "racial malaise, epidemic diseases, general ill-nurture, and immorality." The last three of these factors need no comment here. The first term is defined by Roberts himself as

> a decadence . . . a general social decline . . . an indefinable malaise of the stock itself. . . . Polynesians lived a lotus existence, and dawdled through life in a trance of mental and physical inertia. . . . There could be little virility and less ambition where the beneficent effects of a chastening environment were no longer felt. . . . All was supine and nerveless; and sorcery and superstition were in the ascendant. The stamina was gone from the race. The race, denied the health-giving process of selection and of struggle was passing away.[24]

"*Auwe noho'i e!*" as Hawaiians are wont to say. "My goodness me!" Here we have yet another certitudinous haole upon whom the white man's burden weighs heavy. Roberts is sounding the same disapproving note as did Dr. E. S. Goodhue of Honolulu, whose jeers about Hawaiians appeared in 1900. Both of these disdainful men—and others too, like the redoubtable Arnold Toynbee in the 1930s—seem to have drawn their opinions of Polynesians from the same *Handbook of Phrases for Scornful Appraisal of Lesser Races*. Even so, we must remind ourselves to be more charitable toward them than they allowed themselves to be toward the "dawdling" Polynesians. After all, they, with all their purposeful vigor and arrogant convictions, were products of their times and places—just as we, much more enlightened, are products of our mellowed own.

Roberts' prejudices are cruel enough to provoke shouts of outrage from all hardworking Polynesians, male and female. No haole anthropologist, in the years when Roberts compiled his report (and very few anthropologists since then), ever spent months on end, up to his knees in mud, at the hard labor involved in growing a crop of taro and maintaining the paddy's banks and irrigation ditches that bring a continual flow of fresh water to the plants during the first stages of growth. Nor did a patronizing haole ethnologist ever actually attempt to do the women's hard work of making kapa, "the paper-bark cloth," which requires weeks of preparation, attention, and patient application before a single piece of the fragile stuff is finished. Furthermore, even after Westerners' cheap and gaudy cotton fabrics came to Polynesia to displace kapa, and tins of Argentina's corned beef replaced pork on the hoof, the "idle" and "inert" Polynesians had to work hard at some gainful employment in order to earn the money with which to pay for those expensive imports from foreign countries.

Roberts' simplistic explanation for racial malaise is characteristic of Britons' attitudes, established during the late Victorian era, when all things and all other peoples were measured against Imperial England's standards of competence and performance—and of Christian morality. Darwin's theory of evolution, which he devised for animals, was misused then by England's philosopher-scientists, who applied the processes of natural selection (and, in Herbert Spencer's memorable phrase, the laws governing "the survival of the fittest") to economics and labor and to human members of "the working classes"—not to mention to "aborigines" wherever those might be found. These tenets of imperialist Social Darwinism influenced imperious European and American philosophers and proclaimers of progress far into the twentieth century. Most certainly they helped to shape the attitudes of Stephen Roberts in Australia and those of Arnold Toynbee in England.

These are attitudes far removed, indeed, from George Forster's generous appraisal of Polynesians as "that innocent race of men." But then Forster, who saw Pacific islanders a hundred years earlier, between 1772 and 1775, met them before "the corruption of manners" achieved by Europeans had ruined them—exactly as he feared they might.

None of those closet scholars of the Victorian era who observed Pacific islanders from afar seemed to understand that Polynesians, in their traditional ways of living, had been quite content and productive before Westerners began to intrude upon them. Those islanders could not have survived if they had been idle and inert, supine and nerveless. Nor did the haole savants recognize that Polynesians would have continued to be untroubled, even thriving, if foreigners had not pushed in upon them, bearing sleazy trade goods, new kinds of germs and ideas, firewater, firearms—and demands for payment for their merchandise, in cash or in kind. Nowadays, with our better understanding of the difficulties of merely managing to survive in any culture, especially in those of our advanced Western societies, scholars are not so censorious, so "judgmental," as they prefer to say. In fact, they are more likely to envy the happy, carefree (and imaginary) Polynesian of precapitalist times, supine under his ever-fruitful coconut palm, nibbling at the local equivalent of lotus roots. . . .

By the term "racial malaise" Roberts and his contemporaries seem to have meant the inability of Polynesians to accept, both physically and psychologically, the alien standards of behavior and thought that Westerners wanted them to adopt. If that inability, or unwillingness, to adjust to foreigners' ways was indeed evidence of a "sickness of spirit," then Polynesians were indeed sick, weakened, and vulnerable. Almost every foreigner who saw them in their native settings felt as much. And Roberts was right when he gave primary importance to "racial malaise" as a factor contributing to the decline of Pacific societies.

But why, we ask, should Polynesians be so sick, so universally afflicted? Roberts gave us the answer: "To this world, rotting to the core, and crumbling with the heritage of generations of contributing weaknesses, came the Europeans, destroying the last vestiges of regulation."[25]

杧杧杧杧

Most early European visitors to the Pacific islands, said Roberts, ascribed their diminishing populations to merely physical causes, "such as disease and firearms." But later visitors, he acknowledged, held other opinions. Coming as they did before the time of Freud, Jung, and their colleagues, those observers must have been strongly affected by the signs of psychological distress they noticed in Pacific islanders. Thus, Roberts wrote:

> Dr. Litton Forbes (1874) first clearly expressed the additional psychological cause: "that great unsettling of the native mind, which almost eludes all accurate analysis." Gros (1894) wrote of "a kind of fatalism, an odd submission." Gratiolet [blamed] "ennui: Le Kanaque s'ennuie—comme l'animal captif." Leroy and Broca [proposed] "a sadness due to the neighborhood of the whites—the impossibility of the natives to support the contact of civilization."[26]

With a final quotation, this one from W. H. Rivers, an eminent British psychopathologist-turned-ethnologist, Roberts continued his presentation of the accepted dogma: "Because of the enormous influence of the mind upon the body among lowly people, this psychological despair is the basic cause of depopulation. . . . The natives just die by wasting away."[27]

Having invoked the revered authorities of his time (as all persons who are so presumptuous as to write histories are obliged to do), Roberts added supporting opinions of his own:

The native, under the changed conditions, has neither interest nor hope. . . . Hence arises that despair which colors every native act and which makes him drift, as an unwilling agent, through an existence which has no appeal for him, either as an individual, or as a member of a wider social unit. Religion, society, clan, tribal pride—all have gone: the shadow of the white man, with his incomprehensible code, is over everything: and the native feels that he has but to pass. . . .[28]

When we read such somber appraisals of the malign effects of those White Shadows in the South Seas, we want to doubt them. How could the natives have become so disturbed in spirit so quickly?, we ask. And so universally? Perhaps, we argue, they were sick in body, weakened by all those foreigners' diseases, and therefore too miserable physically to exert themselves? Or were they just being sensible, relaxing rather than working, because they did not feel inclined to labor for the profit of masterful white men rather than for the benefit of their own brown selves? Questions like these arise faster than do answers—and more easily than the one unified theory that will explain the whole tragic collapse of so many Polynesian minds and societies.

We are stopped short in these searchings for evasions of truth by testimony from Pacific islanders themselves. Their sickness of the spirit was genuine. Members of all their societies, without exception, recognized their helplessness under the impact of the haoles' civilization. Many of their poets expressed the people's grief in mournful little prophecies that are positively Japanese in their message of *mono no aware,* the awareness of "the sadness of things."

Thus, Fijians said:

> Death is easy,
> Of what use is life?
> To die is rest.[29]

Tahitians lamented:

> The *fau* leaves shall lie strewn,
> Faded [are] the branching coral's hues,
> Our people shall pass away.[30]

And Hawaiians addressed a long *Prayer to Lono,* of which this is only a small part:

> . . . The leaves of Lono are falling.
> Doomed is the image of Lono to destruction.

> Standing, it falls to the foundation of the land;
> Bending low is the glory . . .[31]

The Europeans' appraisals collected by Roberts, the comments sent home to Europe by Robert Louis Stevenson from Samoa, these valetudinarian expressions from hapless Polynesians, all refer to people late in the nineteenth century. Nonetheless, Roberts' conclusions (and the statements from Freud and Jung) apply equally well to Hawaiians during the years between 1800 and 1825. Hawaiians too lived in peril then, as endangered as were their kinfolk in other islands of the Pacific.

Despite the biases that reflect the culture which shaped his mind, Roberts did sense certain fundamental truths about the imperiled peoples of the Pacific. In one section of his study he composed a veritable threnody for dying Polynesians. In it we can detect a humane man, moved by the saddening tale he is relating:

> The native of the stone age had to bring his institutions into line with those of industrialized Europe: he had to compress the evolution of centuries into a few years; and his only method was by the wholesale abandonment of everything old. . . . Everything went, save his primitive passions. . . . And it is not good for a people to turn its back on its past this way, for that way lies ruin. . . . If the study of native races the world over yields any conclusion, it is that a people bereft of a past . . . must die. . . . The islander had neither the old or the new, but was drifting in a morass of uncertainty, with nothing to cling to, and no lodestone. And the result was death, both physical and racial, for the will to live had gone. The native stood between the world which had gone and that new world in which he could not assimilate himself, and simply gave way.[32]

Roberts published his inquiry in 1927. In 1966 another Australian, Alan Moorehead, would publish, in greater detail, "An Account of the Invasion of the South Pacific, 1767–1840." He gave his book the perfect title: *The Fatal Impact.*

ぐぐぐぐ

All these insupportable forces, both physical and spiritual, combined to assail the psyches of all Polynesians, leading to that "moral catastrophe" about which Jung warned people everywhere and in all times.

In contrast with Hawaiians, placed in double jeopardy, the haoles who came among them, apparently so free and easy and undisciplined, were secure in their social relationships with other people. Those wandering haoles, wherever they went, behaved in accordance with a code of ethics they had evolved through centuries of experience. It may have been a rough and hard code, not as courteous as that of knights errant nor as uplifting as the Rule observed by a set of cloistered monks. But it was a practical working code for groups of relatively violent men, who would have been little more than beasts without its controls. Haoles did not abandon this code, whether they met in Manila or whored in Honolulu. They knew where they had come from, and where they were going. They did not yet stand on the brink of moral catastrophe.

In Polynesians' terms, haoles had their established set of kapus to govern them—rules decreed more by encounters with other men than by the god they tossed overboard while sailing westward around Cape Horn. In general, they remembered those rules in their relationships with each other, in business dealings ashore or while sailing their ships from port to port throughout the seven seas. Unfortunately for Hawaiians, however, haoles were not good teachers of their rules of conduct. They expected that, of course, everybody else thought and acted the way they did. And, naturally, when an innocent Hawaiian did not understand the white man's "incomprehensible code" (as Roberts referred to it), the impatient haoles simply pushed him aside, calling him stupid, or unwilling, or lazy—or worse. Very few Hawaiians could make that sudden transition from the simplicity of their past into the frenetic competitiveness of the haoles' present.

Until the haoles came, bringing the whole world in their train, Hawaiians too had their set of kapus to guard and to govern them. But after 1778 that code of ethics was weakened. And in 1819 it collapsed: "Standing, it falls to the foundation of the land," as the *Prayer to Lono* mourned. After 1819, for too many years, Hawaiians were "a people without law," just when they most needed law—for guidance and governance and protection against assailants from without and within. Needed defenses against not only their own "primitive passions" but also against those of other men.

Naturally, in their associations with Hawaiians, foreigners ignored any of the rules that got in the way of convenience (or of lust). The American missionaries, very soon after they arrived in Honolulu, recognized the flexibility of haole morality—and presented readers at home with a fine example of the conflicting signals being sent out by the two opposing haole factions, the carnal and the puritan:

> Though the people have abolished their idols, they have not abandoned their vices. To the stranger, who enters their habitations of ignorance and depravity,— as a token of respect, the husband offers his wife, the father his daughter, and the brother his sister! When solemnly assured, that there is a God in heaven, who forbids and abhors such iniquity, they reply: "Other white men tell us this is right; but you are strange white men."[33]

Tyerman and Bennet, too, mentioned this conflict of standards after the missionaries began their reforms:

> The traffic of prostitution . . . is most shameless here . . . the gospel and its other triumphs are evil spoken of by many Christians (falsely so called) who visit these seas, and are filled with rage, disappointment, and malice when they find that they cannot riot in licentiousness, as former voyagers did, on these once polluted shores; therefore do *they* abhor the change, and calumniate those who have been instrumental in its production.[34]

Paradoxically, those free and easy haoles, ashore and afloat, who seemed to be so lawless, kept a great many laws to safeguard them, while Hawaiians kept almost none. In consequence, as Hawaiians themselves recognized only too clearly, long before 1860, they were *"huikau"*—lost in the shuffle, confused, bewildered . . .

ᜭᜭᜭᜭ

Little is known about the ways in which commoners and their physicians responded to the new diseases that attacked them during the period from 1800 to 1825. John Papa Iʻi remembered how, after the maʻi ʻokuʻu epidemic in 1804, King Kamehameha I decreed a program for the immediate training of many kāhuna lapaʻau in order to meet expected threats to the people's health. But, in that unlettered society, no records could be kept, to tell later generations about the success (or failure) of the medical profession's efforts, and no oral accounts from that time have been preserved. The devastating decline in the total population between 1805 (when presumably the training program began) and 1832 (when the first official census ended) indicates that kāhuna lapaʻau were unable to save their people.

Nevertheless, we can assume that, in general, kāhuna lapaʻau did try to help their patients with whatever means they could command. Yet their medications, if not their other kinds of treatment, were pitifully inadequate. (But, let us not forget, in those days haole physicians were no better supplied with medicines and other therapies against infectious diseases.) Some commoners may have recovered from infections because of their bodies' natural defenses—"the strength of their constitutions," as Westerners explained, or "by God's will," as both missionaries and Hawaiians declared. But, as census counts revealed in 1831–1832, more Hawaiians had died in the years since 1805 than were born, whether or not the sick ones gained the help of physicians native or foreign.

The Reverend Artemas Bishop, a member of the Second Company of American missionaries (who arrived in Hawai'i in 1823), believed he knew why Hawaiians were perishing in such great numbers:

> They have little knowledge of the means of cure, when attacked by disease, and consequently are either left to the strength of their constitutions for recovery, or, what is more common, to linger and die. They have no diet for the sick except their common one of *poe* and raw *fish,* and no couch but the ground to rest upon. The greater part of those who are taken sick, never recover, especially among the children.[35]

Bishop, and all his fellow missionaries, regarded Hawaiians in their native habitat entirely from the perspective of their own native habitats back home in New England. To them the grass hut was nothing but a hovel under thatch, resembling an aging molding haystack more than a house. The resemblance could not be missed, of course. Captain Cook had noticed it too, in 1778, comparing them with "oblong corn stacks" such as he had seen in Yorkshire. But he, observing rather than judging, accepted Hawaiians' thatched huts for what they were: simple dwellings for a simple people. Puritan disdain sank to the levels of disgust when they saw how some Hawaiian families lived in those hovels amid squalor that no fastidious God-fearing New Englander could possibly condone.

One evening in 1824 the Reverend C. S. Stewart "went strolling along the beach south of the Mission House" (that is, in Kaka'ako) and saw

> a picture of poverty and filthiness too degrading to be real. The largest hut I passed was not higher than my waist; capable only of containing a family, like pigs in a sty, on a bed of dried grass, filled with fleas and vermin. . . . It was the time of their evening repast; and most of the

people were seated on the ground [outside the hut], eating *poe* surrounded by swarms of flies, and sharing their food with dogs, pigs,
and ducks, who helped themselves freely from the dishes of their masters! The *tout ensemble* was almost too disgusting to be witnessed.[36]

Lucy Thurston, wife of the Reverend Asa Thurston, distressed
about native children in Kailua, Kona,

pitied their condition. The doors of their little huts obliged them to
stoop half down to enter them. I looked into several of them. Wretchedness! wretchedness! How can fellow beings thus live? Yet from these
miserable abodes the little children crawl out active and sprightly as
children in America.[37]

Here speak the authentic voices of the rigid haole intellects of their
time, gripped in the vise of their notions about how everyone should
live. For God's sake they had come to the Sandwich Islands, bursting
with compassion no doubt, but, taken aback by the strangeness of
this alien country, had been rendered incapable of perception—and
therefore fretted because Hawaiians did not live as did Americans
back home in New England. Even though motherly Mrs. Thurston
found the corrective to her misgivings in those sprightly children
crawling out from their "miserable abodes," she could not yet accept
the facts of life as they were presented in Hawai'i.

Neither could the other members of the American mission. They
had been instructed, back in Boston in 1819, to lift up all Hawaiians,
as quickly as possible, to the level where, literally, they could crawl
forth from those rude waist-high shelters, to dwell upright (and fully
clothed) in commodious frame houses built in any one of New England's several cozy styles. The goal was a laudable one, no doubt, but
in the 1820s it was rather beyond the reach of a people as impover-
ished and unprepared as the Hawaiians. The missionaries had not
yet understood how even the humblest of their family homes in New
England were far more palatial than was the so-called palace of
Hawai'i's kings. (To their credit, being sensible folk, they learned this
lesson after a few years of exposure to realities in the islands, and
relaxed the standards of housing they expected of natives.)

Even so, from the Hawaiians' point of view, what else did they
really need to shelter them against the usual balmy night airs and the
infrequent showers of rain that fell upon the islands' coastal plains?
(In very heavy rains, to be sure, the thatch leaked, and then things

and bodies within got soaking wet. But, no trouble, no matter, the dwellers shrugged. In a couple of days the sunshine would come back, and everything would dry out again—while the people wondered why they should be seized with sore throats, coughs, and sniffles, the whole range of symptoms that might, or might not, end in lung fever and death.)

Chiefs needed great houses in which to display their possessions and flaunt their lordliness. But commoners needed nothing more than a lowly hut. They required little household furniture save a few lauhala mats and sheets of kapa, an assortment of gourds and calabashes, a couple of poi pounders, adzes, or hatchets, and a heavy board for use in mashing cooked taro into *pa'i 'ai* or poi. They lived in commendable simplicity, not yet having accepted the rule that they must acquire many things. They spent the daylight hours outside the hut, working at chores that brought in food, water, and firewood, or fashioning the articles they would yield to the tax collectors of the chiefs who ruled them. Some families kept both dwellings and surroundings neat; others did not bother about such niceties. For commoners, perforce, materials sturdier than short branches for rafters and purlins, and leaves of ti or hala or bunches of *pili* grass for thatching, were just not available. Therefore, the waist-high hut was the only kind of shelter they could make. Compared with the costly spaciousness in which Americans lived then, as well as today, such simplicity was adequate, if not exactly enviable.

And yet, in a way, the missionaries were right to be shocked by the mere sight of the waist-high hut. It was indeed primitive and demeaning to those forced to huddle in one. And, even to Westerners in the early nineteenth century, not as yet softened by civilization's indulgences, it must have been dismayingly uncomfortable even to people in good health.

As Reverend Bishop's letter revealed, dying Hawaiians must have passed their last days in utmost misery, never soothed by medicines, often abandoned by relatives, always without solace, not even by the hope of heaven.

From Lahaina in 1826, the Reverend William Richards, who succeeded the Reverend C. S. Stewart at that station, declared:

They are all perfectly ignorant of the nature of disease, and do not exercise even the judgment of children in their manner of administering medicine. . . . They are not only destitute of physicians, but of suitable persons to wait upon the sick also, being quite as ignorant of the business of nursing as they are of medicine.[38]

Two years earlier, Stewart himself, while still stationed in Lahaina, reported that almost every day "we are most painfully reminded that we dwell among the habitations of cruelty." He described the stoning of a lunatic on the beach (which he stopped before the victim was killed), "the customary way of treating such objects throughout the islands." He had heard of even worse cruelties:

> The helpless and dependent, whether from age or sickness, are often cast from the habitations of their relatives and friends, to languish and to die, unattended and unpitied. . . . A poor wretch thus perished [near by] after having lain uncovered for days and nights in the open air, most of the time pleading in vain to his family . . . for a drink of water.[39]

When at length the poor man died, his corpse

> was drawn into the bushes . . . and left a prey to the dogs who prowl through the district in the night. . . . The truth of the apostle's description of the heathen, that they are "without natural affection, implacable, and unmerciful," is found most fully here, in the prevalence of the abhorrent and tremendous crime of infanticide. . . . In those parts of the islands where the influence of the mission has not extended, *two-thirds of the infants born, perish by the hands of their own parents, before attaining the first or second years of their age!*[40]

Such merciless cruelty, whether to lunatics, to the dying, or to infants, was reported from many places in Polynesia, but it was by no means widespread. In Honolulu, for example, the same missionaries who despaired over "the dark hearts" of the heathen also noticed how, with some families, relatives and friends gathered around a death-mat, wailing in sorrow and singing plaintive laments during a dying person's last hours. The frequency with which infanticide was practiced is unknown. Certainly, it was scarcely needed after the foreign diseases began their heartless thinning out: most infants died almost as soon as they were born.

"In this land of disease and death . . . of inconceivable corruption and horror," Stewart wrote, dying haole derelicts fared no better than Hawaiians—unless, in those decades before hospitals, they were fortunate enough to be taken into the home of a missionary family. (Because missionaries opposed Sin, and therefore Lechery, they did not take in American boys dying of the venereal diseases. Usually they directed their compassion toward victims of consumption, with which they themselves were all too well acquainted. With these offerings of charity, they added more burdens to already exhausted mission women, and the dangers of infecting everyone in the household, especially the children, with virulent tubercle bacilli.)

On 7 June 1824, in Honolulu, the Reverend Mr. Stewart and his ailing wife went again

> to see a young American sailor who is very ill. . . . He is one of the many infatuated beings, who desert their ships, to wander among the licentious inhabitants of the island, without a home, and with scarce a subsistence. He suffers exceedingly, and is entirely destitute of every comfort: his bed is a dirty mat spread on the ground, with a piece of native cloth for a covering, and a block of wood for a pillow.[41]

Stewart neglected to give all the facts relating to this affecting tale about the sad end to a sinner's misspent life. Whether or not he intended the omission, Stewart did not explain that other people too were caring for the physical needs of the dying sailor. Mr. and Mrs. Stewart no doubt brought him spiritual solace, and possibly vials of useless Western medicines, and packets of haole foods. But certainly, close by, lived a Hawaiian family, poor without doubt, but yet full of aloha, who took pity on the ailing haole boy, dying so far from home and family. Who else made the waist-high hut in which he lay? Who else provided the lauhala mat, the kapa sheet, the log pillow upon which he rested his head? And the sips of tepid water and the mouthfuls of fish and poi that sustained him until the end?

Stewart passed over such homely details in his zeal to conclude this mournful account with the obligatory moral:

> We do all in our power to prevent his suffering for want of medicine, food, and necessary attentions. . . . This lad, like many others who live at ease in sin, while their health and strength are continued, now that he is in a situation of agony and danger, he is overwhelmed with guilt and shame, and with trembling and tears supplicates the counsel and the prayers, which in other circumstances he would have dismissed and perhaps scorned.[42]

Although the missionaries wrote uplifting descriptions of the "happy deaths" of several high chiefs who died "in the bosom of the Lord" after they had been converted to the Christian faith, no one gave any attention to the manner in which commoners—"persons of small account," as Kamakau called them—faced death, "the King of Ter-rors," as Stewart regarded it. Probably, "tired and worn and spent," after being sick for a long time, feeling helpless if not actually unhelped, commoners yearned for death. They were not yet instruct-ed in the torments of Christianity's hellfire, or elevated by the prom-ise of its heaven, to wonder much about what happened to them after death. To the people of old death meant only a long sleep, either in Pō ia Milu, the dark realm of Milu, for the spirits of those who had been as wicked in this world as that evil chief had been, or in the abode of Niolopua, the god of sleep, for the spirits of those who had been reasonably good during their life on earth. Perhaps knowing that they "owed a death to nature" made the going easier, un-til "darkness settled like cobwebs across their eyes," as Kamakau wrote.[43] "*Ku'u ka luhi, ua maha,*" said the watchers beside the death-mat, "weariness is released, peace comes."[44]

Another possible interpretation of Hawaiians' acceptance of the approach of death has been presented by Kekuni Blaisdell: "Death after a meaningful life was welcomed as a reuniting with one's ances-tors in the eternal spiritual realm and completion of a recurring cycle of rebirth and transfiguration into *kinolau* (non-human forms) or reincarnation into other human services."[45] The ease with which cer-tain Hawaiians could achieve "a willed death," whether they were ill or apparently healthy, has always surprised and intrigued haoles who lack this ability. More than likely, when the terminal agony (or the fear of it) became intolerable, such fortunate people simply "turned their faces to one side," and invited Death to come for them. *Na kanaka oku'u wale aku no i kau 'uhane,* "the people dismissed freely their souls and died." Thus did the Reverend Lorrin Andrews define the word *'uhane,* spirit or soul, in his *Dictionary* published in 1865.

For most people, however, death did not come so gently. Among the saddest of the missionaries' accounts are the ones about children —whimpering, crying, tossing feverishly for days and nights on end, before peace came to them at last.

Adults, young or old, must have wondered why they were being made to die in such new and painful ways. "What is my great offense, O god?" some would have asked, as did that chief of olden times when he sought forgiveness for a fault he could not name. Oth-ers would have suspected that the gods they had rejected, after the haoles came, resented being abandoned, and made their anger felt in the form of these alien and terrible sicknesses. Like the dying haole sailor youth who forgot his jealous Jehovah in the years of good health, but could not escape the dread of him as death approached, some Hawaiians too remembered their possessive deities when, too late, they thought of the kapus they had scorned or broken.

This remembrance was a significant influence even as late as 1875:

> There is a very prevalent feeling among the people that because they forsook their ancient gods and adopted the worship of the haole, they are doomed to extinction. To argue with them is in vain. They still feel that their ancient gods have power, if not to save, at least to trouble and punish them.[46]

And, if Malo's story is true, other Hawaiians, especially those who had moved to Honolulu, must have groaned in despair when they thought of the vindictive spirit of Captain Cook, in the shape of Ka Mū nui 'ele'ele, the Great Black Ghoul, stalking them because he was not yet placated.

Even closer to all Hawaiians, and therefore most dreaded of all, were their 'aumākua. "In this new era," Kamakau warned, they had become not protectors but "bitter enemies who punished severely the faults of their descendants . . . who break laws, commit adultery, and disregard the laws of God, of the land, of parents, husbands, wives, children, and relatives."[47] In another manuscript, Kamakau set forth his explanation for the destruction of his countrymen:

> The reason . . . is well known, it is the influx of foreigners, a very destructive element; then the desire to possess honor and wealth, for these are the friends of contagious diseases; and too because the people mixed up with foreigners when they entered houses of prostitution and there caught diseases not before known to them, and which none of their simple remedies could cure. All these diseases were like poisonous draughts to this people, and many have died, thus depopulating these islands.[48]

This idea of the poisoning of his race entered often into Kamakau's thoughts. It was inescapable, as he saw people around him sickening, withering, falling away. "Thriving seedlings the people of old bore; great gourds filled with seeds they were," he mourned in the 1860s. "But today they are poison gourds, bitter to the taste." And barren, without seeds, he might have added, from which came no new vines to spread across the plains.

From Lahaina, in June 1823, the Reverend Mr. Richards and Mission printer Elisha Loomis sent a grim message: "Gross darkness covers the people, and thousands are everywhere perishing in the depths of ignorance and sin."[49]

The ancient customs observed at the time of death were being abandoned also, especially in Honolulu. Seldom did the kahuna 'aumakua of a dead man go to his household to present "the ritual offering of a pig . . . or a chicken . . . to make acceptable the soul of the dead person to live together with his 'aumakua, his ancestral gods."[50] No longer did male relatives of the dead man preserve his body by filling the belly cavity with salt, or care for his bones by hiding them in a secret place. An aged man, remembering the days of old, might ask himself who would care for his bones when he was dead. But, sighing for times past and respect lost, he would not ask the question aloud—because he knew too well that no sons were left to him, to offer him respect in this world and comfort in the next.

No longer did grieving sons and close friends brand their skin with burning coals, or knock out a front tooth, or receive a tattoo by which to remember the loss of a respected elder. Yet sometimes, but only rarely now, for a man or a woman especially beloved, relatives and friends would gather around the death-mat to chant the *kanikau* of grief, to sing the songs of parting, to wail. The old ways too were ending, perishing with the people.

In Honolulu the bodies of the dead, however they may have died, created other problems. A small cemetery southeast of the harbor received the corpses of foreigners. After 1821 missionaries buried many of their infant children (and, in due time, some of their own number as well) in the graveyard they set aside between the Mission compound and Kawaiaha'o Church. But no one tells us where commoners took their dead. Probably they did what their ancestors had always done, consigning some bodies to the cleansing sea, others to the shifting sands of nearby dunes, or to caves and lava tubes, and a beloved few to shallow graves dug in the earth near the homes in which they had dwelled.[51]

From the few priests who still served in the few temples that still observed the old ways, prayers went up, no doubt, addressed to the great gods. But the gods were gone away now, unhelping now, no longer caring for the people in their need.

And among the most learned priests, those who knew the 2,102 lines of the *Kumulipo,* a few would have lifted up their faces to the silent heavens, asking why these new afflictions, these new ways of dying, should have fallen upon the people. But no comfort would come from the remoteness above. Only from within themselves would rise a voice from the past: "Many who came have vanished, lost in the passing night . . ."

☙☙☙☙

Out of this mixture of experiences and influences, good and bad, biological, sociological, and psychological, a new kind of Hawaiian began to appear, with a different set of values and attitudes than the ones his parents and grandparents acknowledged. Although many of the haoles who influenced the natives could not have been the best of examples—for which reason many a Hawaiian who imitated them fell by the wayside, literally and figuratively—a sufficient number of decent haoles did influence a sufficient number of decent Hawaiians to give them some conception of the dignity of an individual and the value of a human life. Not all Hawaiians deserved Jacques Arago's censure, delivered when he saw them in 1819: "The word licentiousness has no meaning here; every one runs after pleasure, and no one finds the least fault."[52]

Indeed, if the accounts of the early foreigners in Hawai'i are to be accepted, the ideal virtues that romantical Europeans attributed to a "Noble Savage" (wherever he might be encountered) were found more often among Hawaiians than the equivalent virtues expected of a Civilized Man were found among those visiting haoles. With a foundation of sensibility and intelligence to build upon, then, the process of transforming a primitive native to a civilized Hawaiian was achieved with relative ease. For some, as with Kamehameha I, Kalanimoku, and Ke'ōpūolani, it was achieved gracefully, in their maturity if not in earlier years. For others, such as Queen Ka'ahumanu, Chiefess Kapi'olani, and Chief Kuakini, it was well begun and needed only the salving grace of the Christian religion, into which they could put both their belief and their hope, before the transformation could be brought to a consoling conclusion. These exemplars are drawn only from the great chiefs. For every chief who flourished in the changing society, a dozen or a score of commoners must have lifted themselves up from hopelessness to dignity.

But the help of a new religion must wait for the future. During the period from 1800 to 1825, "good" and "virtuous" Hawaiians did exist, despite the innumerable temptations to which they were exposed, despite the crumbling away of their culture and the weakening of the kapus that had been devised to tell them what to do and how to behave. Not all Hawaiians gathered around the fleshpots in the port towns, to carouse with haoles. Not all Hawaiians picked up the vices and the diseases that the foreigners shared so affably.

One unquestioned proof that some Hawaiians were not drawn into the cesspits of civilization lies in the fact that they and their children survived the many dangers of those difficult decades. Another proof lies in the generosity with which Hawaiians received their foreign visitors. Later, much later, haoles themselves would extol it as "the Aloha Spirit." Yet aloha was here, under many other guises, from the beginning. Occasionally a few individuals might forget or betray the rules of hospitality, but the people in general were remarkably friendly to everyone who came from abroad. Because they were a homogeneous group, in both thoughts and manners, the extreme heterogeneity of their visitors must have impressed them as further evidence of the power to be found in the haoles' great world beyond the seas.

But with that concession to power Hawaiians' interest in a man's origins stopped. Race, color, creed, and station in a foreigner meant nothing to them, although they were acutely conscious of rank and station among themselves. In their responses to foreigners Hawaiians were not snobbish, not vicious. They accepted a foreigner exactly as he presented himself to them. White, black, yellow, red, brown, or tan; rich or poor; ugly, handsome, or plain; clean or dirty; healthy or sick; whole or maimed; virtuous or wicked; diligent or lazy: whatever he was when he arrived, some Hawaiians somewhere made him welcome, making room for him in their hospitality as well as in their country. Foreigners never ceased to be surprised by Hawaiians' capacity for kindness. And very few foreigners were so unmoved by this kindness as to take advantage of its givers. This is the secret of the aloha spirit. The man who receives aloha, as well as the one who gives it, is a better man because of the exchange.

In 1900 another critic, having observed the same cast of characters giving the same show, came forth with a less complimentary review of the performance. Dr. E. S. Goodhue had lived in Hawai'i long enough to decide that he knew all about the place and its people. So he wrote a book about them, for the instruction of fellow Americans "back in the States," who might be wondering what they had acquired with the annexation of the Territory of Hawai'i. Looking at

Hawaiians down his long haole nose, anticipating Stephen Roberts by twenty-seven years, Goodhue judged them rather uncharitably:

> For hundreds of years, they had wanted nothing enough to strive for it. They had all they wished to eat, and, if they fought, it was not with a patriotic will, but because they were forced into service by the ambitious chiefs.
>
> This want of purpose had grown into a Polynesian character, which was to be interested by sensational objects of worship, stuffed with suggestion, patched with adhesions of duty, and remade periodically, then, after all, sustained through any particular ordeal, by somebody else's backbone. At the same time, the indifferent, good-natured, run-down morality, was given a vicious phase by the influence of lawless foreigners that infested the islands of the Pacific, and satisfied their sensual desires among the attractive, but non-resistant, people.[53]

Hawaiians' generosity to newcomers was not a sign of weakness but an evidence of strength. For almost the first hundred years after Captain Cook's arrival, Hawaiians outnumbered their visitors and, until the late 1880s, outnumbered even all the foreigners who came to live permanently in their islands. From the beginning, then, Hawaiians were cast in the role of hosts, were confirmed in that role by right of long possession, and played it with the confidence of habit. In the early years of contact with foreigners, Hawaiians as a group, secure in their numbers, did not feel threatened. They acted much as did the helpful Indians of Massachusetts when the needy Pilgrims settled in that bleak region. And they never reacted in the hostile manner that North American Plains Indians were forced to assume against waves of pioneers intruding upon their tribal lands.

Captain Vancouver gave Hawaiians high praise in 1794: "Our reception and entertainment here by these unlettered people, who in general have been distinguished by the appellation of savages, was such as . . . is seldom equalled by the most civilized nations of Europe."[54]

The bounty of their islands and of their sea allowed Hawaiians to be generous without fear of privation. Except in times of warfare or prolonged drought they had enough to eat and to drink. Although providing foodstuffs in such vast quantities as King Kalani'ōpu'u sent out to Captain Cook's ships during their long stay at Kealakekua Bay undoubtedly drained the countryside of victuals, that was an extraordinary occasion. The usual request to provision a single ship

carrying a crew of twenty to twenty-five men would not have depleted a district's supply of foods. Far from resenting the request,
natives happily complied, and not only in order to receive the things
their visitors offered in exchange.

A feeling of responsibility for the welfare of others, expressed in
some cases merely out of a sense of duty, in others by the ability to be
genuinely kind, was present in lowly commoners as well as in lordly
chiefs. It was one of the important components in the mixture of
motives that characterize Hawaiian hospitality. Hawaiians did not
need Christians to teach them about aloha. After all, they had
evoked the word, with all its gentle meanings, out of their own experiences. Christian missionaries, when they arrived in 1820, found
that aloha had prepared the way for them as effectively as had their
guiding Jehovah.

Of course exceptions to the gentle man and the generous woman
could be found among Hawaiians, especially so after their society
with its rules of behavior began to disintegrate under the impact of
foreigners. And of course other forces contributed to the pleasing
sum of motives that called forth their hospitality: the wish to possess
some of the new things that foreigners brought with them; the
human inclination to have a good time, uncomplicated by troubles
with new-made friends; and in some districts, but not in all, either
orders from above—given by chiefs and priests who had always told
their people what to think and what to do—or the very examples of
those rulers in their relationships with foreigners.

The visitors helped themselves too: most of them, common sailors,
even though they may have been a debauched and sinning lot according to Puritan standards, asked nothing more than hospitality from
islanders. Sailors gave of their good nature—and their meager possessions—as willingly as did their hosts. The attractiveness of Hawaiians, in general and in particular, in person and in manner, would
have been another factor. It has impressed foreigners from the beginning—except for those Frenchmen who touched at La Pérouse Bay.
Beyond any doubt it affected the responses of most haoles. Even
Puritan missionaries could be smitten: "They are a lovely youth,
Obadiahs in miniature," Samuel Whitney reported from Kaua'i in
1820, soon after he reached his station at Waimea.[55] Moreover,
unlike cannibal Marquesans, haughty Maoris, and truculent
Samoans, Hawaiians, as Dampier wrote, were "blest with the most
mild and tractable natures possible."[56] Many mariners felt that only
the people of Tahiti matched those of Hawai'i in these attributes.

Their good nature can be attributed primarily to the social code which regulated relationships among themselves, and secondarily to their belief that they were not endangered by foreigners or degraded by the services haoles wanted them to provide. Their social relationships, typical of people living in island communities, were founded upon the principle that, in time of need, every member of a family, clan, or district could call for help from relatives and neighbors. Then, too, the sharing of some kinds of foods by the people in a neighborhood was a frequent experience—and a very sensible way to avoid waste in those days before refrigerators for preserving foods from spoiling. In addition, the sharing of labor in communal projects —such as moving stones to be used in constructing temple foundations and walls or for lining paths and irrigation ditches—had long since accustomed Hawaiians to being considerate and cooperative.[57]

More than mere cooperation entered into their personal relationships, however. They added the important ingredients of generosity and good humor to the tasks that duty required of them. Taught by example, rather than coerced by kapus, they gave of what they had—as many still do—cheerfully and ungrudgingly, knowing full well, of course, that what they gave would be returned to them many times over, like bread cast upon the waters. When Christian missionaries went among them with this message (which, after all, is not confined to Christians), Hawaiians already knew the meaning of charity, and the admonition to regard thy neighbor as thy self. Christianity built on that firm foundation, giving Hawaiians the chance to find through the new religion a new kind of sustenance: hope in the future.

Simple and selfish self-interest, naturally, also entered into their relationships with foreigners. But no one can cast a stone at them for sharing this most basic of human motives. "Aloha abides," Hawaiians said, to other Hawaiians and to haoles alike.

ぐぐぐぐぐ

Auwē! Alas! . . . Good nature, goodwill, the good fun of having a good time, the many ways of expressing aloha—these could not save all Hawaiians from the afflictions that had been set loose among them. Already Miss Beverley's curse was claiming hecatombs of victims, not only in Hawai'i. Already Diderot's prophecy was being fulfilled, not only in Tahiti. The "corruption of manners" that George Forster feared was progressing at a rate that neither kings nor gods could stop.

If those corrupters of manners, the foreigners who came swarming in, had been better men, worthier of the people they were exploiting, Hawaiians would have been less endangered. Unfortunately, most of the world's small supply of better men preferred to stay at home, in their churches, mansions, academies, and counting houses. The few good and decent men who did venture so far from home were overwhelmed by the determinedly evil, the merely wicked, and the ineffectually indifferent many who shipped out with them. "Born to be bad," the wicked bragged, and lost no chance to prove it.

Captain Golovnin, in 1818, praised Hawaiians as being "a free and strong race." If only they could be converted to the Christian faith, said this prescient man, and instructed in the art of writing, "they would in a century reach a state of civilization unparalleled in history."[58] The prophecy was generous (and would be realized long before the century had passed), but conditions in Hawai'i prevented its being even begun before 1820. The Hawaiian race was endangered then—and the instructors they needed, in both literacy and morality, were not to be found in the islands.

Honolulu, where most haoles gathered, was sordid and foul, with grogshops and brothels aplenty but not a thing to stir the mind or uplift the spirit. Already this Sheltered Haven was gaining a reputation as the most debauched place between Canton and Valparaiso. Like London, in Hester Thrale's unkind summation, Honolulu was "a Sink for every Sin." Hilo and Lahaina were only slightly better, simply because they were smaller towns, less frequented by profiteering traders and profligate sailors, all "living at ease in sin."

With such teachers to observe, and more like them arriving aboard every ship, Hawaiians were imperiled, in spirit as in body. They too had their share of evil men, of wild wild women, of weak and unthinking many. Without their guardian kapus, they had nothing now to protect them, least of all a sense of sin, because they had not yet learned about sin. They knew nothing about "free will" and "freedom of choice," those achievements of men and women who have never been enslaved and who willingly accept the restraints of an elevated moral code. How could Hawaiians have known about choices, free will, and all the other privileges of free men, when gods, priests, chiefs, and kings had been dictating their every action and almost every thought since the moment of their birth? The grip of many habits from the past was still too strong, their innocence in the present too pervasive, their ability to hope for a future scarcely awakened.

As, a hundred years later Roberts would say of all Polynesians, almost every form of self-control that regulated Hawaiians' behavior was dropped, and only their "primitive passions" remained—unchecked.

Persuaded by those passions, too many Hawaiians went to the port towns, in pursuit of happiness as they imagined it. They found it —for a while—in good times, in pittances to spend, in the pleasing pretty things that their few coins could buy. No one told them about the other prices they would have to pay.

In choosing Fun, Pleasure, Good Times, the present joys of "Wela ka Hao," with no thought for the morrow, too little concern for the spirit, they invited Death to enter in to claim them.

John Papa I'i, in his "Expression of Aloha for Matthew Kekuana'oa," gathered all of these metaphors for life and love and death in one short mournful poem:

> Death . . . is like love
> That flees at my angry reply.
> It reels, it staggers,
> When it comes, it comes like a sudden sickness.
>
> It pulls and jerks open the door,
> Like the blowing of a Kona gale,
> Then it is still, without a stir.
> It comes in silence before me, a love that is hurt,
> Tired and worn and spent.[59]

The foreigners, who neglected their own bodies, minds, and spirits, presented Hawaiians with the worst of all possible models to follow. This, beyond any doubt, was the greatest of all misdeeds that those friendly unthinking haoles ever committed against their unthinking friendly hosts, so full of aloha, so innocent in the needs of the mind and of the spirit.

Hawaiians needed help, if they were to survive, whether as individuals or as a people. Yet none of them realized how desperate was their plight. Neither did the few haoles who lived among them, nor the many foreigners who sailed in to the islands' ports for purposes of trade and, worse, for recruitment and refreshment, before they sailed off again. In 1819, neither in Hawai'i nor in any other part of the great world, no one knew, or bothered, or cared about the dying of the Hawaiian people.

Then, just in time, from across the seas, the helpers came.

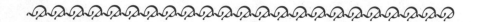

NINE

Many Who Came Have Vanished

No one can say how many Hawaiians lived on their isolated islands at any time before 1832. Only in 1831–1832 was the first census taken, at the suggestion of American missionaries and with their help. The head count of 130,313 obtained during that census, inefficiently though it may have been conducted by present standards, gives demographers a relatively dependable figure to compare with enumerations made in later years.

Before 1832, therefore, all population numbers given by visitors, starting with the officers of Captain Cook's expedition in 1778–1779, could have been nothing more than guesses. These ranged all the way from the high of "half a million" offered by Lieutenant James King[1] in 1779 (who later revised his estimate to 400,000); through carping William Bligh's reduction of that published second guess to 242,000 (reckoned according to a method revealed only to himself);[2] to George Youngson's asseveration that the population of Hawai'i in 1805 was precisely 264,160.[3] Obviously, one man's guess was not as good as another's.

In the twentieth century less daring scholars have settled on a figure "between 250,000 and 300,000" as a "reasonable estimate" for the population in 1778. Even so, as R. C. Schmitt has pointed out, this compromise has been erected on "evidence of the flimsiest kind."[4] For want of information, most demographers have adopted this range of 250,000 to 300,000 as a point of departure for discussions about the numbers of native Hawaiians since 1778. In 1989, however, David Stannard expressed a decidedly different opinion: the Hawaiian population in 1778, he declared, was "roughly between 800,000 and a million."[5] Also in 1989, Dye and Komori proposed a much lower figure: about 100,000 people in 1778.[6]

Observations made by a number of foreigners who visited Hawai'i soon after 1778 provide indirect support for accepting a figure lower than 400,000. Thus, Captain George Dixon, visiting with Captain Nathaniel Portlock in 1786, thought that King's estimate was too high "by half."[7] Archibald Menzies, surgeon and naturalist with Captain George Vancouver's expedition, which visited these islands in 1792, 1793, and 1794, believed that either King had miscalculated the number of natives (a possibility which the pragmatic lieutenant had been the first to suggest) or that "the population since his time must be greatly diminished on all the islands."[8] Many similar challenges to King's estimate can be found in the literature of the early nineteenth century.

Nonetheless, if we lack a definite reference count for native Hawaiians in 1778, at the beginning of their recorded history, we have ample data with which to plot the sad swift progress of their decline after that fateful year. The graph presented in Figure 1, prepared from census reports taken from 1831-1832 until 1960, shows all too clearly the slide toward extinction to which contact with foreigners doomed the Hawaiian people.

Figure 1 plots the logarithm numbers of the "pure Hawaiian" population against time, just as microbiologists would do with successive counts of the living cells in a bacterial culture. For bacteria the "growth curve" obtained by such a method would represent the several successive phases in the life cycle of a culture. The graph depicted here is characteristic of "the phase of logarithmic decrease," the penultimate stage near the end of a culture's life cycle, when the number of cells that are dying or dead, compared with the number of living cells that are being formed, increases in a logarithmic progression. The slope of the curve indicates the rate at which death is triumphing over life. When this phase ends, and the last cell has died, the final stage of the culture is reached: all life in it is extinct. That ultimate stage, however meaningless it may be for the cells in the dead culture, is a necessary endpoint, both practically and philosophically, for the student of that culture.

Translated into terms of human experience, the graph reveals several important facts about the culture of the "pure-blooded" Hawaiian people. Most immediate in its message is the implacable course of the destruction of the Hawaiian race. As that rapidly descending line shows, Hawaiians did not succeed in withstanding the impact of foreign people and the germs they introduced. Once that destruction

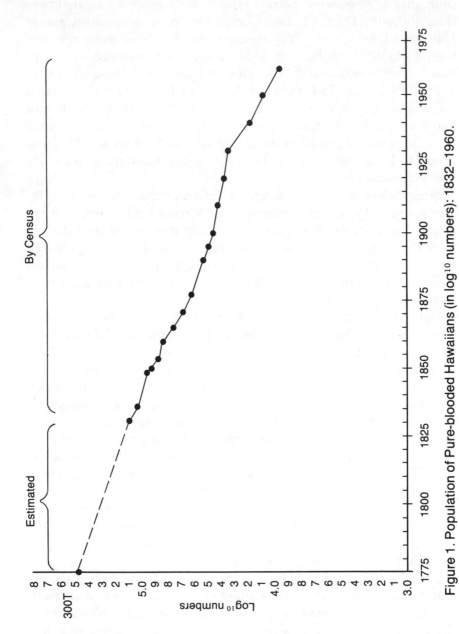

Figure 1. Population of Pure-blooded Hawaiians (in log₁₀ numbers): 1832–1960.

had begun, nothing could stop it: not civilization, not Christianity, not Americanization, sanitation, medication, or immunization, neither faith nor prayer nor acts of government, could swerve it from that predestined plunge. For Hawaiians as a race, no matter what they did or what was done for them, death was inescapable.

In 1900, when the United States annexed these islands, only 29,799 pure-blood Hawaiians were counted. In 1991, no one knew how many were left. Best guesses ranged from the necessary statistical 1 to "about five or six thousand."

The slope of the curve indicates that, during the time from 1832 to 1960, the death rate—or, better, the "disappearance rate"—for native Hawaiians has been remarkably constant. This constancy has continued despite the fact that only in a few special years (notably in 1848 and 1853) did severe epidemics claim many more lives than were lost during years in which no serious epidemics occurred.

This relatively constant rate of disappearance in itself reflects:

 • A vulnerability of Hawaiians to death or disappearance not only from introduced infectious diseases but also from other causes.
 • The presence in each generation of a fairly constant proportion of the population which was unable to withstand the assorted factors contributing to their decline.
 • No significant improvement, at any time after 1832, under any form of government or religion or socioeconomic auspices, in the total milieu in which native Hawaiian people lived. In other words, the trend established early in the nineteenth century continues today, near the end of the twentieth century.
 • Since 1832, and probably beginning before that year, a genocidal decline in birth rates—or, at the very least, in the survival rates of infants—and probably an accompanying decline in fertility-fecundity of adults.
 • The existence of other factors, which in themselves did not lead directly to mortality but assisted the gradual decrease in numbers of Hawaiians of unmixed blood. For example, the slightly steeper slope to the curve since 1930 probably reflects an artificial depletion in the numbers of people formerly placed in the census category for "pure Hawaiians." This kind of depletion can be attributed to marriage of native women to non-Hawaiians, migration, denial of ancestry under social pressures, and so on, rather than to actual death. It can reflect also, as Schmitt has pointed out, the decreasing number of people classified by census-takers since 1920 as "pure Hawaiians." The data after 1970 are even more confused, and much less helpful, inasmuch as the

U.S. Census regulations for that year "eliminated the traditional distinction of (full) Hawaiian and Part Hawaiian, since pure-blooded Hawaiians were very few in number and of questionable identity. The Part Hawaiians were merged into the single category of 'Hawaiian' or classified with other races."[9] (For this reason, Figure 1 ends with the census of 1960.)

᠙᠙᠙᠙

As anyone acquainted with statistics will know, when census counts for Hawaiians are plotted, severe epidemics of diseases (even though they occurred frequently between 1804 and 1920) do not impose precipitate spikes on the curve. (They would appear as dramatic dips, of course, if annual population figures were plotted.) In other words, census counts, by showing the sum of all experiences leading to the decrease in the native population, tend to "smooth out the curve." But the *slope* of the curve does reveal that the sum of all these experiences was unrelentingly destructive for Hawaiians. The consistency of this trend indicates that factors other than epidemic diseases alone were acting at all times on a population which was sensitive to a variety of influences.

Beyond denying, however, is the evidence that Hawaiians did not learn much about ways of staying alive. They did not learn either from their own troubles or from the experiences of foreigners who tried to teach them how to adapt to new customs and new perils. In other words, by being unable or unwilling to change their mores, Hawaiians committed themselves to continuing mortality. Regrettably, this intransigence persists among many families of Hawaiians even today.

The *Honolulu Advertiser,* in an editorial published on 3 May 1989, felt compelled to make this point once again, as it has done so often in the past:

> Heart disease is the No. 1 killer of native Hawaiians. Native Hawaiians also are more likely than others, statistically, to be struck by other killers—cancer, diabetes, hypertension, and infectious diseases.
>
> Much of this suffering is preventable through diet, exercise, and early medical care.

In contrast, the editorial stated, deaths from heart disease among residents belonging to all other ethnic groups are so few that Hawai'i "has the lowest rate of heart disease deaths among all states." Unfortunately, few of the Hawaiian and part-Hawaiian people whom the editorial was trying to advise will read it, and even fewer will bother to take any action to help themselves to avoid being included in these dismaying statistics.

On 9 July 1989, in the *Sunday Honolulu Star-Bulletin and Advertiser,* Dr. Jack Lewin, director of the State of Hawaii Department of Health, emphasized this fact: "Hawaiians have the poorest health status of any group in the United States. It is a tremendous irony," he added, after comparing their plight with the good health enjoyed by members of all other ethnic groups in Hawai'i.

If the curve of the graph in Figure 1 is projected backward in time from 1832, it intersects the ordinate for population in 1775 at approximately 300,000. This is as good a confirmation as we are likely to get for the "reasonable compromise" of historians. (On the other hand, we must remember that, while this kind of playing with numbers may be applied to microbes in a culture medium, it is not as safely applied to human beings. Even more so than microorganisms, people are subject to so many other environmental factors, and are apt to be so full of the ingenuities of adaptation, that projections of this sort, either forward or backward, should be considered as being little more than statistical games.)

Unless Hawaiians of unmixed blood make a deliberate effort to increase their numbers by mating only among themselves (an effort earnestly to be wished, if only for sentimental reasons, and one not likely to be achieved, for reasons even more dictated by sentiment), and unless the rate of decrease since 1832 should change for the better, and assuming that any human beings at all will be alive in this endangered world by then, the last pure-blooded Hawaiian probably will have disappeared within two more generations—that is, by the year 2025.

Here is another of those dire prophecies that alarmists are always making about one "endangered species" or another. Yet it is likely to be realized sooner than predicted, if only because Hawaiians, so full of aloha, are utterly incapable of making so selfish an effort to perpetuate themselves as a race apart.

Even so, with respect to Hawaiians as a sociopolitical group, the prediction is already fulfilled: pure-blooded Hawaiians, who represented only about 1 percent of the population in the islands in 1970, have long ceased to exist as a significant political-social entity. This conclusion was reached by officialdom before 1970, when U.S. Census bureaucrats decided to "eliminate" the category for full-blooded Hawaiians because "they were few in number and of questionable identity," as Nordyke stated. Once again, pride of race and of lineage, in living warm-blooded human beings, fell before the decrees of statisticians.

Thus not too far in the future the number of full-blooded Hawaiians will approach so close to zero that statisticians will consider it "not significant." Hurtful as this fact of statistics will be, the truth must be told, in sorrow and regret, for it informs the mind of the death of a noble people. The psychological, economic, and social plight of many pure-blooded Hawaiians and part-Hawaiians who survive today can be traced to the fact that they have not learned this most fundamental of all facts about themselves.

The only comfort we can extract from their confusion in the present lies in the great number of "part-Hawaiians" who, when the last "pure Hawaiian" is gone, will be preserving some of the genes, if not the whole lineage, of their Polynesian ancestors. In 1986, "using Department of Health definitions of ethnicity," 203,355 part-Hawaiians were counted, "or almost 20 percent of the total population."[10]

Depending on our sentiments and prejudices, we can conclude that, in less than 200 years after their discovery by representatives of Western civilization, Hawaiians either have been completely assimilated into the new culture, or they have been completely eliminated from it. Given the histories of native peoples in other countries, and the factors determining the adaptability of humankind in all parts of the world (not to mention the flexibility of prejudices), both conclusions can be supported, although perhaps only one will be acceptable.

Unaware though they must have been about so many of the conditions that determine the welfare of an indigenous society in any part of the world, early visitors to Hawai'i could see that contact with foreigners was affecting Hawaiians in a number of adverse ways. Some of the more perceptive voyagers seem to have sensed the changes rather than measured their extent. Yet, feeling uneasy about the consequences of contact, they relieved their discomfort with rhetoric. Captain George Dixon, for example, who in 1786 really could not have known enough about the subject of public health from which to derive any dependable conclusions, must have been responding to impressions of unfortunate changes when (with the aid of a ghost-writer) he delivered this bland pronouncement:

> The inhabitants of these islands appear subject to very few diseases; and though they doubtless have been injured by their connections with Europeans, yet so simple is their manner of living, that they pay little regard to this circumstance, and seem to think it an affair of no consequence.[11]

Without much doubt, that coy circumlocution about having been "injured by their connections" refers to the venereal diseases, presented to their hosts by at least a few sailors from every ship that visited these islands. Other foreigners, however, having observed more definite instances of Hawaiians' responses to discovery and exploitation, did write accounts that seem to be trustworthy. They are the witnesses who provide the information upon which this essay is based.

In Hawai'i, as in all places subjected to similar attrition, two sets of factors led to a decrease in population: the first, those that provoked an actual loss of people from any cause; the second, those that induced a lowered birth rate.

Loss of People

Hawaiians who survived the travail of birth were subjected immediately to all the influences that take the lives of human beings everywhere.

Major Causes

A number of circumstances peculiar to these islands and their indigenous people made certain of those influences very important in the effects they had on the health and the society of Hawaiians.

Warfare and Attendant Hardships. Long before 1778 ambitious chiefs had begun to wage campaigns of aggrandizement against adversaries in districts far from home. Where once a narrow valley or a small community had been prize enough, eventually a whole island became the goal. Some of the most powerful warlords, such as Kalani'ōpu'u of Hawai'i and his arch-rival, Kahekili of Maui, looked even farther afield than the island each had subdued: they directed their aggressions across the narrow channel between the two islands, in a desultory and costly conflict that brought victory to neither leader. In the assaults of total war that they ordered, not only soldiers died in battle or as sacrifices upon the altars of Kū, the bloodthirsty war god. Women, children, and elders, too, were slaughtered, in villages overrun by invaders; or they died, not so brutally perhaps but just as surely, from starvation during the famines caused when plundering enemies destroyed homes, crops, and taro patches, and ate or took away all the foodstuffs they could carry.

Foreigners when they came added new dimensions to the ancient methods of warfare. Hawaiian tacticians, too, quickly understood the increased killing power of muskets and cannons, while they envied foreigners the mobility afforded by sailing vessels. Henceforth, those quarreling chiefs could not rest until they had acquired firearms and ships, regardless of price. No one heeded Vancouver's fatherly advice ("Stop making war; live in peace; be friends with each other"); and few foreign captains followed his example in refusing to sell weapons and gunpowder to the vying chieftains. Vaulting ambition and a mad zeal to win or lose everything they owned impelled the fighting kings, from Hawai'i to Kaua'i, and they did not cease their contestings until all were subdued save one. In 1795 Kamehameha I, the only conqueror, was acknowledged the sovereign lord of still-smoking villages, and of the people who had survived the battles, the sequels of pacification, rituals of sacrifice to Kū-the-Snatcher-of-Lands, and the famines that followed pillaging armies as thirst follows a drought. "The earth must have sighed," wrote Samuel Kamakau in 1876, "because of the blood of men shed without cause, all to honor and elevate the chiefs, and to give lands and riches to those who were the instruments which had caused the shedding of human blood."[12]

And yet even before the war between Kalanikūpule of O'ahu and Kamehameha of Hawai'i began, the prophet Ka'opulupulu foretold the consequences of their rivalry. Rarely has a prophet in any land been as farseeing as was Ka'opulupulu when he warned Kamehameha

> that the nation will be taken by white men, and that the people would dwell landless in the houses of the fish, that there would be an end to the line of kings, leaving but the bare shelves, and that a stubborn disobedient generation was coming, which would cause the native race to dwindle . . .[13]

Historians, native as well as foreign, have not agreed upon the sizes of the armies which took part in those climactic engagements between 1770 and 1795, or upon the number of people who died either during the conflicts or while the Conqueror established his dominion after the fighting ended. Nonetheless, the cost in lives must have been significant: as Kamakau declared, "Many had been slaughtered, baked in the *imu* [earth oven], and pounded out of existence."[14]

In 1792 Vancouver noticed that "Mowee and its neighboring islands were reduced to great indigence by the wars, in which for many years they had been engaged." In his opinion, the burdens of maintaining opposing armies, the neglect of agriculture because the men had been called to war, and "vast supplies" taken by

> half-famished trading vessels . . . have left a very scanty portion for the remaining inhabitants of Mowee. . . . Rannai and [Kahoʻolawe] which had formerly been considered as fruitful and populous islands, were nearly over-run with weeds, and exhausted of their inhabitants; nor has Owyhee escaped the devastation consequent on her foreign and intestine disputes, which had been numerous and severe.[15]

Contagious Diseases. Infectious microorganisms have been the most serious and the most persistent agents contributing to the reduction of the Hawaiian people since 1778. Wars and catastrophes have come and gone, like the men and the occasions which provoked them, but the attrition of contagious diseases has been a constant factor in the destruction of Hawaiians. Newly introduced pathogenic microorganisms killed inordinately large numbers of people in the explosive attacks known as epidemics. Then, when the initial violence subsided, some pathogens disappeared entirely, at least for a time, while others continued to smolder in the populace as endemic infections. These insidious organisms gnawed away at the people, killing several here, a few more there, for decade after decade, until, in the course of more than 200 years, the total number of victims claimed by any one pathogen was greater than the number killed in the primary sweep of that disease. Among these chronic diseases the several kinds of gastrointestinal infections, syphilis, gonorrhea, tuberculosis, and, later, leprosy, would have been only the most diligent of killers.

Hawaiians were not the only people to be so affected by microbial invaders from Asia, Europe, and the Americas. Natives of Oceania's scattered islands learned very early to associate outbreaks of sickness with visits from foreigners. In 1800 an anonymous English missionary wrote, in his *Historical Sketch of the Otaheitian Islands:* "Many of their diseases are of European extraction: nay, the natives remark, that with every ship they receive a cargo of new diseases."[16]

The American missionaries in Hawai'i knew exactly whom to blame for introducing diseases when, in their *Annual Account for 1828,* they wrote from Honolulu to the American Board of Commissioners for Foreign Missions' officers in Boston: "The seeds of disease and death are scattered in profusion by the licentious visitants of these islands; and multitudes of unhappy sufferers pine in sickness, and need the benevolent agency of a skillful physician to apply suitable remedies."[17]

Yet not all "visitants" were licentious, and not all Polynesians were unchaste. What today we call "childhood diseases," for example, socially acceptable even then in New England, could take a dreadful toll among the most innocent of islanders, the children, even the children of missionaries themselves, as well as among the adult members of a population. Nor could the "benevolent agency" of several regiments of physicians ever put a halt to the destruction of Polynesia's people.

Before the American missionaries reached Hawai'i in 1820, to become for the next thirty years the most reliable reporters about the health and well-being of Hawaiians, some of those earlier "visitants" were the ones who provided the best information about the impact of introduced diseases on the native population. The records they left us are sporadic and incomplete, giving little more than hints about what was happening. The reason for this is not hard to understand: most of those travelers were neither physicians nor demographers, and all of them stayed in the islands for only a short time. Almost invariably, however, and usually in a counterpoint of dithyramb and dismay, after extolling the comforts and charms of the Sandwich Islands these mariners seemed to feel compelled to make some reference to the disturbed health of their inhabitants. This practice began with the very first of Hawai'i's visitors: many members of Captain Cook's expedition, when they looked back on their two sojourns in the islands, realized how seriously their presence had affected the Hawaiians.

The same anonymous missionary who, in writing a *Historical Sketch of the Otaheitian Islands,* included in his book a short digression on the Sandwich Islands, arraigned Britain's sailors for what they had done to Hawai'i's people:

Notwithstanding all the precautions which Captain COOK had taken to prevent it, these friendly islanders were contaminated with the venereal disease, of which great numbers had already died [before February 1779, he claimed, basing his statement upon evidence not transmitted to us]. Cruel memorial of the British name! the first boon of *civilization* to the *Barbarians* of the South Seas![18]

That conscience-stricken Englishman, because of his prejudices, and Cook's companions, because of the shortness of their visits, would have been more impressed by the symptoms of the venereal diseases than by those of any other infections the explorers might have imparted to Hawai'i's people. The venereal diseases in their early stages, especially gonorrhea, show symptoms that even a layman can recognize; whereas certain other ailments, such as the dysenteries and scabies, "the itch," would have been so common to sailors as to be undeserving of mention. But the chronic diseases, such as tuberculosis, leprosy, or the late stages of syphilis, would have been so slow to develop that their symptoms would not have been detectable until long after the mariners had put out to sea again.

Captain Dixon, recalling his visit to the Sandwich Islands in 1786, could give expression only to a vague unease about the impact of discovery on Hawaiians. More than likely Dixon was correct in his appraisal of Hawaiians' health in 1786. Although diseases may not have been "very common among them"—except for the venereal infections, of course—their reprieve was coming to an end.

By 1786 tuberculosis had begun its devastation. Every ship's crew must have included several consumptive mariners who would cough and spit and spew virulent tubercle bacilli about them wherever they went. Captain Charles Clerke, Cook's colleague and successor, and Surgeon William Anderson, both "far advanced in the consumption" when they landed at Waimea, Kaua'i, in 1778, were only the more notable of that expedition's infectious invalids.

By 1792, when Captain George Vancouver's ships made their first visit to the islands, Surgeon Archibald Menzies saw that Kalanikūpule, King of O'ahu, was ailing with "the wasting disease." On the afternoon of 22 March, while the ships lay off Waikīkī, Kalanikūpule went out to call on Vancouver

lying on a litter in a double canoe. A chair was lowered down for him in which he came into the ship, and appeared very weak and emaciated from a pulmonary complaint that now produced hectic symptoms, for which I gave him some medicines, accompanied with some general directions how to manage his complaint.[19]

And Edward Bell, Vancouver's clerk on HMS *Chatham*, at Lahaina on 14 March 1793, noticed a wife of Kahekili, king of Maui:

> Only a few years ago [1787] when the *Prince of Wales* was at Atooi [she] was one of the handsomest little girls on the island, she was now indeed wonderfully altered, she was in appearance far gone in consumption and the bearing of two or three children had wrought such a change in her features for the worse . . .[20]

Hawaiians were not the only Polynesians to be so affected by the white man's tuberculosis. In 1791 or 1793, according to Father Ildefonse Alazard, it reached Vaitahu of the Marquesas Islands in the person of a Tahitian named Tama. "The [Catholic] missionaries have never ceased to make war against this dreadful malady, the great reaper of young natives," Alazard wrote in 1905. "They have recommended to the natives thousands and thousands of times, all of the hygienic measures and methods of prevention which are imposed upon similar cases."[21]

But in the Marquesas, as elsewhere, the foreigners' diseases could not be stayed. Between 1804 and 1838, under the impact of all those conqueror germs—not only of the tubercle bacilli—the population of the single Marquesan island of Nukuhiva decreased from 17,700 to 8,000; and between 1838 and 1848, it further declined to 5,000. In 1905, when Father Alazard compiled his mournful account, "La diminution continue sans que rien soit capable de l'arrêter." And by 1938, in all their green and beautiful islands, only 2,283 Marquesans remained.[22]

Not many years had passed, however, before Hawaiians (as well as other Polynesians) who suffered from foreigners' microbes began to return the favors in kind, by means of polluted water, contaminated foodstuffs, and bodies for hire that were rotten with disease. Thus, on 8 October 1789, just after leaving the island of Hawai'i, George Mortimer, lieutenant of marines aboard the brig *Mercury*, told about the consequences of his ship's stay at Kealakekua Bay from 23 to 25 September 1789:

> At 10 o'clock . . . died Thomas Smith, ship's cook. As we had no surgeon aboard, we could not ascertain the nature of the disorder which proved fatal to him; but we supposed it to have been an inflammation of the bowels, occasioned by a violent bilious colic, a complaint that our first and third mates, myself, and several of the seamen, laboured under at the time.[23]

By that time, too, a few Hawaiians were trying to understand not only the nature of their new ailments but also the most understandable reason why they were being so sorely tried. In 1791 crusty Captain James Colnett wrote of "the toll taken by contagions" and concluded: "Being unable to comprehend either the nature or the severity of the new diseases, every one attributed the decline in population to warfare rather than to sicknesses as well."[24]

In 1792 Captain Vancouver and Surgeon Menzies, too, having noticed a decrease in the population, blamed it on war and its sequels:

> At Whyteetee . . . although the town was extensive, and the houses numerous, yet they were thinly inhabited, and many appeared to be abandoned. The village of Whymea [on Kaua'i] is reduced at least two thirds of its size since . . . 1778–1779. In those places where . . . the houses were most numerous, now [there is] a clear space, occupied by grass and weeds. [Most of the chiefs had died, too] nor did we understand that many had died a natural death, most of them having been killed in these deplorable contests.[25]

Captain William R. Broughton, visiting at Waikīkī in June 1796, soon after Kamehameha won O'ahu, wrote that "the situation of the natives was miserable, as they were nearly starving; and, as an additional grievance, universally infected with the itch."[26]

Yet even in such "miserable" communities some visitors found only what they wanted to see. Foremost among those determined romantics was a young Frenchman, François Peron. He, too, visited the Sandwich Islands in 1796, most improbably as first officer of the Boston merchantship *Otter,* but during the month of his stay noticed nothing as sordid as a diseased body. Or, if perchance he did see such a reminder of real life, he had suppressed all recollection of it when, about twenty-five years later, at home again in France, he wrote his *Memoires . . . sur ses voyages.* In his impressions of Hawai'i, set down in the sort of stars-in-the-eyes travel-writer's prose that stay-at-home readers demanded even then (and mariners happily provided), Peron remembered only the beauties of this New Eden.

A few foreigners, to be sure, managed to be very practical men, both in the observations they made and in the behavior they expected of visitors and Hawaiians alike. Unfortunately, these realists could do little to safeguard islanders against the manifold dangers to which they were being exposed. The best of them, like Captain Cook in

1778 and Captain Amasa Delano in 1801, tried to protect the natives from foreigners' diseases as well as from their greed. Cook failed in his purpose, for "the venereal distemper" was transmitted by people and lusts beyond the control of his regulations; whereas Delano gained a notable success, if on a small scale: the vaccinating of his few Hawaiian sailors in order to immunize them against Canton's smallpox was a procedure over which he could impose adequate control.

Another realist was John Turnbull, supercargo aboard the British trader *Margaret,* which spent the period from 17 December 1802 to 21 January 1803 in Hawaiian waters. Turnbull noticed many aspects of native life both in Hawai'i and Tahiti. His account of the more serious contagions suffered by Tahitians at the time is clear and pertinent: venereal disease (which "has swept off thousands since Europeans arrived" in 1767); intermittent fever ("very fatal"); the dysentery ("seldom fails to be fatal"); scrofula ("which breaks inwardly and wastes them like a consumption"); rheumatism and agues; and "many others."[27]

Turnbull's remarks about these maladies in Tahiti show that, even though he may have erred in estimating their effects, he was aware of their relationship to the well-being of a population. The fact that he wrote nothing at all about diseases of any kind among Hawaiians suggests that in 1802 they were not yet so seriously affected as to call his attention to their ailments. In any event, Turnbull was the last of the interested foreigners who would not see overwhelming evidence for the effects of introduced diseases on Hawai'i's people. The relative respite from alien plagues they had enjoyed since 1778 was about to end.

The full force of a devastating epidemic, apparently the first great pestilence Hawaiians would experience in modern times, struck them in 1804. Once again Kamehameha was preparing his forces for the conquest of Kaua'i. His first attempt to acquire that island in 1795 or 1796, soon after he gained O'ahu, had been foiled when a divine wind drove his fleet of war canoes back to O'ahu's shores. Since that time, from headquarters on the island of Hawai'i, he had devoted more than six years to building a fleet of *peleleu* canoes and in training the warriors who would man those vessels.

Just before the expedition was about to depart from the island of Hawai'i, still another daring prophet, this one named Lono-hele-moa, appeared before Kamehameha, entreating him not to undertake this needless war. When Kamehameha would not heed him, Lono-hele-moa predicted that "a great pestilence would come among the King's people."[28] Despite this warning, Kamehameha assembled his warriors on Oʻahu, readying them for the first stage of his assault upon Kauaʻi—the crossing of the channel between the two islands.

In that mob gathered in a staging-area unprepared to accommodate them, the prophecy of Lono-hele-moa was fulfilled. As with so many other armies in the history of other warring nations, Kamehameha's troops provided the circumstances for inviting an epidemic of gastrointestinal disease. The great volume of excrement released by all those people, whether or not they tried to dispose of their wastes according to the prescribed kapus, soon polluted with fecal microorganisms the meager supplies of water and foodstuffs that the waiting army could acquire. An epidemic was inevitable. Kamakau described it:

> At the end of this time [of mobilization] the pestilence appeared called ʻokuʻu. It was a very virulent pestilence, and those who contracted it died quickly. A person on the highway would die before he reached home. One might go for food and water and die so suddenly that those at home did not know what had happened. The body turned black at death. A few died a lingering death, but never longer than 24 hours [sic]; if they were able to hold out for a day they had a fair chance to live. Those who lived generally lost their hair, hence the illness was called "Head stripped bare" (Poʻo-kole).[29]

Ever since that time historians, physicians, and demographers have tried to identify this terrible disease. Guesses range all the way from the impossible, through the unlikely, to the most probable suspects. Yellow fever, for example, could not possibly have occurred because mosquitoes had not yet been introduced to serve as vectors of the virus. Bubonic plague was unlikely because, if the infection really had been "the Black Death," the plague bacilli would have survived among rodents to cause cases among humans in the years after 1804, just as they did for many years after 1899, when the islands' first authentic epidemic of bubonic plague did affect people and rats on Oʻahu, Maui, and Hawaiʻi. The most probable suspects for the maʻi ʻokuʻu, "the squatting sickness," are typhoid fever, bacillary or amoebic dysentery, and (a poor third) Asiatic cholera.

Our best clues are offered not in the symptoms described by Kamakau and others, which are too vague and variable (if not imagined) to be diagnostic, but from the names by which Hawaiians referred to the epidemic: *'ōku'u, ma'i 'ōku'u, ahulau 'ōku'u, kau 'ōku'u, ma'i ahulau, po'okole,* and *ikipuahola*. *'Ōku'u* means "to squat, to crouch, to sit hunched up, as at stool," and obviously suggests a dysentery of some kind. *Po'okole,* "a full bald head," refers to the loss of hair which can follow the high fever that often accompanies the severest forms of typhoidal enteritis.

The blackening of the body at death (if it did occur) could be attributed to subcutaneous hemorrhages caused by many kinds of viruses and bacteria, including those of typhoid-paratyphoid fevers and, of course, those of bubonic plague and other pasteurelloses. The lack of any reference to the dreadful, violent purgation, the "rice-water stool," and the subsequent dehydration that are so characteristic of Asiatic cholera—and which could scarcely have escaped the notice of native chroniclers—remove that disease from the position of most likely suspect. If we can recognize anything in these vague descriptions and earthy native names, it is a set of symptoms best associated with typhoid fever (or with some other salmonellosis of comparable seriousness). The great mortality attributed to the epidemic does indicate its severity, at least for Hawaiians, even though the figures seem to have been very much exaggerated.

Naturally, no one knew where the disease had come from, or by what means it arrived in Hawai'i. But long before 1804, hundreds of sailors aboard dozens of ships arriving from all the world's quarters had had ample opportunity to introduce the microorganisms which eventually caused the epidemic of 'ōku'u. Those virulent microorganisms, gradually spreading among residents, taking an unnoticed toll at first, would have been widely distributed, polluting drinking water and victuals, until they exploded with destructive violence among susceptible warriors and camp followers crowded in their unsanitary bivouacs along the beaches of southern O'ahu.

Whatever its nature, whenever it happened, the epidemic did affect the course of Hawaiian history in several important ways. Most immediately, it compelled Kamehameha to call off once again his invasion of Kaua'i. Uncounted numbers of his chiefs and warriors had sickened and died. Kamehameha himself, according to Kamakau, "contracted the disease, but managed to live through it." When "his counsellors all died, and many of their chiefs and families," Kamehameha suffered irreparable losses.[30]

When he lost such stalwart supporters, Kamehameha had to turn to their sons and to other younger chiefs for assistance in managing his kingdom. Almost without exception these younger men brought little of their fathers' interests and abilities to the needs of government. Possibly they lived in awe of the potent king, but more probably they had already been so corrupted by contact with foreign visitors, ideas, and things that they could no longer see the problems complicating the king's rule or attempt to resolve them (as he sought to do) for the best interests of the nation as a whole. They were, rather, so feckless in their concern for ease and dissipation, so unbridled in their selfishness, that they would be the worst possible influences upon the rising generation, and especially upon the young heir-apparent, both before and after he became King Kamehameha II.

Fortunately for Kamehameha I, among the survivors was Kalanimoku. From the time of the ma'i 'ōku'u until 8 May 1819, when the Conqueror died, Kalanimoku served his liege-lord as prime minister, with absolute devotion, great ability, and unparalleled modesty. And when the founder of the dynasty had gone, Kalanimoku served the second and third Kamehameha kings just as loyally, until in 1827 his time came to die. For twenty-three years he had been, as his people said, "the iron cable which held fast the nation; at his death that stay was broken." With Kalanimoku—and, after 1819, with Queen Ka'ahumanu also—to control the affairs of government, perhaps no other high chiefs were needed.

From the point of view of Kamehameha and Kalanimoku, the two who actually governed the kingdom after 1804, the epidemic's sudden removal of a number of contentious companions-in-arms, several of whom might have challenged the king's preeminence, may have been an advantage in consolidating his rule over the islands he had so recently conquered. Yet, as the future would show, the nation lost much of value when so many of those hard and virile warrior chiefs—and their patrician *virtu*—were swept away in so short a time. If most of them had lived—to be conservative, reactionary defenders of the old ways against the encroachments of foreigners, especially during the period from 1812 to 1840—who can deny that the history of the Hawaiian people would have been different? If only some of them had survived, to sow their seed and breed more of their kind, would not the foreigners have been prevented from exploiting the islands as easily as they did?

And what of the commoners in the kingdom? Because no one ever paid much attention to them, no one noted how they fared during the ma'i 'ōku'u. R. C. Schmitt, who in 1970 published the definitive study of this epidemic, gave some idea of the confusion with which a succession of writers have viewed it:

> Many writers have contended that one-half, or even a majority, of the population died in this epidemic, but others have been more conservative. Some applied these rates to the entire kingdom, while a few limited them to Oahu. One source confined mortality to two-thirds of an army of 8,000, another gave it as one-eighth of the total population, and a third suggested annual crude death rates of either 441 or 482 per 1,000 inhabitants in the year of the plague. A few have proposed absolute figures: 22,000 (on "Oahu alone"); 112,000–128,000 (net decline for all islands); and 175,000. Others have been satisfied with broad descriptive terms, such as "a vast number," "multitudes," or "dreadful havoc." One skeptic attributed the higher figures to "legendary exaggeration," and many later writers have remained cautiously noncommittal. General agreement as to the great severity of the epidemic has thus been accompanied by widely varying opinions in respect to actual mortality levels.

After analyzing the conflicting information relating to the ma'i 'ōku'u —most of which can only be inferred from comments that in themselves can be little more than hearsay and gossip—Schmitt decided:

> The foregoing evidence makes it almost impossible to escape the conclusion that the 'oku'u has been greatly exaggerated. If, as seems likely, the epidemic was limited to Oahu, the death toll was probably well under 15,000 (out of perhaps 35,000 or 40,000 on the Island at the time). If only Kamehameha's troops suffered, the mortality was considerably less, certainly not over 5,000. Such death totals are still high by anyone's standards, but they hardly compare to some of the astronomical figures found in the literature.[31]

With this judgment all sensible demographers (and historians) must concur. Uncertain as we today must be about the details of the epidemic, we can agree in believing that a pestilence of shocking proportions did occur. Even if half the population did not succumb, even if "not over 5,000" people died, that was still a great number of deaths to happen within a relatively short period among a people not previously acquainted with such a catastrophic experience. Until then the population probably had been declining steadily although inconspicuously, under the double impact of foreigners' diseases, introduced almost continuously since 1778, and civil warfare, all but continuous since a time before Captain Cook visited the islands.

Regardless of the actual number of lives claimed by the maʻi ʻokuʻu, the mortality it caused was so high, and the horror associated with it was so profound, that the memory of this first massive assault upon the Hawaiian people persisted through several generations, even after other plagues had come to assail them.

Whether or not they did so with reasons founded on facts, survivors blamed the maʻi ʻokuʻu for many of the calamities that subsequently befell the nation; and they sensed in it the beginning of "the Sliding Way of Death," down which their race was slipping. Without benefit of statistics or the long perspective of time, with only their empty households and crowded burial pits to tell them what was happening, their instinct was correct. The graph of the population of the Hawaiian race shown in Figure 1 is a mathematical representation of that slide toward extinction.

In 1862 a letter written by W. Kahala of Puna, Hawaiʻi, to the editor of *Ka Nupepa Kuokoʻa*, presented the beliefs of many Hawaiians at that time:

> I was the one who inquired of an old man of the time of Kamehameha I, relative to the universal sickness called Okuu, and he told me . . .
>
> 1. The okuu was the plague which caused the death of men, of women, and of children, and this sickness took the larger half of the people. There was no other sickness like this one spoken of.
>
> 2. The number of deaths at this and that place through the group, on one day was forty in some places, 80 in some places, 120 in others, and several fours in some places; in places thickly populated were the larger number of deaths. [These figures are not meant to be taken literally; they are the old Hawaiian way of indicating "large numbers."]
>
> 3. The length of time of this plague scouring the people . . . was three months or perhaps more, with fatalities day after day.
>
> 4. That was the prime cause of the decimation of this race. In this way are we certain. The larger half of the people died, and the remainder was a very small part, and those remaining are those to spread this race, and if there had been many well preserved, the race would increase.

The ʻokuʻu epidemic achieved at least one other important effect which had both immediate and long-lasting consequences: the native medical profession's "crash program" for training more kāhuna lapaʻau. This was the time when "Peleula was covered with healing heiaus, where offerings were made and methods of healing were taught," as John Papa Iʻi remembered, and when "promising members of the court" were assigned to the heiaus to be trained as physicians.[32]

This intelligent response to new dangers on the part of the medical profession was destined to be futile. No medical profession anywhere in the world, least of all in isolated Hawai'i, was prepared either in philosophy or in therapeutics to combat microorganisms as the causative agents of diseases. Nonetheless, the kāhuna lapa'au who received their training in the years after the ma'i 'ōku'u continued the principles and practices of native medicine far longer into the nineteenth century than might have been possible without that program of intensive preparation.

ℰ℩ℰ℩ℰ℩ℰ℩

For those who survived, life went on. For several decades after the ma'i 'ōku'u Hawaiians seem to have been spared another great epidemic of that devastating kind. Minor outbreaks of imported diseases troubled them often enough, as Don Francisco Marin and Stephen Reynolds of Honolulu noted in their journals; and always the endemic contagions, lurking among them now, carried off a few people here, a few there, year after year. Death, held in abeyance for so long in the days of old, had settled among them now, as much at home as were the foreigners who had come to stay, as ineradicable as the weeds and the bugs and the germs the haoles had brought with them across the seas.

Vasilii Mihailovich Golovnin, as captain of Russia's sloop of war *Kamchatka,* visiting the islands in 1818, noticed the most obvious, and probably the worst, of the chronic ailments that were killing Hawaiians:

> Another vice, also introduced by Europeans [prostitution], causes great harm to this good people by spreading that infectious disease which is such a detriment to people of loose morals. . . . I enquired among the Europeans who have lived here for a long time and their opinion is that this disease was unknown here before Cook. The Europeans who visit or reside in the Islands, not only make no attempt at destroying or decreasing it, but maintain and spread it themselves.[33]

Physicians with a French scientific expedition provided the most extensive account of Hawaiians' health in the period from 1800 to 1820. Aboard the corvette *Uranie,* commanded by Captain Louis Claude Desaulses de Freycinet, the expedition visited the Hawaiian

Islands from 8 to 30 August 1819. The conclusions about Hawaiians' diseases reached by *Uranie*'s three "doctor-naturalists" appeared in the official account of the voyage, published under Freycinet's name between 1827 and 1839. As undeterred by the difficulties of making assorted diagnoses at sight as all their predecessors had been, Messieurs Gaimard, Quoy, Guerin, and Freycinet presented ten pages of discussion pertaining to matters of health in the Sandwich Islands.

To them the most universal medical problem was "the itch," or scabies.[34] Syphilis continued upon its deadly course, said M. Gaimard. He had not seen any "definitive cases" on Oʻahu, but islanders to whom he talked "claimed that syphilis is much more prevalent on Wahou than on Owyhi. . . . I learned from a European living on Mowi that on that island the venereal disease manifested itself frequently by buboes in the groin and the arm pits and by chancres."[35]

Dysentery "seldom spared those who are attacked by it. Recently . . . it has killed off a large number of people."[36] Very much a man of his time in the theories he expressed, M. Quoy thought that

catarrhal infections appeared to be very frequent. They affect . . . the pulmonary mucus, causing frequent coughing, which, developing into phthisis, kills patients. I noticed one, under a shed, a young girl stretched out on some mats, and near death from this terrible disease. One has to . . . attribute the cause of this to, first, changes in the atmosphere which suddenly changes from heat to extreme cold, as a result of strong winds; second, to the lack of warm clothing which could protect the body from the influence of these variations; third, also to the habit of the natives to spend several nights in succession in the open, etc. We happened to see some tall strong vigorous men having these obstinate coughs which would end up by becoming fatal to them.[37]

M. Quoy had no reservations about the harmfulness of tobacco:

The use of tobacco, introduced . . . by the Anglo-Americans, has become general. . . . The natives like it not any less than strong liquor. . . . A single pipe serves several people, chieftains as well as their servants; it is passed from one person to another, and each is satisfied to take a few hasty puffs.[38]

To their distress about the toxic effect of the American sotweed, we can add our more modern form of revulsion over the sharing of pipes (not to mention the utensils used in eating and drinking) and the direct method of communicating germs that they provided.

Although smallpox had not yet reached the islands (and would not arrive until 1853), the French visitors heard of a Spartan method used by O'ahu's people for preventing its spread: "When a child is thought to have smallpox, he is suffocated."[39](But we can wonder how the Hawaiians knew that the disease was smallpox, if they had never encountered it.) Cases of insanity in people and madness in dogs, employing the same vocabulary, were dismissed in the same sentence: "There are no mad dogs here . . . [but] some insane people . . . exist; the maniacs are tied up and sometimes they are left to die of hunger."[40]

They mentioned just two instances of congenital deformities: "a boy with only four fingers on each hand, whose left arm [was] very thin and the right one atrophied" and a weak, stunted man, only fifty inches tall, "hunched in front and in the back," whom they classified as a case of rickets.[41]They also saw something they called "the terrible leprosy," less common and less varied perhaps than in the Marianas, but "nonetheless fatal to those who are attacked by it. An individual suffering from elephantiasis [Elephantiasis Graecorum, a nineteenth-century term for leprosy] had one leg covered with reddened ulcers; and one woman whose nose bones no longer existed was making that kind of whistling noise which is a true symptom of the advanced stage of that disease."[42]If those were indeed cases of genuine leprosy—as they could have been, just as they might also have been cases of advanced syphilis, tuberculosis, scabies, or several other kinds of mutilating diseases—then this report from *Uranie*'s physicians indicates that Hawaiians had contracted leprosy much sooner than historians have suspected.

In concluding their observations on health and disease, Freycinet and his colleagues "had the general impression that since a few years ago, the population of the Sandwich Islands has been strangely reduced." Seeking explanations for this decrease, they invoked the same reasons that so many visitors, both before and after them, would state:

> the frequent wars . . . under the reign of Kamehameha I . . . the introduction of alcoholic drinks by Europeans . . . the catastrophes caused by terrible earthquakes; diseases not known previously, brought in by foreign ships; the unaccustomed fatigue resulting, for

the lower classes, from gathering and transporting to the beaches the sandalwood meant for trade; finally, licentiousness and infanticide, terrible consequences of poverty and privation. . . .[43]

Conditions Favoring the Spread of Infectious Diseases. Except for the "terrible earthquakes" (which in truth have not as yet been very destructive), the reasons proposed by those French physicians, as well as others they could not have known, did contribute to the increasing mortality among Hawaiians. But by far the most important agencies were the newly introduced pathogenic microorganisms together with the changing social circumstances which helped to disseminate them among the susceptible populace.

Since 1778 the new microorganisms had been swarming in from all quarters, and Hawaiians, with their lives in forfeit, were being forced to accommodate to them or perish. Unfortunately for Hawaiians, their ignorance about microorganisms was not the only factor which interfered with their ability to adapt to the invisible invaders. A great number of other influences, most of them sociological and economic, others physiological, and some perhaps psychological— but all of them interrelated in an extremely vicious cycle—also contributed to the spread of infectious microorganisms among this vulnerable people.

- Dislocation of the Hawaiian people as they moved from sheltered (and usually healthful) households or communities to the deadly port towns. There they could have been subjected to all the hazards of disruption: inadequate housing, crowding, squalor, filth, poverty; careless disposal of personal and household wastes; utterly inadequate provision for potable water and clean foods; and ignorance of what, lately, we have learned to call "safe sex."
- Breakdown of the traditional kapus of hygiene and sanitation, thereby aggravating all forms of pollution.
- Deterioration of the family system, especially those rules and sanctions concerning responsibility for the care of children. When the indulgence of pleasure for adults outweighed the claims of the young, children were abandoned, or killed, or willfully denied the chance to be born (by methods of contraception or abortion).
- Prostitution and promiscuity, with the attendant evils of venereal diseases, abortion, infanticide, and sterility.
- Lack of understanding among natives of the manner in which contagious diseases are transmitted or by which the sick should be treated. Being uninstructed, they were too often unafraid if not actu-

ally feckless: they did not take care of themselves when they were sick; did not avoid the company of others who were sick; did not learn from foreigners how they might ease their illnesses or, indeed, prevent them in some instances. Worst of all, they were unwilling to give up traditional habits and customs. Of these the most dangerous would have been the hoʻopūʻā method of feeding infants, whereby someone, anyone available, sick or well, would chew a bit of solid food until it became fluid enough to dribble into the mouth of the baby being fed.

• Lack of physicians, either native or foreign, with consequent lack of medical advice, treatment, and solacing for the people, whether sick or well. Inadequate though these may have been, when compared with modern methods, they would have been better than nothing, if only for their psychological benefits.

• Malnutrition during much of the time, exacerbated to the point of famine during seasons of war, drought, or labor for chiefs. Nutritional deficiencies, compounded by physical and psychological traumata imposed by the environment, would have lowered the resistance of many natives, leaving them almost defenseless against even slightly virulent microbes.

• Psychological distresses, although much more difficult to identify and to assess, must be mentioned as possible agencies for assisting the infectious process and—as more than one foreigner remarked—for the ease with which natives could die.

Hardships Related to Trade with Foreigners. Hunger; exposure to rain, wind, and cold; exhaustion; accidents; neglect of children; the infectious diseases those predisposing conditions invited: all these influences, and perhaps others as well, took their toll in Hawaiian lives when commoners were ordered by their chiefs to provide the amounts of foodstuffs, water, and firewood needed by visiting foreigners. Although the greatest exactions of the chiefs upon the labor of their people would not come until the sandalwood trade reached its height, during the decade from 1820 to 1830, some "unmurmuring" commoners suffered some of the ill effects of exploitation every time a foreign vessel arrived.

Maternal and Infant Mortality. Figures are lacking, understandably, which would indicate how many women practiced contraception, abortion, and infanticide at any time in Hawaiʻi's history. American missionaries, after their First Company arrived in 1820, expressed utmost horror over both the methods used and the frequency with which they thought "iniquitous" females employed them. On the other hand, native historians and informants, while agreeing that some women resorted to these practices, maintained that most did not. The exemplary fondness for children shown by the majority of Hawaiians since 1778, the fact that visiting foreigners saw hunchbacks, cripples, and other deformed adults who obviously had not been killed at birth, seem to support the statements of the native historians rather than those of the missionaries.

Nonetheless, the number of deaths among Hawaiians each year exceeded the number of births. From what we know of Hawaiian mothers and their infants in later years, from 1820 to the present, we can guess that, for many reasons, maternal and infant mortality rates in the period before 1820 must have been as high as they were shown to be, by actual statistics, in the years subsequent to 1840.

The causes of death threatening infants were almost too numerous for a newborn child to escape: improper diet, malnutrition, the ghastly method of feeding by ho'opū'ā; neglect, filth, cold; and, of course, pouncing upon it from all sides, myriads of pathogenic microorganisms. The marvel is that any infant at all survived these assaults on its weak defenses.

Those same factors, and more, would have been responsible for the death of mothers, although with less reason. But Hawaiian women were slow to learn, and slower to change. They neglected to care for themselves even more than they neglected to care for their babies. And, all too often, if they managed to emerge from the travail of childbirth itself without too much physical damage, they succumbed a few days later to childbed fever, or to erysipelas, or to other postparturition infections.

Minor Causes

While a few Hawaiians still died in ways that would not have surprised them—by being drowned at sea, for example, or being burned in sudden fires, even by being offered in sacrifice at a neighborhood heiau—after 1778 foreigners brought the means and the incentives for depleting the national gene pool that would have been absolutely new to islanders. Foremost among the influences contributing to the decrease of the population were migration, occupational hazards, urban living, and native physicians.

Migration. Hawaiian men made good sailors, and Hawaiian women provided most agreeable companionship for lonely captains at sea. These wanderers went away in the prime of their lives, and most of them did not return to the land of their birth. Whether or not they died abroad (as the majority of them did), their departure represented a double loss for the kingdom: it deprived the nation of the presence of their individual selves; and it denied the race the children they might have engendered had they stayed at home.

Occupational Hazards. Primitive though they were, compared with monstrous engines that maim, mangle, and kill people today, the new machines employed by foreigners claimed Hawaiian limbs and lives at an increasing rate. Hawaiians who had never seen a wheel, who had known no other machines than staves, adzes, levers, and pump-drills, now had to learn how to use—and to respect—all the devices which artisans in the rest of the world had invented during the passage of thousands of years. Bursting muskets, exploding cannons, flaring gunpowder, scalding whale oil, snapping hawsers, crushing cratefuls of cargo, not to mention kicking horses, stampeding cattle, goring bulls, frenzied "runaways" dashing through the towns, each year took their unwary victims by the dozen.

Urban Living. Grogshop brawls and waterfront riots, vendettas for love or hate, lonely suicides, murders premeditated or fortuitous, accidents, manslaughters, drunkenness, family fights: all enlivened the local scene, giving residents subjects for gossip, giving burial grounds further reasons to expand.

Native Physicians. According to clucking foreigners, who scarcely could have been in a position to know what they were talking about, kāhuna lapaʻau and their ministrations killed many a trusting patient, while the maleficent attentions of kāhuna ʻanāʻanā carried off quite a few other healthy members of the native populace. Beyond any doubt, those scoffing appraisals were exaggerated, both in the effects they attributed to kahunas of any specialty and in the numbers of victims they imagined. Most native patients lived or died regardless of the treatments their kāhuna lapaʻau prescribed. And we can safely say that foreign physicians, had they been in attendance, would have compiled no different records of successes and failures. Nonetheless, we must accept the probability that a very few hypersusceptible natives were eased out of this world either by the ineptitude of physicians or by the attentions of sorcerers.

Lowered Birth Rates

Even today, despite modern medicine's extensive knowledge about the body's parts and their functions, and a growing awareness about the role the psyche plays in influencing some of these functions, scientists have not yet defined all the factors which affect the complex processes that control fertility and conception in the human species. In order to avoid presumption on the one hand, and oversimplification on the other, this account will be confined to a consideration of the regulators of birth rates which demographers do accept.

Birth Control

The extent to which Hawaiian women practiced birth control, by employing methods known to them or to their kāhuna hoʻohāpai keiki (or obstetricians), is not known. Some women at least, by their own testimony, did prevent the birth of children.

Contraception and abortion may be accepted as means of limiting population growth in a thriving or overcrowded society, as we are realizing in the overcrowded world of today. But they are literally genocidal methods to employ when a society is endangered because the number of its people is decreasing. Hawaiians, wasteful of their lives in the best of times and wanton in the sowing of their seed, seem to have been reckless in ways that led to destruction of the harvest even when bad times came upon them.

Infertility

The causes of infertility—or barrenness and sterility, to use the older terms—appear to be numerous. They seem to be expressions of inhibiting agencies which can be either physicochemical or psychological in origin, or, indeed, can be manifestations of both sets of agencies operating concomitantly.

Of the physicochemical interferences, those caused by contagious diseases would have been extremely important. The venereal diseases, especially syphilis and gonorrhea, notorious for their effects on the reproductive organs, probably would have been the maladies primarily responsible for infertility, as the Reverend Artemas Bishop maintained in 1838. But other chronic infections—such as those caused by certain viruses, by the tubercle bacilli and other species of bacteria, and by yeasts, fungi, protozoa, and certain worms—might also have caused infertility. After all, not every Hawaiian was syphilitic or gonorrheic, despite accusations to that effect made by a few foreigners who reviled everything "native" and therefore traduced all natives. Relatively few Hawaiians were so debauched and so dissolute as to be beyond caring about what happened to them or their families. And a great number of Hawaiians were clean and decent folk, even by Puritans' exacting standards, although missionaries might take exception to the flexible definitions of "virtue" that some natives adopted.

There were, as well, other physical-physiological influences that might have led to infertility: prostitution and promiscuity; premarital sex begun at the earliest possible age; malnutrition and consequent deficiencies of essential metabolites; chronic alcoholism; organic dysfunctions; anatomical anomalies; and, possibly, especially among chiefs, genetic defects as a result of prolonged inbreeding.

Psychological influences, also, too subtle to detect but nonetheless adverse in effect, could have upset potential mothers if not the male gene donors. Chief among the psychological tensions and pressures elicited during this early period would have been the stresses of the anxiety-fear complex, conscious or subconscious, induced by watching gods, spying priests, domineering chiefs, disapproving parents, glowering mates, and exploiting foreigners. Less immediate, but more deep-rooted, perhaps, would have been the spiritual confusion, the *accidie* and *ennui,* "the malaise," that followed upon the disintegration of the established social system under the impact of representatives from a "superior" society.[44]

In any event, whatever the possible causes may have been, the fact of infertility among Hawaiians was all too evident. Despite a prodigious amount of uninhibited sexual activity by almost everyone capable of indulging in it, the birth rate began to decline. Children, formerly so plentiful, were no longer produced in numbers sufficient to increase the population, or even to maintain it at a stable level. A few Hawaiian women, to be sure, bore many children, a few had only one or two offspring, but most of them bore none at all. And most of the children who were born died before they were ten years old. In 1838 the Reverend Artemas Bishop said that "the great majority of children born in the islands die before they are two years old."[45]

Barrenness, although it was especially remarked among the chiefs, extended to commoners as well. And it affected not only matings of native Hawaiian couples. All too often, matings between foreign men and native women proved to be just as barren. Why this should be so we cannot say, even today. We can only wonder at the implacability with which agencies we cannot define, by processes we cannot comprehend, prevented imperiled Hawaiians, the lowly as well as the great, from continuing their lines.

By the period from 1834 to 1841, when "the earliest reliable statistics of births and deaths" became available, "the depopulation effect of lowered fertility" was apparent. In 1971 R. C. Schmitt calculated that "the crude birth rate was only 19 and the crude death rate was near 77. This low birth rate is about 60 percent lower than rates characteristic of societies that have no effective contraceptive methods; hence this low rate of fertility was a significant factor in the steep decline of the number of Hawaiians."[46] This depressing generalization applies not only to the period 1834–1841: even more important, it applies to the entire history of the Hawaiian people after 1778.

ʻ ʻ ʻ ʻ

The new germs, aided and abetted in their attack by all these other factors, and perhaps by others as well which have not yet been recognized, exacted an appalling mortality among Hawaiians. Adults as well as children and infants sickened and died. And, even worse, babies were not born in sufficient numbers to replace the people who had died or sailed away.

By 1819, as Freycinet's physicians reported, "a number of villages formerly well populated, recently abandoned, are now reduced to ruins." And in 1857, Charles Gordon Hopkins, editor of *The Polynesian,* could write: "The people are ignorant, and they are dying."[47]

Even so, in 1820 no one quite realized, yet, the extent of the reduction in population. Not even Hawaiians knew, yet, what the price of their having been discovered by the world was going to be. But among the elders who had not succumbed, among those few who could look back and compare, the suspicion grew that too many members of the race had been lost. *"Ua hala, ʻaʻole hoʻi hou mai,"* the elders said, "they have gone, never to return."[48]

NOTES

The following abbreviations are used in the notes and references:

ABCFM   American Board of Commissioners for Foreign Missions, Boston
AH   Archives of Hawai'i, Honolulu
HHS   Hawaiian Historical Society, Honolulu
HMCS   Hawaiian Mission Children's Society, Honolulu
HMsMisc. Hawaiian Manuscript Miscellaneous, Bishop Museum
MH   *Missionary Herald,* Boston
PRO   Public Records Office [Admiralty], London

1. Life and the Land

1. Kirch 1985:67.
2. *Sunday Star-Bulletin and Advertiser,* 22 Oct. 1989, pp. A-3 and A-7.
3. Stannard 1989:32–58.
4. Zimmerman 1948:63, 107.
5. Freud 1938:37.
6. Stokes 1936:36.
7. Dibble 1843:109.
8. Alexander 1899:24.
9. Toynbee 1947 (I):165.
10. Alexander 1899:19.
11. Braudel 1981:412.
12. Ibid.:99; Roberts 1927:282.
13. Personal communication; Hanner MS.
14. Carter, in Barrau 1963:2–14.
15. Alexander 1899:99.
16. Ibid.:99.
17. Malo 1951:245.
18. Ibid.:246.
19. Kamakau 1964:25.
20. Zimmerman 1948:94.
21. Ibid.:106.
22. Ibid.:107.
23. Ibid.:111, 116.
24. Ibid.:119.
25. Ibid.:119.
26. Ibid.:106.
27. Stannard 1989: 37, 79.
28. Zimmerman 1948:173.

2. Two Unprovable Hypotheses

1. Houghton, in Kirch 1985:63.
2. King 1778–1779 (122):146; brackets added.
3. Bowers 1966.
4. Larsen 1966.
5. PBS's *Nova,* 25 Jan. 1978.

6. Joklik et al. 1984:362.
7. *WHO Chronicle* 23 (7)(1969): 321–323.
8. Chappel 1927; Lai 1960; Bowers.
9. Chappel 1927:8–9.
10. Dubos 1965:190.
11. Davis et al. 1973:618–619.
12. Castiglioni 1975:925.
13. *Honolulu Star-Bulletin,* 28 July 1969, p. D-20.
14. King 1778–1779 (122):121.
15. Buxton 1928:83.
16. Rosen 1954:743; brackets added.
17. Kamakau 1964:109.
18. La Pérouse 1798 (II):46–47.
19. Ibid. 1798 (III):167–169; brackets added.
20. Pukui et al. 1972:159.
21. Alexander 1899:45.
22. Joklik et al. 1984:578.
23. La Pérouse 1798 (III):169.
24. Willetts 1958:109.
25. Bowers 1966.
26. Larsen 1966.
27. Chung et al. 1969:566.
28. Blaisdell 1989:5.
29. Miller 1940; Bowers 1966; Chappel 1927; Lai 1960.
30. Miller 1940.
31. Chappel 1927:7.
32. Judd 1974:95.
33. Hardy, personal communication, 1989.
34. *Polynesian,* 17 July 1852.
35. Cutting, in Alicata 1964:2.
36. Alicata 1964:31, 35.
37. Bayly 1778–1779:16.
38. Pogue 1978:61.
39. Roberts 1927:58.
40. Fenton 1942:510.
41. Squire 1877:72–75.
42. Hawaii Dept. of Health, *Physician Alert,* 7 March 1989.
43. *Honolulu Advertiser,* 25 Feb. 1989, p. D-6.

3. The Native Medical Profession

1. Kamakau 1964:95–115.
2. I'i 1959:65.
3. Pukui and Elbert 1965:11.
4. Malo 1951:113.
5. Bryan 1951:4.
6. Pukui et al. 1979 (II):154.
7. Kamakau 1964:95.
8. Ibid.:109.
9. Handy 1936:123–125.
10. Handy et al. 1934:11.
11. Handy 1927:242.
12. Kamakau 1964:98.
13. Ibid.:95–96.
14. "Fragments of Hawaiian Methods of Treating the Sick," ca. 1870:77.
15. Pukui et al. 1979 (II):145–146.
16. Ibid.:147.
17. Knipe 1989:89.
18. Handy 1927:233.
19. Kamakau 1964:107.
20. Ackerknecht 1942:504.
21. Kamakau 1964:95–96; brackets added.
22. Ibid.:106.
23. Ibid.:108; an elegant illustration of a *papa 'ili'ili,* by Joseph Feher, appears on p. 94 of this edition of Kamakau.
24. Ibid.:99.
25. Ibid.:99.
26. Ibid.:99; brackets added.
27. Ibid.:100.
28. Handy et al. 1934:7.
29. Kamakau 1964:101.
30. Handy et al. 1934:9.
31. Kamakau 1964:101.
32. Ibid.:114.
33. Pukui 1942:372.
34. Kamakau 1964:102.
35. Ibid.:102.
36. Ibid.:115.
37. Ibid.:103.
38. Ibid.:104, 115.

39. Ibid.:104; brackets added.
40. Ackerknecht 1943:66.
41. Handy 1927:233.
42. K, personal communication, about 1975.
43. Ackerknecht 1942:504, 513.
44. Kamakau 1964:107.
45. Pogue 1978:50.
46. Alexander 1899:66.
47. Handy 1927:245.
48. King 1989:28.
49. Handy 1927:247.
50. Kamakau 1964:98.
51. Handy and Pukui 1958:144.
52. Ibid.:143.
53. Kalaniana'ole Collection, HMS KI, 1735–1742, in B. P. Bishop Museum.
54. Handy and Pukui 1958:143.
55. Ibid.:142.
56. Ibid.:143.
57. Ibid.:144.
58. Dubos 1965:440.
59. I'i 1959:47–48.
60. Kamakau 1964:111.
61. Holman, letter to ABCFM, 21 Nov. 1820.
62. Handy et al. 1934:18.
63. Pogue 1978:43.
64. Taylor, *Honolulu Star-Bulletin*, ca. Feb. 1953; brackets added.
65. Handy et al. 1934:23.
66. Ibid.

67. Pukui et al. 1972:156.
68. Kamakau 1964:112.
69. Handy et al. 1934:22.
70. HMS K, I'i 1626–1634, in B. P. Bishop Museum.
71. Newman 1948: 59 (3):118–135; 59 (4):145–156.
72. HMS Misc. no. 52, in B. P. Bishop Museum.
73. Fenton 1942:503–526.
74. Handy and Pukui 1958:145.
75. Handy et al. 1934:25.
76. Handy and Pukui 1958:145.
77. Pogue 1978:41.
78. Kamakau MS, *Ka Mo'olelo o Hawai'i*, II, in B. P. Bishop Museum, p. 2.
79. Andrews 1865:97.
80. Cooke, *Honolulu Advertiser*, 24 June 1976, pp. C-1, C-2.
81. Akana et al. 1922:8.
82. Kamakau 1964:111.
83. Ackerknecht 1942:513.
84. Pogue 1978:43.
85. Kamakau 1964:97–98.
86. Ibid.:96.
87. Taylor, *Honolulu Star-Bulletin*, ca. Feb. 1953.
88. Pogue 1978:41; Pogue 1978:50.
89. Ohule MS, Archives of Hawaii; and HMS K (I):1500–1581, in B. P. Bishop Museum.

4. Kāhuna Lapa'au After 1778

1. Blaisdell 1983 (I):102.
2. Law, *Journal*, in Cook Collection, no. 94, Archives of Hawaii.
3. Samwell 1917:24.
4. Ellis 1783:151.
5. Shaler 1808:93.
6. Kamakau 1964:109.
7. I'i 1959:46–47.
8. Akana et al. 1922:55
9. Handy et al. 1934:17–18.
10. Choris 1822:15–16.
11. Ellis 1963:250.

12. Holman, letter of 21 Nov. 1820 to ABCFM in Boston; in HHS Library.
13. Chapin 1838:264.
14. Pogue 1978:50.
15. Kamakau 1964:96.
16. Ibid.:29.
17. Ohule, HMS K (I):1500–1581; MS in B. P. Bishop Museum.
18. Kawai Li'ili'i, HMS K (I):1994–1997; MS in B. P. Bishop Museum.

19. Pukui et al. 1979 (II):149.
20. Ibid.:150.
21. Ibid.:151.
22. Halford 1954:223.
23. Pukui et al. 1979 (II):159.
24. Ibid.:160–167.
25. *Kuokoʻa,* 16 Dec. 1866.
26. Ibid.: 11 June 1870.
27. Ibid.: 2 April 1870.
28. Ibid.: 2 March 1867.
29. Bushnell 1969:107–121.
30. Pogue 1978:53.

31. Larsen 1966:27–44.
32. Hänsel 1968:293–313.
33. Judd, 1839, MS in HMCS
    Library; brackets added.
34. Ibid.
35. Judd, 1871, HMs.Misc. no. 52,
    in B. P. Bishop Museum.
36. Chun 1986:xii–xiv.
37. Blaisdell, in Chun 1986:ix.
38. Pukui, personal communication,
    1960.
39. Blaisdell 1989:6.

5. 1778: An End, and a Beginning

1. Malo 1951:187.
2. Kamakau 1961:48.
3. Ibid.:61.
4. Ibid.:92–83.
5. Ibid.:92.
6. Malo 1951:190.
7. Beaglehole 1967 (I):264, 279.
8. Ibid.:264–265.
9. Ibid.:265; brackets added.
10. Ibid.:265; brackets added.
11. Ibid.:265–266; brackets added.
12. Edgar, in Beaglehole 1967
    (I):226, n. 1.
13. Ibid.
14. Roberts, in Beaglehole 1967
    (I):266, n. 1.
15. Charlton, *Journal,* MS, Admiralty
    51/4557; typescript in AH,
    Cook Collection no. 114.
16. Beaglehole 1967 (I):596.
17. Ellis 1783:152.
18. "Historical Sketch of the Sand-
    wich Islands," 1800:17; brackets
    added.
19. Beaglehole 1967 (I):269.
20. Ibid.

21. Ibid.
22. Ibid.:276.
23. Ledyard 1783:68.
24. Beaglehole 1967 (I):474.
25. King 1778–1779 (122).
26. Beaglehole 1967 (I):474.
27. Ibid.
28. Ibid.:485.
29. Ibid.:479, n. 1.
30. Ibid.:490.
31. Ibid.:490–491.
32. Kamakau 1961:98.
33. Beaglehole 1967 (I):576.
34. Ibid.:576, n. 1.
35. Ibid.:576; brackets added.
36. Buxton 1928:83–84; Joklik et al.
    1984:730.
37. Kamakau 1961:103–104.
38. Samwell 1917:24.
39. Ibid.
40. Beaglehole 1967 (I):lxxxvi.
41. Restarick, n.d.
42. Beaglehole 1967 (I):593.
43. Kamakau 1961:101.
44. Ibid.
45. Beaglehole 1967 (I):578.

6. Exploration and Exploitation: 1786–1825

1. Beaglehole 1974 (I):620.
2. Cook and King 1784 (II):549.
3. Beverley 1792:106–108.
4. La Pérouse 1798 (I):36.

5. Ibid.:167, 169.
6. Portlock 1789:77.
7. Kamakau 1961:144.
8. Pogue 1978:91.

9. Boit 1792:9–13.
10. Howay 1930:20.
11. Turnbull 1813:199.
12. Meares 1790:350; brackets added.
13. Lisiansky 1814:101.
14. Campbell 1816:209.
15. Kamakau 1866–1868:548.
16. Pukui et al. 1974:262.
17. Campbell 1816:167.
18. Pukui and Elbert 1965:281.
19. Kamakau 1961:189.
20. Kuykendall 1938:41.
21. Manby 1929:44.
22. M'Konochie, 1816, in HHS Ann. Rpt. 14, 1906:29–43.
23. Kuykendall 1938:21.
24. Meares 1790:31.
25. Ibid.:35.
26. Bell 1929 (I):20.
27. Kamakau 1961:164.
28. Wyllie 1850:46.
29. Reynolds 1850:51.
30. Vancouver 1798 (V):107.
31. Reynolds 1850:51.
32. Kuykendall 1938:317.
33. Zimmerman 1948:177.
34. Berger 1970:29.
35. *Honolulu Star-Bulletin,* 14 May 1970, p. G-13.
36. *Honolulu Advertiser,* 26 June 1989, p. A-6.
37. Ten Bruggencate, *Sunday Star-Bulletin and Advertiser,* 11 June 1989, p. D-4.
38. Emerson 1928:132.
39. Alexander 1899:152.
40. Reynolds 1850:51–52.
41. Stewart 1828:301.
42. Chamberlain, *Journal,* 12 April 1827.
43. Reynolds 1850:52.
44. Menzies 1920:12–13.
45. Bennett 1840:246.
46. Illingworth 1923:8.
47. Wight 1909:49.
48. Ten Bruggencate, *Sunday Star-Bulletin and Advertiser,* 19 March 1989, p. D-4.
49. I'i 1959:143.
50. John Cook 1927:6.
51. Beaglehole 1967 (I):273.
52. Dibble 1843:29, 31.
53. Chamisso 1939:60.
54. Ibid.:80.
55. Arago 1823:144–145.
56. Dibble 1843:21; brackets added.
57. Personal experience.
58. Hawaii Dept. of Health, Communicable Disease Report, Mar. / Apr. 1989, p. 4.
59. Campbell 1816:104.
60. I'i 1870:10.
61. Kanahele 1986:365.
62. Bingham 1848:78.
63. Daws 1968:58.
64. Ibid.:59.
65. Freud 1938:572.

7. The Time of Troubles

1. Diderot [1796], in Bougainville 1958:328.
2. Forster 1777 (I):303.
3. Menzies 1920:30.
4. Bell 1929:86.
5. Campbell 1816:119.
6. Ibid.:118.
7. Golovnin 1979:212.
8. Ibid.:206.
9. Kamakau MS 54, p. 17, in B. P. Bishop Museum; a slightly different version is in Kamakau 1961:245.
10. I'i 1959:94.
11. Mouritz 1935:11.
12. Turnbull 1813:201.
13. Golovnin 1979:208.
14. Dampier 1971:47.

15. Ibid.:38.
16. Ibid.:38.
17. Ibid.:47.
18. Ibid.:47.
19. Braudel 1981 (I):437.
20. Meares 1790:1, 10, 28, 36.
21. Buck 1953:39.
22. Bishop 1795.
23. Delano 1818:393.
24. Dampier 1971:13.
25. Nordyke 1989:23.
26. Greer 1969:37–88.
27. Dana 1969:141.
28. Hull 1915:263.
29. Tyerman and Bennet 1831 (I):415.
30. Gulick, *MH*, 1831:382.

31. A. Bishop, *MH*, 1832:156.
32. Braudel 1981 (I):560.
33. Goodhue 1900:124.
34. Dibble 1843:109.
35. Kuykendall 1938:98.
36. Matheson 1913:557.
37. Macrae 1922:118.
38. Iʻi 1959:143.
39. Reynolds 1850:52.
40. Ibid.
41. Kuykendall 1938:73.
42. Ibid.:73; brackets added.
43. Blackman 1906:222.
44. Turnbull 1813:224.
45. Alexander 1899:151.
46. Golovnin 1979:202.

8. The Time of Dying

1. Golovnin 1979:211.
2. A. Bishop 1838 (1):52–66.
3. *MH*, Oct. 1834, p. 371.
4. Mouritz 1935:96.
5. Pogue 1978:112.
6. Freycinet 1839:574.
7. Dampier 1971:44.
8. Freycinet 1839:574–575.
9. Joklik et al. 1984:729.
10. Chapin 1838:50–51; brackets added.
11. Braudel 1981 (I):48.
12. Ibid.:81.
13. King 1778–1779 (116).
14. Townsend 1905:6.
15. Duhaut-Cilly 1834–1835 (II):318.
16. Mouritz 1935:142.
17. Frear 1934:7.
18. Stewart, *MH* 1825:70.
19. Tyerman and Bennet 1831:59; emphasis in original.
20. W. P. Alexander, letter of 17 Oct. 1835, in *MH*, 1836:?.
21. *MH*, April 1823, pp. 105–106; brackets added.
22. Oliver 1974 (I):33.
23. Jung 1958:117.

24. Roberts 1927:60.
25. Ibid.:63.
26. Ibid.:64; brackets added.
27. Ibid.:74.
28. Ibid.:75.
29. Ibid.:74.
30. Ibid.:58.
31. Fornander 1969 (II):355.
32. Roberts 1927:69.
33. Letter of 28 June 1820, in *MH*, June 1821.
34. Tyerman and Bennet 1831 (II):19.
35. A. Bishop, letter of 7 Dec. 1823, in *MH*, May 1824, p. 140.
36. Stewart 1828:153.
37. Thurston, *MH*, June 1821, p. 177.
38. Richards, letter of 27 June 1826, in *MH*, June 1827.
39. Stewart 1828:250.
40. Ibid.; emphasis in original.
41. Ibid.:296.
42. Ibid.
43. Kamakau 1964:53.
44. Pukui and Elbert 1965:174.
45. Blaisdell 1983:101.
46. *Islander* (1875) 31:201.

47. Kamakau 1964:79.
48. Kamakau 1866–1868:27.
49. Richards and Loomis, letter of 5 June 1823, in *MH,* Feb. 1825, p. 42.
50. Kamakau 1964:33–34.
51. Keene, personal communication, 1989.
52. Arago 1823:146.
53. Goodhue 1900:124.
54. Vancouver 1798 (V):35.
55. Whitney, letter in *MH,* 14 Oct. 1820.
56. Dampier 1971:47.
57. Kanahele 1986:361–364.
58. Golovnin 1979:206.
59. I'i 1870:18.

9. Many Who Came Have Vanished

1. Schmitt 1968:19–20.
2. Gould 1928:35.
3. Freycinet 1839 (II; 1):585.
4. Schmitt 1971:340.
5. Stannard 1989:37, 79.
6. Borg, *Sunday Honolulu Star-Bulletin and Advertiser,* 22 Oct. 1989, pp. A-2–A-7.
7. Dixon 1789:267.
8. Menzies 1920:131 fn., 136.
9. Nordyke 1989:34–35.
10. Ibid.:35.
11. Dixon 1789:276–277.
12. Kamakau 1961:64.
13. Ibid.:167.
14. Ibid.:163.
15. Vancouver 1798 (III):301.
16. "Historical Sketch of the Sandwich Islands," 1800:121.
17. *Annual Account,* 13 August 1828, in *MH,* December 1829, p. 373.
18. "Historical Sketch of the Sandwich Islands," 1800:17; brackets added.
19. Menzies 1920:125.
20. Bell 1929:88.
21. Alazard 1905:5–6.
22. Villaret 1938:16.
23. Mortimer 1791:8.
24. Colnett 1940.
25. Vancouver 1798 (I):405.
26. Broughton 1804:40.
27. Turnbull 1813:367–368.
28. Kamakau 1961:187.
29. Ibid.:188.
30. Ibid.:189.
31. Schmitt 1970:359–364.
32. I'i 1959:46.
33. Golovnin 1979:67.
34. Freycinet 1839 (II; 2):574.
35. Ibid.:574.
36. Ibid.:575.
37. Ibid.:574.
38. Ibid.:583.
39. Ibid.:575.
40. Ibid.
41. Ibid.
42. Ibid.; brackets added.
43. Ibid.:584.
44. Roberts 1927.
45. Bishop 1838:54.
46. Nordyke 1989:21.
47. *Polynesian,* 20 Jan. 1857.
48. Menzies 1920:52.

GLOSSARY

(Based on the *Hawaiian Dictionary* by Mary Kawena Pukui and Samuel H. Elbert)

'aihue. Thief, robber

aikāne. Catamite (in 1778); a friend (at present)

'ai noa. Free-eating, without observing taboos

āiwa. Mysterious taboo

akua. God, goddess, spirit, ghost

ali'i. Chief, chiefess, noble, aristocrat, ruler

'anā'anā. Black magic, evil sorcery

'aumakua. Personal or family god; a deified ancestor

auwē. Alas! My Goodness!

'awa. Narcotic infusion prepared from root of *Piper methysticum.* Also known as *kava*

'ea. General term for many infectious diseases

hana. Work, labor, job

haole. A foreigner (formerly); a white person, a Caucasian, especially an American or Briton (at present)

heiau. Temple or shrine

heiau ho'ola. Temple where physicians were trained, or sick people were treated.

ho'ohāhā. To feel, to palpate

ho'oho'iho'i. To cause to go back or to come back

ho'omalu. To gain peace, to make peaceful

ho'opahe'e. To make slippery

ho'oponopono. To correct, to put things aright

ho'opū'ā. To feed by passing chewed food directly from mouth to mouth

huikau. Bewildered, confused, all mixed up

kāhili. Feathered standard, insigne of royalty

kahu ma'i. Nurse to a sick person

kahuna. Priest, expert in a profession. *Kāhuna* is the plural form

kahuna lapaʻau. Physician, healer

kahuna lapaʻau lāʻau. Physician who used medications, usually derived from plants, sometimes from animals or minerals

kālā. Dollar; money in general

kanaka. Man, person, individual. *Kānaka* is the plural form

kanaka maoli. Full-blooded Hawaiian; generically, *maoli* means real, true

kanikau. Chant of mourning, wail of grief, lament

ka poʻe kahiko. The people of old

kapu. Taboo, prohibition, forbidden, sacred; to invoke or enforce a *kapu*

kaukau. Pidgin English, meaning food or to eat; derived, according to tradition, from sailors' term "chow"

kilu. Game using quoits fashioned from coconut shells

kino lau. Physical manifestations of a supernatural being

koali (or *kowali*). Some kinds of morning glory vines, *Ipomoea* spp.

kōʻele. Work done for chiefs

Kūʻokoʻa. *The Independent* (a newspaper)

kupuna. Grandparent, or elder

kupuna lapaʻau. Elder healer

lāʻau. Plant or tree, or materials derived from such, used in medications prescribed by *kāhuna lapaʻau*

laukahi. *Plantago major,* a broad-leafed plantain, often used as a medicine

māhū. Homosexual, of either gender

maʻi. Sickness, ailment, disease

maʻi aliʻi. The chiefs' disease: leprosy

maʻi ʻōkuʻu. "The squatting sickness," the dysentery epidemic that occurred in 1804

maʻi Pākē. The Chinese disease: leprosy

makaʻāinana. Commoner, populace, people in general

makahiki. A period of relief from war and labor, lasting about four months, from our mid-October until mid-January, celebrated with sports contests and religious ceremonies

makai. Directional: toward the ocean, seaward

malo. Loincloth, worn by males

mana. Divine power, spiritual power, derived from the gods, present in varying amounts in every created thing, from people to pebbles, from clouds to grains of sand

mauka. Directional: inland, toward the mountains

menehune. Legendary race of small people, who worked at night *moa.* Small leafless plant, *Psilotum nudum,* used in medications

nī'aupi'o. Offspring from the mating of high-born siblings, or of half-brother and half-sister

noni. The Indian mulberry, *Morinda citrifolia,* a small tree, a source of dyes and medicines

'ohana. Family, kin-group, relative

'ōkolehao. Alcoholic beverage prepared from distillate of fermented *ti* roots

'ōpala haole. Foreign trash, or rubbish, applied to half-Hawaiian children

pā'ao'ao. A latent, weakening ailment of children

pa'i 'ai. Cooked taro, without water added, pounded into a hard mass

Pākē. A Chinese person

pale keiki. Midwife

pani. Literally, closing; the bit of food given a patient at the end of a period of treatment

panipani. A vulgar word, defined in genteel glossaries as "coition"

papa li'ili'i. "Table of Pebbles," laid out in the form of a human body, used to instruct students in medicine

pau. All done, finished, ended, over

po'e kahiko. The people of old

pōpolo. The black-berried nightshade, *Solanum americanum,* used in medications

pu'uhonua. A place of refuge, a sanctuary

'uhaloa. A small weed, *Waltheria indica,* used in preparing medicines

'uhane. Spirit, soul, ghost

ule. Penis

'ulu maika. Bowling

wai ea. Sea water, used in ritual of purification

References

Ackerknecht, Erwin H. 1942. "Problems of Primitive Medicine." *Bulletin of the History of Medicine* 11 (5):503–521.

———. 1943. "Psychopathology, Primitive Medicine, and Culture." *Bulletin of the History of Medicine* 14 (1):30–67.

———. 1948. "Medicine and Disease among Eskimos." *Ciba Symposium* (July–August):917–918.

Akana, Akaiko (trans.), D. M. Kaaiakamanu, and J. K. Akina. 1922. *Hawaiian Herbs of Medicinal Value*. Honolulu: Territorial Board of Health.

Alazard, Ildefonso. 1905. *Réponse au Calomnies de M. Dejeante*. Paris: Chadenat.

Alexander, W. D. 1899. *Brief History of the Hawaiian People*. New York: American Book Co.

Alicata, J. 1964. *Parasitic Infections of Man and Animals in Hawaii*. Tech. Bull. 61. Honolulu: Hawaii Agricultural Experiment Station, College of Tropical Agriculture, University of Hawaii.

Andrews, L. 1865. *Hawaiian Dictionary*. Honolulu: Mission Press.

Arago, Jacques. 1823. *Narrative of a Voyage around the World, 1817–1820*. London: Treutel & Wurtz, Treutel.

Barrau, Jacques (ed). 1963. *Plants and the Migrations of Pacific Peoples*. Honolulu: Bishop Museum Press.

Bayly, William 1778–1779. MS. Extract from Manuscript Journal. Typescript in Hawaiian-Pacific Collection, University of Hawaii–Manoa.

Beaglehole, J. C. 1967. *Journals of Captain James Cook on His Voyages of Discovery: The Voyage of the Resolution and the Discovery, 1776–1780*. 2 vols. Cambridge: Cambridge University Press (for the Hakluyt Society).

———. 1974. *Life of Captain James Cook*. Stanford: Stanford University Press.

Bell, Edward. 1929. [1792–1794.] "Log of the Chatham." *Honolulu Mercury* 1 (Sept. 1929):80 and 2 (Jan. 1930).

Bennett, Frederick D. 1840. *Narrative of a Whaling Voyage Round the Globe 1833–1836*. London: Richard Bentley.

Berger, A. J. 1970. "The Present Status of the Birds of Hawaii." *Pacific Science* 24:29–42.

Beverley, Charlotte. 1792. *Verses on the Death of Captain Cook*. 3rd ed. Hull: E. Foster.

Bingham, Hiram. 1848. *Residence of Twenty-one Years in the Sandwich Islands. . . .* Hartford, Conn.: H. Huntington; New York: S. Converse.

Bishop, Artemas. 1838. "Inquiry into the Causes of Decrease in the Population of the Sandwich Islands." *Hawaiian Spectator* 1 (1):52–66.

Bishop, Charles. [1795.] MS. Log of the *Ruby*. Typescript in B. P. Bishop Museum.

Blackman, William F. 1906. *Making of Hawaii*. New York: Macmillan.

Blaisdell, Richard K. 1983. "Health Section." In *Native Hawaiian Study Commission Report on the Culture, Needs, and Concerns of Native Hawaiians*, Vol. 1. Honolulu.

———. 1989. "Historical and Cultural Aspects of Native Hawaiian Health." *Social Process in Hawaii* 32:1–21.

Bloxam, Andrew. 1925. *Diary of Andrew Bloxam, Naturalist of the "Blonde," on Her Trip to the Hawaiian Islands from England, 1824–1825*. Spec. Pub. 10. Honolulu: B. P. Bishop Museum.

Boit, John, Jr. [1792.] "Remarks on the Ship Columbia's Voyage from Boston (on a Voyage Round the Globe)." *Proceedings of the Massachusetts Historical Society* 53 (1920):217–275.

Bowers, Warner F. 1966. "Pathological and Functional Changes in 864 Pre-European Contact Polynesian Burials from the Sand Dunes at Mokapu, Oahu, Hawaii." *International Surgery* 45 (2):206–217.

Braudel, Fernand. 1981. *Structures of Everyday Life: Civilization and Capitalism, Fifteenth to Eighteenth Centuries*. Vols. 1 and 2. New York: Harper & Row.

Broughton, William R. 1804. *Voyage of Discovery to the North Pacific Ocean . . . Performed in His Majesty's Sloop Providence, and Her Tender, in the Years 1795–1798*. London: T. Cadell & W. Davies.

Bryan, E. H., Jr. 1951. "Kahunas' Means for Curing on Exhibition." *Honolulu Advertiser*, Nov. 18, 1951. P. 4.

Buck, Peter H. 1953. *Explorers of the Pacific: European and American Discoveries in Polynesia*. Spec. Pub. 43. Honolulu: B. P. Bishop Museum.

Bushnell, O. A. 1969. "Hawaii's First Medical School." In *Hawaii Historical Review: Selected Readings*. Honolulu: Hawaiian Historical Society.

Buxton, P. A. 1928. *Studies Relating to Human Diseases and Welfare in Samoa, Tonga, the Ellice Islands, and the New Hebrides*. Researches in Polynesia and Melanesia, Memoir 2. London: London School of Hygiene and Tropical Medicine.

Campbell, Archibald. 1816. *Voyage Around the World, from 1806–1812*. Edited by James Smith. Edinburgh: Archibald Constable & Co.

Carter, George F. 1963. "Movement of People and Ideas Across the Pacific." In *Plants and the Migrations of Pacific Peoples*, ed. Jacques Barrau. Honolulu: Bishop Museum Press.

Castiglioni, A. 1975. *History of Medicine*. New York: J. Aronson.

Chamberlain, Levi. 1822–1849. MS. Journal. HMS H24, in B. P. Bishop Museum.

Chamisso, A. von. 1939. *Account of the Voyage Around the World on the Rurik, 1815–1818*. Annual Report for 1939. Hawaiian Historical Society: 55–81.

Chapin, Alonzo. 1838. "Remarks on the Sandwich Islands, Their Situation,

Climate, Diseases, and Their Suitableness as a Resort for Individuals Affected with or Predisposed to Pulmonary Diseases." *Hawaiian Spectator* 1 (July):248–267.

Chappel, H. G. 1927. *Jaws and Teeth of Ancient Hawaiians.* Memoirs, vol. 9, no. 3. Honolulu: B. P. Bishop Museum.

Choris, Louis. 1822. *Voyage Pittoresque autour du Monde.* Paris: Firmin Didot.

Chun, Malcolm Naea. 1986. *Hawaiian Medicine Book: He Buke Laau Lapaau.* Honolulu: Bess Press.

Chung, G. H. S., C. S. Chung, and R. W. Nemecheck. 1969. "Genetic and Epidemiological Studies of Clubfoot." *American Journal of Human Genetics* 21:566.

Clerke, Charles. [1778–1779.] MS. Excerpts from the Log of HMS *Discovery.* PRO Admiralty 55, vol. 22. Typescript in Archives of Hawaii.

Colnett, James. 1940. *Journal of Capt. James Colnett aboard the Argonaut from April 26, 1789 to November 3, 1791.* Toronto: Champlain Society.

Cook, James. 1784. *Voyage to the Pacific Ocean. . . .* Vol. 2. London: G. Nichol & T. Cadell.

Cook, James, and James King. 1784. *Voyage to the Pacific Ocean. . . .* Vol. 3. London: G. Nichol & T. Cadell.

Cook, John. 1927. *Reminiscences of John Cook, Kamaaina and Forty-niner.* Honolulu: New Freedom Press.

Corney, Bolton G. 1884. "Behaviour of Certain Epidemic Diseases of Natives of Polynesia, with Especial Reference to the Fiji Islands." *Transactions of the Epidemiological Society of London,* n.s., 3:76–95.

Dahlgren, E. C. 1916. *Were the Hawaiian Islands Visited by the Spanish Before Their Discovery by Captain Cook in 1778?* Stockholm: Almqvist and Wiksells.

Dampier, Robert. 1971. *To the Sandwich Islands on H.M.S. Blonde.* Honolulu: University Press of Hawaii.

Dana, Richard Henry, Jr. 1969. *Two Years Before the Mast. . . .* Harvard Classics, vol. 23. New York: Collier.

Danielssen, D. C., and W. Boeck. 1847. *Om Spedalsked.* Privately printed. Christiania.

Davis, B. R., R. Dulbecco, H. N. Eisen, H. S. Ginsberg, W. B. Wood, and M. McCarty. 1973. *Microbiology.* 2nd ed. New York: Harper & Row.

Daws, Gavan. 1968. *Shoal of Time: A History of the Hawaiian Islands.* New York: Macmillan.

Delano, Amasa. 1818. *Narrative of Voyages and Travels.* Boston: E. G. House.

Dibble, Sheldon. 1843. *History of the Sandwich Islands.* Lahainaluna: Press of the Mission Seminary.

Diderot, Denis. 1796. "Supplement au Voyage de Bougainville." In *Voyage autour du Monde par la Frégate La Boudeuse et la Flute L'Etoile.* Reprint 1958. Paris: Club des Librairies de France.

Dixon, George. 1789. *Voyage Around the World, 1785–1788.* London: George Goulding.

Dubos, René. 1965. *Man Adapting*. New Haven: Yale University Press.

Duhaut-Cilly, A. B. 1834–1835. *Voyage autour du Monde, principalement à la Californie et aux Îles Sandwich*. Paris. Typescript of translation in B. P. Bishop Museum.

Edgar, Thomas. [1778–1779.] MS. Excerpts from His Log. PRO Admiralty 55/21. Typescript in Archives of Hawaii, Cook Collection, no. 111.

Ellis, William. 1783. *Authentic Narrative of a Voyage Performed by Captain Cook and Captain Clerke, 1776–1780*. London: G. Robinson.

Ellis, William. 1963. *Narrative of a Tour through Hawaii in 1823*. Reprint of 1827 edition. Honolulu: Honolulu Advertiser.

Emerson, Oliver Pomeroy. 1928. *Pioneer Days in Hawaii*. New York: Doubleday.

Fenton, William N. 1942. "Contacts Between Iroquois Herbalism and Colonial Medicine." *Smithsonian Report for 1941*. Washington, D.C.: Smithsonian Institute.

Fornander, Abraham. 1969. *Account of the Polynesian Race. . . .* 3 vols. Reprint of 1886 edition. Rutland, Vt.: Tuttle.

Forster, George. 1777. *Voyage Around the World. . . .* 2 vols. London.

"Fragments of Hawaiian Methods of Treating the Sick." Ca. 1870. HMsMisc. K, I:1626–1634. B. P. Bishop Museum.

Frear, Mary Dillingham. 1934. *Lowell and Abigail*. New Haven: Yale University Press (private printing).

Freud, Sigmund. 1938. *Basic Writings*. New York: Modern Library.

———. 1961. *Future of an Illusion*. London: Hogarth Press.

Freycinet, Louis de. 1839. *Voyage autour du Monde . . . pendant les années 1817–1820*. Hawai'i section translated by Marian Kelly and Ella Embree Wiswell. Typescript in B. P. Bishop Museum.

Gast, R. H., and A. Conrad. 1973. *Don Francisco de Paula Marin and Letters and Journals of Francisco de Paula Marin*. Honolulu: Hawaiian Historical Society.

Golovnin, V. M. 1979. *Around the World on the Kamchatka, 1817–1819*. Translated and edited by Ella Lury Wiswell. Honolulu: University of Hawaii Press.

Goodhue, E. S. 1900. *Beneath Hawaiian Palms and Stars*. Cincinnati: Editor Publishing Co.

Gould, Rupert. 1928. "Some Unpublished Accounts of Cook's Death." *Mariner's Mirror* 14:301–319.

Green, Laura, and Martha Beckwith. 1926. "Hawaiian Customs and Beliefs Relating to Sickness and Death." *American Anthropologist* 28 (1):176–208.

Greer, Richard A. 1969. "Oahu's Ordeal—the Smallpox Epidemic of 1853." *Hawaii Historical Review: Selected Readings*. Honolulu: Hawaiian Historical Society.

Halford, F. 1954. *Nine Doctors and God*. Honolulu: University of Hawaii Press.

Handy, E. S. C. 1927. *Polynesian Religion*. Bull. 34. Honolulu: B. P. Bishop Museum.

———. 1936. "Dreaming in Relation to Spirit Kindred and Sickness in Hawaii." In *Essays in Anthropology in Honor of Alfred Louis Kroeber*. Berkeley: University of California Press.

Handy, E. S. C., and Mary Kawena Pukui. 1958. *Polynesian Family System in Ka'u, Hawai'i*. Wellington: Polynesian Society.

Handy, E. S. C., M. K. Pukui, and K. Livermore. 1934. *Outline of Hawaiian Physical Therapeutics*. Bull. 126. Honolulu: B. P. Bishop Museum.

Hänsel, R. 1968. "Characterization and Physiological Activity of Some Kawa Constituents." *Pacific Science* 22 (3):293–313.

Hayley, William. 1812. *Life and Letters of William Cowper*. London: J. Johnson.

"Historical Sketch of the Sandwich Islands." 1800. In *History of the Otaheitian Islands*. Edinburgh: Ogle & Aikman.

Howay, F. W. 1930. "Early Relations between the Hawaiian Islands and the Northwest Coast." Pub. 5. Honolulu: Archives of Hawaii.

Hull, George C. 1915. "Chinese in Hawaii." *Mid-Pacific Magazine* 9:263–267.

I'i, John Papa. Ca. 1869. MS. "Kanaenae aloha no Ka'imi-haku" [An Expression of Affection for Ka'imi-haku, or Matthew Kekuana'oa]. Translated by Mary Kawena Pukui. MS in B. P. Bishop Museum. (P. 17 of typescript.)

———. 1959. *Fragments of Hawaiian History*. Honolulu: Bishop Museum Press.

Illingworth, J. F. 1923. *Early References to Hawaiian Entomology*. Bull. 2. Honolulu: B. P. Bishop Museum.

Joklik, W. K., H. Willett, and B. Amos. 1984. *Zinsser Microbiology*. 18th ed. Norwalk, Conn.: Appleton-Century-Crofts.

Judd, Bernice. 1929. *Voyages to Hawaii Before 1860*. Honolulu: Hawaiian Mission Children's Society.

Jung, C. G. 1958. *Psyche and Symbol*. Edited by Violet S. de Laszlo. Garden City: Doubleday.

Kamakau, S. M. 1961. *Ruling Chiefs of Hawaii*. Honolulu: Kamehameha Schools Press.

———. 1964. *Ka Po'e Kahiko: The People of Old*. Spec. Pub. 51. Honolulu: B. P. Bishop Museum.

———. 1866–1868. "Ka Mo'olelo o Kamehameha I" and "Ka Mo'olelo o na Kamehameha II ame III." Manuscripts in B. P. Bishop Museum.

Kanahele, George Hu'eu. 1986. *Kū Kanaka: Stand Tall*. Honolulu: University of Hawaii Press.

King, James. [1778–1779.] MS. Log of Lieutenant King, on the *Resolution*. PRO Admiralty 55, vols. 116 and 122. Typescript in Archives of Hawaii.

King, James (with James Cook). 1784. *Voyage to the Pacific Ocean*. Vol. 3. London: G. Nichol & T. Cadell.

King, Serge. 1989. "Principles of Shamanism." *Quest* 2 (3):20–28.

Kirch, P. F. 1985. *Feathered Gods and Fishhooks*. Honolulu: University of Hawaii Press.

Knipe, Rita. 1989. *The Water of Life: A Jungian Journey Through Hawaiian Myth*. Honolulu: University of Hawaii Press.

Kotzebue, Otto von. 1821. *Voyage of Discovery in the Years 1815–1818 . . . in the Ship Rurik. . . .* 3 vols. London: Longman, Hurst, Reese, Orme, & Brown.

Kuykendall, Ralph S. 1938. *Hawaiian Kingdom, 1778–1854: Foundation and Transformation.* Honolulu: University of Hawaii.

Lai, Leonard J. L. 1974. "Report on the Oral Examination of the Pre-European Hawaiians." In Snow, 1974: Appendix C, pp. 159–163.

La Pérouse, J. F. G. de. 1798. *Voyage of La Pérouse Round the World, in the Years 1785, 1786, 1787, and 1788. . . .* 2 vols. London: John Stockdale.

Larsen, Ivar J. [1966.] "Ancient Hawaiian Medicine." Manuscript in B. P. Bishop Museum.

Ledyard, John. 1783. *Journal of Captain Cook's Last Voyage to the Pacific Ocean . . . in the Years 1776, 1777, 1778, and 1779.* Hartford, Conn.: Nathaniel Patten.

Lisiansky, Urey. 1814. *Voyage Round the World, in the Years 1803, 1804, 1805, and 1806 . . . in the Ship Neva.* London: John Booth.

Macrae, James. 1922. *With Lord Byron at the Sandwich Islands in 1825.* Honolulu: W. F. Wilson.

Malo, David. 1951. *Hawaiian Antiquities (Moolelo Hawaii).* Translated by N. B. Emerson. Spec. Pub. 2. 2nd. ed. Honolulu: B. P. Bishop Museum.

Manby, Thomas. 1929. "Journal of Vancouver's Voyage to the Pacific Ocean (1791–1793)." *Honolulu Mercury* 1 (July 1929):44.

Matheson, R. O. 1913. "Old Honolulu." *Mid-Pacific Magazine* 5 (1): 549–553.

Meares, John. 1790. *Voyages made in the Years 1788 and 1789 . . . to which are prefixed . . . a Voyage performed in 1786 . . . in the Ship Nootka. . . .* London: Logographic Press.

Menzies, Archibald. 1920. *Hawaii Nei 128 Years Ago.* Edited by W. F. Wilson. Honolulu: New Freedom Press.

Miller, C. D. 1957 and 1974. "The Influence of Foods and Food Habits Upon the Stature and Teeth of the Ancient Hawaiians." MS, B. P. Bishop Museum. [Published in Snow, 1974: Appendix E, pp. 165–175.]

Mortimer, George. 1791. *Observations and Remarks made during a Voyage . . . in the Brig Mercury. . . .* London: T. Cadell.

Mouritz, A. 1935. *Our Western Outpost: Hawaii.* Honolulu: Printshop Co.

Newman, Leslie F. 1948. "Some Notes on the Pharmacology and Therapeutic Value of Folk Medicines. *Folk-Lore* 59 (3):118–135, and 59 (4):145–186.

Nordyke, Eleanor C. 1989. *Peopling of Hawaii.* Honolulu: University of Hawaii Press.

"Notebook of a Hawaiian Student in Dr. Judd's Medical School." [1871]. MS. Translated by Mary K. Pukui. H Ms Misc. no. 52. Honolulu: B. P. Bishop Museum.

Oliver, Douglas. 1974. *Ancient Tahitian Society.* 3 vols. Honolulu: University Press of Hawaii.

Pogue, J. F. 1978. *Moʻolelo of Ancient Hawaii.* Translated by Charles W. Kenn. Honolulu: Topgallant Press.

Portlock, Nathaniel. 1789. *Voyage Round the World . . . Performed in 1785, 1786, 1787, and 1788. . . .* London: John Stockdale & George Goulding.

Pukui, Mary Kawena. 1942. "Hawaiian Beliefs and Customs During Birth, Infancy, and Childhood." B. P. Bishop Museum, Occ. Papers 16 (17):357–381.

Pukui, Mary Kawena, and Samuel H. Elbert. 1986. *Hawaiian Dictionary.* Honolulu: University of Hawaii Press.

Pukui, Mary Kawena, E. W. Haertig, and Catherine A. Lee. 1972 and 1979. *Nānā I Ke Kumu* [Look to the Source]. 2 vols. Honolulu: Liliʻuokalani Trust.

Pukui, Mary Kawena, Samuel H. Elbert, and Esther T. Mookini. 1974. *Place Names of Hawaii.* 2nd ed. Honolulu: University Press of Hawaii.

Restarick, H. B. n.d. [ca. 1928.] "Cook's Ships Did Not Bring Venereal Disease to Islands, Says Restarick." *Honolulu Star-Bulletin.* [Page and date unavailable.]

Reynolds, Stephen. [1850.] Journal. Manuscript in B. P. Bishop Museum.

[Rickman, John.] 1781. *Journal of Captain Cook's Last Voyage. . . .* Dublin: Price, Whitestone.

Roberts, S. H. 1927. *Population Problems of the Pacific.* London: G. Routledge & Sons.

Rosen, Leon. 1954. "Human Filariasis in the Marquesas Islands." *American Journal of Tropical Medicine and Hygiene* 3 (4):742–745.

Samwell, David. 1917. *Narrative of the Death of Captain James Cook.* Reprint 2. Honolulu: Hawaiian Historical Society.

Schmitt, R. C. 1968. *Demographic Statistics of Hawaii, 1778–1965.* Honolulu: University of Hawaii Press.

———. 1970. "The Okuu: Hawaii's Greatest Epidemic." *Hawaii Medical Journal* 29 (5):359–364.

———. 1971. "New Estimates of the Pre-censal Population of Hawaii." *Journal of the Polynesian Society* 80:240.

Shaler, William. 1808. "Journal of a Voyage between China and the North-Western Coast of America, made in 1804." In *American Register. . . .* Vol. 3. Philadelphia: C. & A. Conrad and Co.

Snow, Charles E. 1974. *Early Hawaiians: An Initial Study of Skeletal Remains from Mokapu, Oahu.* Lexington: University Press of Kentucky.

Squire, William. 1877. "Measles Epidemic in the Fiji Islands." *Transactions of the Epidemiological Society of London* 4:65.

Stannard, David E. 1989. *Before the Horror.* Honolulu: Social Science Research Institute, University of Hawaii.

Stewart, C. S. 1828. *Private Journal of a Voyage to the Pacific Ocean, and Residence at the Sandwich Islands in the Years 1822, 1823, 1824, and 1825.* New York: John P. Haven.

Stokes, J. F. G. 1936. "Dune Sepulture, Battle Mortality, and Kamehameha's Alleged Defeat on Kauai." *Annual Report for 1936.* Honolulu: Hawaiian Historical Society.

"Susceptibility to Infection Among Amerindians." 1969. *WHO Chronicle* 23 (7):321–323.

Townsend, Ebenezer. 1905. "Extract from the Diary . . . 1798." *Annual Report for 1905*. Honolulu: Hawaiian Historical Society.

Toynbee, Arnold J. 1953–1957. *Study of History*. Abridged ed., 7 vols. Oxford: Oxford University Press.

Turnbull, John. 1813. *Voyage Round the World . . . 1800–1804*. London: A. Maxwell.

Tyerman, Daniel, and George Bennet. 1831. *Journal of Voyages and Travels . . . between the Years 1821 and 1829*. London: Frederick Westley & A. H. Davis.

Vancouver, George. 1798. *Voyage of Discovery to the North Pacific Ocean . . . in the Years 1790–1795 . . . in the Discovery . . . and . . . Chatham*. 3 vols. London: C. G. and J. Robinson and J. Edwards.

Villaret, B. 1938. *Climatologie Médicale des Établissements Français d'Océanie*. Paris: Vigot Frères.

Wight, Elizabeth L. 1909. *Memoirs of Elizabeth Kinau (Judd) Wilder*. Honolulu: Paradise of the Pacific Press.

Willetts, William. 1958. *Chinese Art*. New York: G. Braziller.

Wyllie, R. C. 1850. "Address." *Transactions of Inaugural Session*. Honolulu: Royal Hawaiian Agricultural Society.

Zimmerman, E. C. 1948. *Insects of Hawaii*. Vol. 1: *Introduction*. Honolulu: University of Hawaii Press.

INDEX

ABCFM, 176, 276
Abortifacients and abortion: before 1778, 23, 122; since 1778, 241, 290, 293
Ackerknecht, E. H.: and primitive medicine, 70, 80, 91
Adams, Capt. Alexander, 199
Aedes scutellaris, 38; *A. (Stegomyia) aegyptii,* 50; *A. (Stegomyia) albopictus,* 50
AIDS, 31, 32, 35, 58
'Aihue, 226
Aikāne, 137, 138, 236
'Ai noa, 195–196, 199, 242
Akua, 63; in diagnosis, 71; in sickness, 108–109
Alazard, Father Ildefonse, 278
Alcoholic beverages: *'ōkolehao,* 193, 228; others, 226, 288
Aleurites moluccana, 85, 122
Alexander, Rev. William P., 239
Alexander, W. D.: and Kahiki, 17; and *pu'uhonua,* 45; and Spanish mariners, 18–19
Ali'i: and inbreeding, 29; and *kapu* system, 196–197; as rulers, 11–12, 25; since 1778, 186, 194, 202–205. *See also* Chiefs
Aloha Spirit, 260–263
American Board of Commissioners for Foreign Missions. *See* ABCFM
Amerindians: and HLAs, 28; susceptibility to measles, 28
Anderson, Surgeon William, 102, 149, 277
Andrews, Rev. Lorrin, 256
Angiostrongylus cantonensis, 52
Animals, introduced: feral, 175; by foreigners, 170–174, 177–179; as hosts, 178; by Polynesians, 8
Anopheles spp., 51
Anson, Capt. George, 210

Arago, Jacques, 189, 259
Arts and crafts, 10, 13, 185
Ascarids, 51, 178
Assis, Machado de, 238
Astrolabe (ship), 41, 157
'Aumakua: causes of sickness, 8, 11, 109–110; at death, 257; in diagnosis, 63, 65–66, 79; in therapy, 83–84, 90–91, 93; in training, 104
'Awa (kava), 26, 40, 121–122, 193

Baldwin, Rev. Dwight, 114
Balena (ship), 217
Barkley, Capt. and Mrs. Charles W., 206
Barrenness, 29, 190, 293
Barrère, Dorothy, 74–77
Battles: 'Aiea, 166; Nu'uanu, 166, 208
Bayly, William, 53
Beckley, Capt. George, 199
Beckwith, Martha, 76
Bell, Edward, 200, 277
Bennet, George, 213, 239, 250
Beverley, Charlotte, 156–157, 263
Bingham, Rev. Hiram, 221
Bird malaria, 50, 178
Birds: indigenous, 174–175; introduced, 175
Birth control, 293
Birth pains, 74
Birth rates, 269, 292–295
Bishop, Capt. Charles, 208
Bishop, Rev. Artemas: on care of sick, 251; on conspicuous consumption by chiefs, 214; on decrease in population, 228, 293; on mortality in children, 294
Bitter gourd, 85, 122, 124
Black magic, 70, 81
Blaisdell, Dr. R. K.: and fate of native physicians, 49, 101, 125; on meaning of death, 256
Blatchely, Dr. Abraham, 107